Atlas of

ANESTHESIA

Volume IV

Principles of Anesthetic Techniques and Anesthetic Emergencies

Atlas of ANESTHESIA

Series Editor
Ronald D. Miller, MD
Professor and Chairman of Anesthesia
Professor of Cellular and Molecular Pharmacology
University of California, San Francisco, School of Medicine
San Francisco, California

Volume IV

Principles of Anesthetic Techniques and Anesthetic Emergencies

Volume Editor
Kevin K. Tremper, PhD, MD, FRCA
Robert B. Sweet Professor and Chair
Department of Anesthesiology
University of Michigan Health System
Ann Arbor, Michigan

With 16 contributors

CHURCHILL LIVINGSTONE

Developed by Current Medicine, Inc., Philadelphia

Current Medicine, Inc.
400 Market Street
Suite 700
Philadelphia, PA 19106

Managing Editor:	Lori J. Bainbridge
Developmental Editor:	Marian A. Bellus
Editorial Assistant:	Deborah Singer
Art Director:	Paul Fennessy
Design and Layout:	Christine Keller-Quirk
Illustration Director:	Ann Saydlowski
Illustrators:	Liz Carrozza, Wieslawa Langenfeld, Ann Saydlowski, Beth Starkey, Larry Ward, Lisa Weischedel, Debra Wertz
Production:	Lori Holland, Sally Nicholson
Indexing:	Alexandra Nickerson

Principles of anesthetic techniques and anesthetic emergencies / volume editor, Kevin Tremper.
p. cm. — (Atlas of anesthesia ; v. 4)
Includes bibliographical references and index.
ISBN 0-443-07903-X
1. Anesthesia—Atlases. 2. Sugical emergencies—Atlases. I. Tremper, Kevin II. Series.
[DNLM: 1. Anethesia—methods—atlases. 2. Anesthesia—adverse effects—atlases. 3. Emergencies—atlases. 4. Anesthetics—atlasses. WO 517 P927 1997 v.4]
RD81.P745 1997
617.9'6—dc21
DNLM/DLC
for Library of Congress 97-28243
CIP

ISBN 0-443-07903-X

Although every effort has been made to ensure that drug doses and other information are presented accurately in this publication, the ultimate responsibility rests with the prescribing physician. Neither the publishers nor the author can be held responsible for errors or for any consequences arising from the use of the information contained therein. Any product mentioned in this publication should be used in accordance with the prescribing information prepared by the manufacturers. No claims or endorsements are made for any drug or compound at present under clinical investigation.

Printed in Hong Kong by Paramount Printing Group Limited.
10 9 8 7 6 5 4 3 2 1

SERIES PREFACE

This multi-volume series *Atlas of Anesthesia* organizes the largest and most comprehensive collection of teaching visuals in the field of anesthesiology. The publisher, volume editors, and I have invited the most prominent members of the anesthesiology community to provide the most up-to-date information in a format that offers not only the finest images available but also unique schematic presentations of how and why we feel pain. Combined with the slide atlas and CD-ROM, *Atlas of Anesthesia* provides teaching materials of the finest quality in easily accessible formats and allows anesthesiology to become a visual specialty in a way that has never been attempted previously. The topics of the volumes include Critical Care, Scientific Principles, Preoperative Preparation and Intraoperative Monitoring, Principles of Anesthetic Techniques and Anesthetic Emergencies, Subspecialty Care, Pain Management, Cardiothoracic Anesthesia, and Pediatric Anesthesia.

The specialty of anesthesia originally was restricted to operating room anesthesia with some involvement in preoperative evaluation. Furthermore, in the past, patients with severe medical conditions were considered too high risk to be anesthetized (*eg*, those who had suffered a myocardial infarction within the previous 3 to 6 months or those with severe obstructive pulmonary disease). In the last 25 years, it has become possible for patients with extensive medical disease (*eg*, acute myocardial infarction, failure of one or more organs, immunosuppression) to be successfully anesthetized for major invasive surgery.

With far more challenging situations, the specialty has responded by the development of new drugs, monitoring techniques, and subspecialties. The new drugs act on receptors that were not even known a few years ago, necessitating extensive knowledge of receptors (*eg*, opioid) of various functions and selection of drugs for specific effects. Improvements in monitoring include the development of the pulmonary catheter, transesophageal echocardiography, evoked potentials, pulse oximetry, and multiple gas analysis. New techniques such as hemodilution, infusion and warming devices, and fiberoptic endotracheal intubation have also been introduced. Cardiac, neurologic, pediatric, transplant, ambulatory, and obstetric subspecialties have expanded to encompass the entire perioperative period, including extensive preoperative evaluation and therapy, critical care medicine, and pain management, in both acute and chronic settings.

In response to the impressive expansion of the specialty, many educational devices (including books and journals) have been developed. The educational transmission of the combined cognitive and technical aspects of anesthesia can be markedly facilitated by illustrations including images, graphs, decision-making trees, and algorithms.

In bringing this series to publication, credit is due to the volume editors and to the many contributors who have shared their expertise and their time. Credit is also due to Abe Krieger, President of Current Medicine, who conceived the atlas, to Marian Bellus, Senior Developmental Editor, and to Jackie Dunn, who coordinated work on this project in my office.

Ronald D. Miller, MD

PREFACE

The practice of anesthesiology may be characterized as the acute management of the physiologic consequences of injury through the use of drugs and specialized equipment. The latter fall into two categories: that used to provide various types of anesthetics and that used to monitor the physiologic consequences of the surgical stimulus and the anesthetics. Because anesthesiology has been in the forefront of developing physiologic monitoring equipment, we often can be seen by other specialists as employing a variety of "gadgets." Most of these monitoring devices first employed in the operating room quickly migrated to all acute care areas of the hospital. In addition to being seen as specialists on the forefront of monitoring techniques, we are clearly the only specialists that have an understanding of an anesthesia machine. This device is truly a mystery to other specialists, but just as clearly must be thoroughly understood by a competent anesthesiologist. Although this requirement should be obvious, it is sometimes easier said than done. Modern anesthesia machines have incorporated many automatic safety features and consequently have become more complex. With the addition of ultra short acting anesthetics and the advent of total intravenous anesthesia, a series of intravenous drug regulatory systems has also been incorporated into our practice.

In addition to a thorough understanding of the tools of our trade, we must also understand the specific techniques of our trade. Conduction blockade has always been an integral part of an anesthesiologist's armamentarium. In recent years regional anesthetics have migrated to the postoperative period in the form of postoperative analgesia. This migration of anesthetic techniques into postoperative analgesic techniques has been advocated not only to improve postoperative pain management but also to reduce morbidity, mortality, and hospital length of stay. For these reasons regional techniques have seen a rebirth in popularity over the past decade. Other techniques routinely employed require less manual dexterity but a thorough understanding of risk associated with the specific therapies. Patient positioning and peripheral nerve injury associated with positioning have always been risks associated with anesthesia. In recent years with the reduction of mortality associated with anesthesia, the morbidity attributed to positioning problems has become a common cause for litigation. It is therefore important to be current on the potential etiologies of the injuries and the required postoperative follow-up.

The advent of HIV infection has dramatically heightened the public's concern over blood transfusions. Ironically, as the concern increased, so has the safety. Over the past decade the screening and testing of the blood supply has reduced the risks of viral contamination dramatically. Unfortunately, the consequences of contracting one of these viruses can be devastating and the source is easily determined. It is therefore paramount that the transfusion of each component of blood be done for a justifiable reason that falls within published guidelines or the reasons for transfusing outside of recognized guidelines be well documented in the patient's medical record. One of the best methods to minimize the need for transfusions is to minimize blood loss. Deliberate hypotension has been documented for over thirty years to significantly reduce blood loss. This technique is not without risk, and a thorough understanding of the technique and how it should be modified according to a patient's pathophysiology is imperative.

A final principal aspect of our field is the ability to manage acute physiologic emergencies. Since the practice of anesthesia is by definition cardiopulmonary resuscitation, it is clear that we must be expert in the diagnosis and treatment of hemodynamic and respiratory emergencies. Finally, there is a metabolic emergency that is unique to anesthesia, malignant hypotherrnia. We are the experts and all other physicians look to us for the management of this life-threatening disease.This volume of *Atlas of Anesthesia* is dedicated to anesthesia techniques and emergencies. The chapters have been divided into groups, the first involving equipment (Chapters 1–3),the second involving techniques (Chapters 4–8), and the last describing emergencies (Chapters 9–11). The purpose of this atlas is to enhance understanding and to function as a reference for specific techniques and procedures of interest. It is not intended to replace a comprehensive text and for that reason references are kept to a minimum. The *Atlas of Anesthesia* and a standard comprehensive text complement each other as references for the modem practice of anesthesiology.

Kevin K. Tremper, PhD, MD, FRCA

CONTRIBUTORS

Steven J. Barker, PhD, MD
Professor and Head
Department of Anesthesiology
The University of Arizona College of Medicine;
Director, Perioperative Services
University Medical Center
Tucson, Arizona

Manbir Batra, MD, FRCPC
Clinical Associate Professor
Department of Anesthesiology
Universtiy of WashingtonSchool of Medicine
Staff Anesthesiologist
Virginia Mason Medical Center
Seattle, Washington

Ronald J. Faust, MD
Professor of Anesthesiology
Mayo School of Medicine;
Consultant in Anesthesiology
Mayo Clinic
Rochester, Minnesota

Peter S. A. Glass, MB, ChB, FFA, (SA)
Associate Professor
Department of Anesthesiology
Duke University School of Medicine;
Director, Clinical Research
Department of Anesthesiology
Duke University Medical Center
Durham, North Carolina

Steven M. Karan, MD
Assistant Professor of Anesthesiology
Department of Anesthesiology
F. Edward Herbert School of Medicine
Uniformed Services University of the the Health Sciences
Bethesda, Maryland;
Staff Anesthesiologist
Department of Anesthesiology
Walter Reed Army Medical Center
Washington, DC

Paul E. Kazanjian, MD
Clinical Assistant Professor
Department of Anesthesiology
University of Michigan School of Medicine
Ann Arbor, Michigan

Edwin W. Lojeski, DO
Assistant Professor of Anesthesiology
Department of Anesthesiology
F. Edward Herbert School of Medicine
Uniformed Services University of the Health Sciences
Bethesda, Maryland;
Staff Anesthesiologist
Department of Anesthesiology
Walter Reed Army Medical Center
Washington, DC

Edward D. Miller, Jr., MD
Professor
Department of Anesthesiology and Critical Care Medicine
Johns Hopkins University School of Medicine;
The Frances Wall Baker, MD, and Lenox D. Baker, Jr, MD, Dean of the Medical Faculty
Chief Executive Officer
Johns Hopkins Medicine
Baltimore, Maryland

Sheila M. Muldoon, MD
Professor and Chair
Department of Anesthesiology
F. Edward Herbert School of Medicine
Uniformed Services University of the Health Sciences
Bethesda, Maryland;
Staff Anesthesiologist
Walter Reed Army Medical Center
Washington, DC

Vildan Mullin, MD
Associate Professor
Department of Anesthesiology
University of Michigan School of Medicine;
Director of Neuroanesthesia
University of Michigan Medical Center
Ann Arbor, Michigan

Michael F. Mulroy, MD
Clinical Associate Professor
Department of Anesthesiology
University of Washington School of Medicine
Seattle, Washington;
Clinical Assistant Professor
Department of Anesthesiology
University of California, San Francisco, School of Medicine
San Francisco, California;
Staff Anesthesiologist
Department of Anesthesiology
Virginia Mason Medical Center
Seattle, Washington

Joseph Neal, MD
Clinical Associate Professor
Department of Anesthesiology
Universtiy of Washington
Staff Anesthesiologist
Virginia Mason Medical Center
Seattle, Washington

James F. Szocik, MD
Clinical Assistant Professor
Department of Anesthesiology
University of Michigan School of Medicine;
University of Michigan Medical Center
Ann Arbor, Michigan

Joseph W. Szokol, MD
Clinical Instructor
Northwestern University School of Medicine
Chicago, Illinois;
Attending Staff
Evanston Hospital
Department of Surgery (Division of Anesthesia)
Evanston, Illinois

Jeffery S. Vender, MD, FCCM
Professor
Department of Anesthesia
Northwestern University School of Medicine
Chicago, Illinois;
Chief, Anesthesia
Evanston Hospital
Evanston, Illinois

Brian J. Woodcock, MBChB, MRCP, FRCA
Assistant Professor
Department of Anesthesiology
University of Michigan School of Medicine
Ann Arbor, Michigan

CONTENTS

Chapter 6

Patient Positioning

Ronald J. Faust

Chapter 7

Transfusion Therapy

Paul E. Kazanjian

Chapter 8

Deliberate Hypotension

Edward D. Miller, Jr.

Chapter 9

Malignant Hyperthermia

Steven M. Karan, Edwin W. Lojeski, and Sheila M. Muldoon

Chapter 10

Airway Emergencies

Joseph W. Szokol and Jeffery S. Vender

Chapter 11

Hemodynamic Emergencies

Brian J. Woodcock

1

Intravenous Drug Delivery Systems

Peter S. A. Glass

For a drug to be effective it must enter the body and reach its biophase (*ie*, the site at which the drug produces its effect). The way a drug is introduced into the body can be considered the drug delivery system. This chapter discusses drug delivery systems used by anesthesiologists to administer drugs that conventionally have been administered intravenously in the perioperative period.

The concept of administering drugs intravenously was initiated when William Harvey first described the arterial circulation in 1628. In 1656, Christopher Wren injected opium intravenously into dogs and humans by means of a quill and bladder, rendering the subjects unconscious, and therefore probably providing the first intravenous anesthetic. The first use of an intravenously administered drug to provide anesthesia for surgery was by Pierre-Cyprien Ore in 1874 using chloral hydrate.

Drug delivery systems for the administration of intravenous drugs have been vastly improved since the original quill and bladder. The development of the hypodermic needle by Frances Rynd and a functional syringe by Charles Pravaz led to the first use of a needle and syringe to administer a drug intravenously by Alexander Wood in 1853. This was a significant improvement in the original intravenous delivery device used by Wren. Present-day syringes, catheters, and needles are descendants of these early devices.

Technologic developments in this century led to the next major advance in intravenous drug delivery systems: infusion pumps that can accurately control the rate of drug administration. In addition, the development of microchip and computer technology has led to the introduction of calculator and smart pumps. Calculator pumps are capable of automating simple calculations from information entered into the pump by the user. Smart pumps solve complex mathematic equations to implement sophisticated administration schemes that could not be achieved manually by the user. Closed-loop controllers and target-controlled infusion pumps are examples of smart pumps.

In contrast to the development of sophisticated pumps for intravenous drug delivery, systems to deliver traditional intravenous drugs by very simple, noninvasive means are also being developed. These systems include transdermal and transmucosal delivery of opiates and hypnotics.

HISTORICAL CONSIDERATIONS

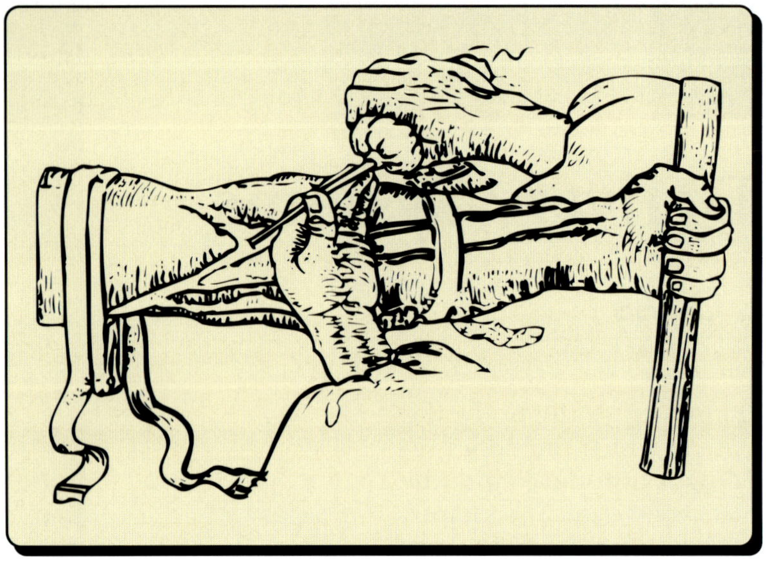

Figure 1-1. The impetus for intravenous drug delivery was initiated by the description of the circulation by Harvey in 1628. Christopher Wren and coworkers at Oxford University in 1657 tested the concept of access to distant target areas in the body through the circulation (as opposed to other then more conventional routes, *eg*, enteral) by initial injection into the venous system. Wren injected opium and other substances ("liquors") into the circulation of dogs and humans with a quill and bladder. (*Adapted from* Major [1].)

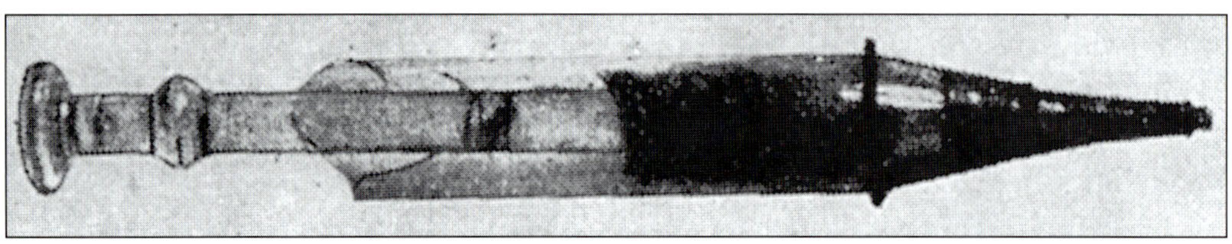

Figure 1-2. Nearly two centuries later, Alexander Wood used the hollow needle and syringe illustrated here to administer medications into a vein, setting the stage for the evolution of intravenous anesthesia. (*Adapted from* Dundee and Wyant [2]; with permission.)

DELIVERY SYSTEMS USED FOR THE ADMINISTRATION OF INTRAVENOUS ANESTHETICS IN THE PERIOPERATIVE PERIOD

- Syringe
- Devices to control flow
  - CAIR clamp
  - Dial-a-Flo
  - Pumps
- Gravity-controlled devices
- Positive displacement devices
  - Calculator pump
  - Smart pumps (automated delivery system)
    - Preprogrammed
    - Pharmacokinetic model driven
    - Closed loop
- Novel delivery systems
  - Transmucosal
  - Transdermal
  - Inhalational
- Manual intravenous drug delivery

Figure 1-3. Delivery systems used for the administration of intravenous anesthetics in the perioperative period.

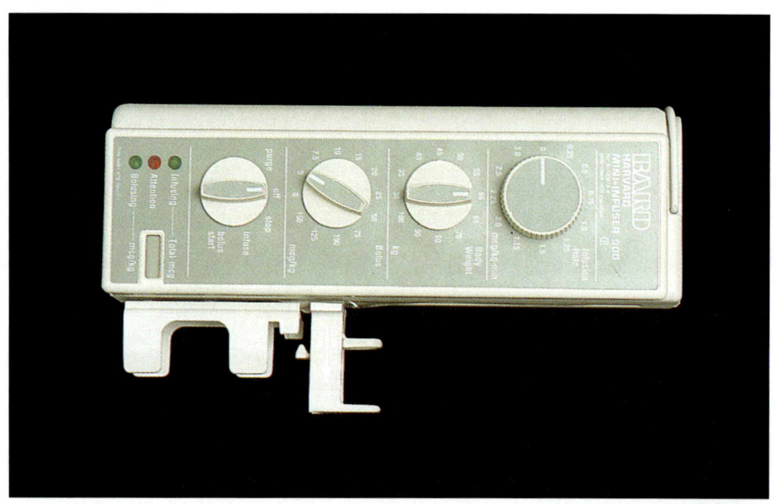

Figure 1-4. The Bard Alfentanil Infusor pump (Baxter Anesthesia Group, Andover, MA). This was the first infusion device with a calculator function dedicated to the administration of an intravenous anesthetic drug. The calculator function simplifies the calculation of infusion rates and enables drug dosing to weight or unit time and will provide administration of a bolus or infusion. This pump thus encouraged for the first time the manual incorporation of pharmacokinetic principles in the delivery of an intravenous anesthetic. Numerous calculator pumps are now available and have become the primary infusion pumps for intravenous anesthetic drug delivery. (Courtesy of Baxter Anestheia Group, Andover, MA.)

MANUAL INFUSION SCHEMES FOR ANESTHESIA, SEDATION, OR ANALGESIA

	Anesthesia		Sedation or Analgesia	
Analgesics	Loading dose, *μg/kg*	Maintenance Infusion, *μg/kg/min*	Loading dose, *μg/kg*	Maintenance Infusion, *μg/kg/min*
Alfentanil	50–150	0.5–3	10–25	0.1–0.25
Fentanyl	5–15	0.03–0.1	1–3	0.01–0.03
Sufentanil	1–5	0.01–0.03	0.1–0.5	0.002–0.01
Remifentanil	0.5–2	0.1–0.4	*	0.025–0.1
Hypnotics				
Ketamine	1500–2500	25–75	500–1000	10–20
Propofol	1000–2500	50–150	250–1000	10–50
Midazolam	50–150	0.25–1.5	25–100	0.25–1
Methohexital	1500–2500	50–150	250–1000	10–50
Neuromuscular Blockers				
Succinylcholine	500–1000	50–150		
Atracurium	200–400	4–6		
Vecuronium	40–80	0.5–1.5		
Pancuronium	70–100	0.25–0.75		
Mivacurium	100–200	4–8		
Rocuronium	300–600	8–12		
Cisatracurium	100–200	1–2		

Figure 1-5. Manual infusion schemes for anesthesia, sedation, or analgesia. The loading doses and infusion rates recommended for anesthesia are those that are used in combination with 60% to 70% nitrous oxide. Following the loading dose, a high infusion rate should initially be used to compensate for distribution to peripheral tissues. The infusion should then be vigilantly titrated to the lowest infusion rate that will maintain the desired endpoint. *Asterisk* indicates that because of a steady-state concentration with an infusion of remifentanil and the possible risk of rigidity with a bolus dose, a loading dose is not recommended for analgesia. (*Adapted from* Glass and coworkers [3].)

INFUSION SCHEMES FOR TOTAL INTRAVENOUS ANESTHESIA

Hypnotic			Opiate		
Drug	Loading dose, *mg/kg*	Maintenance infusion, *μg/kg/min*	Drug	Loading dose, *μg/kg*	Maintenance infusion, *μg/kg/min*
Propofol	1–2	150–80	Fentanyl	3–6	0.05–0.01
Midazolam	0.1–0.2	1–0.25	Alfentanil	20–40	1.5–0.25
Methohexital	1–2	150–80	Sufentanil	0.5–1	0.01–0.002
			Remifentanil	0.5–2	0.4–0.1
			Kentamine	1000–2000	40–10

Figure 1-6. Infusion schemes for total intravenous anesthesia. Following the loading dose, an initially high infusion rate to account for redistribution should be used and then titrated to the lowest infusion rate that will maintain adequate hypnosis and analgesia. (*Adapted from* Glass [4].)

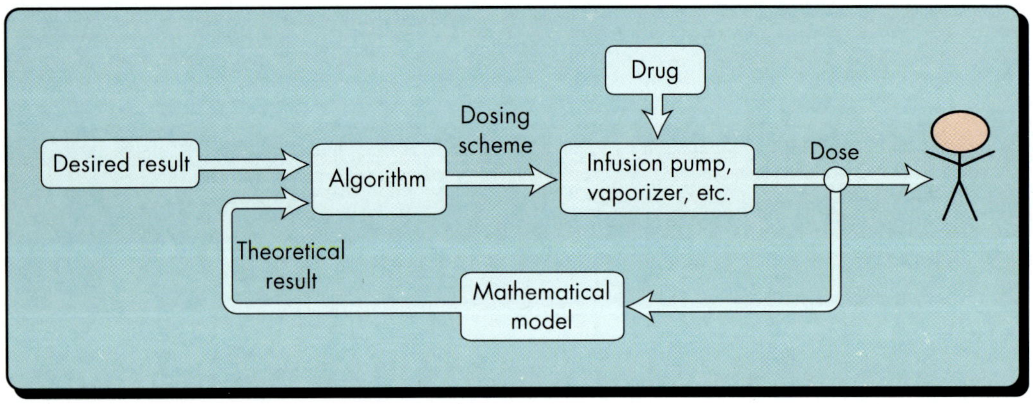

Figure 1-7. The components of a pharmacokinetic model–driven infusion device providing an automated physician closed-loop drug delivery system. In such a system the physician chooses a target concentration of the drug and, using the known pharmacokinetics of the drug, automatically calculates and delivers the required dose to achieve the target concentration. (*Adapted from* Jacobs *et al.* [5].)

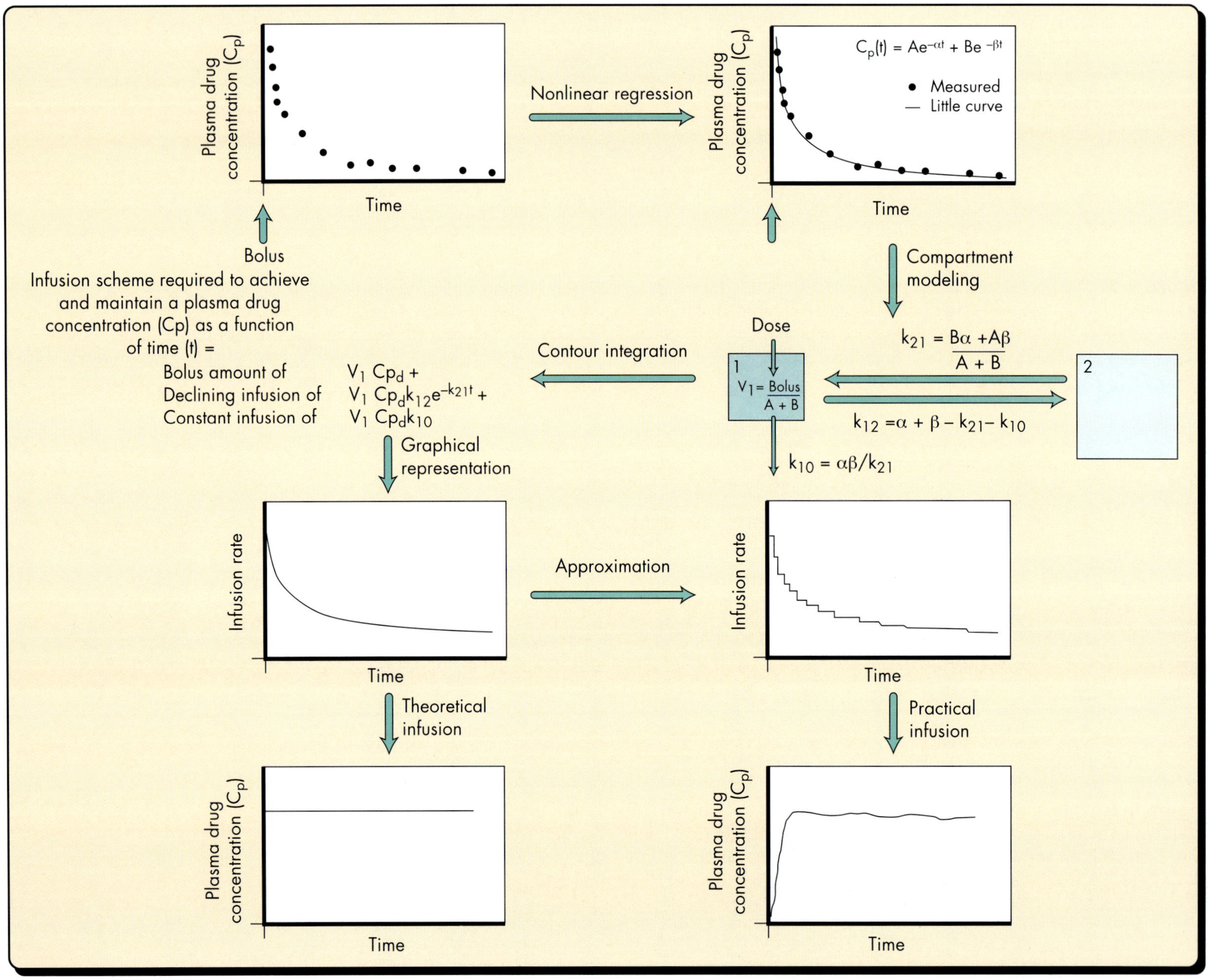

Figure 1-8. Steps involved in pharmacokinetic model–driven infusion. Typically, pharmacokinetic models are derived from experiments in which plasma drug concentration (Cps) are measured at intervals following bolus administration of the drug. Nonlinear regression is used to fit a mono-, bi-, or triexponential curve to the resulting concentration versus time data. There is an algebraic relationship between the exponential decay curves and a one-, two-, or three-compartment pharmacokinetic model. The BET (bolus, elimination, transfer) infusion scheme is derived from the two-compartment model using contour integration. A BET infusion results in the maintenance of a constant specified Cp. Practical implementation of the BET scheme using real infusion pumps and infusion rates that change only at discrete intervals of time results in a Cp profile that approximates that resulting from a BET infusion. (*Adapted from* Glass [4].)

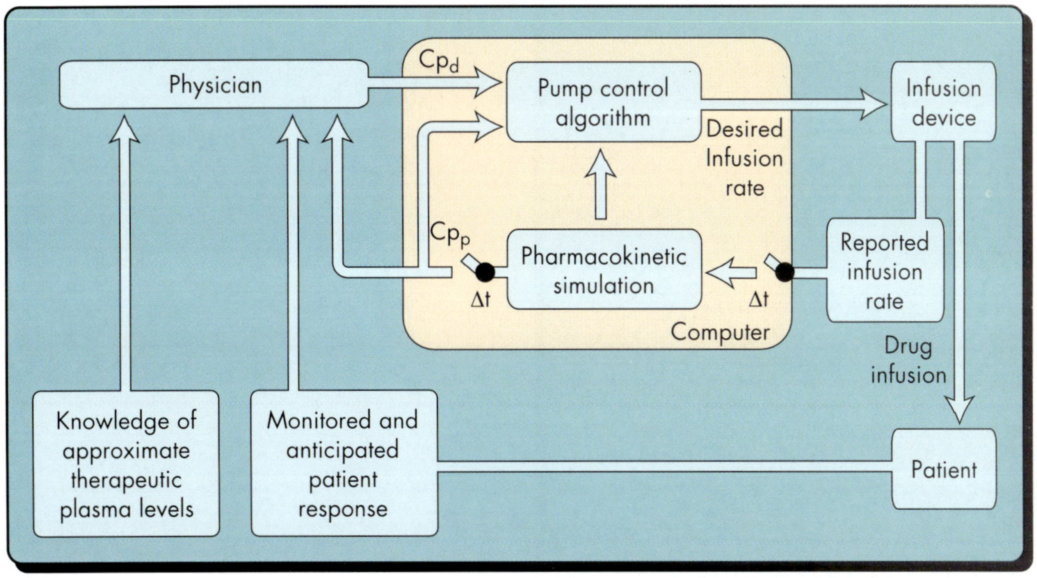

Figure 1-9. Schematic illustration of the authors' approach to pharmacokinetic model–driven drug delivery or target-controlled infusion systems. With these devices, the physician enters the desired plasma drug concentration (Cp_d). An infusion device control algorithm uses a pharmacokinetic model for the drug being infused to determine what the infusion rate should be for the next infusion interval (*eg*, 10 sec). The infusion device delivers drug to the patient, and the infusion rate is fed into a simulation of the pharmacokinetic model to compute the current predicted plasma drug concentration (Cp_p). The infusion rate required for the next time interval to enable Cp_p to equal Cp_d is then calculated and administered. On the basis of monitored and anticipated patient response and knowledge of approximate therapeutic plasma drug concentrations (*eg*, Cp50 [*see* Figs. 1-4, 1-5, 1-6]), the physician can titrate Cp_d as necessary. (*Adapted from* Jacobs and coworkers [6].)

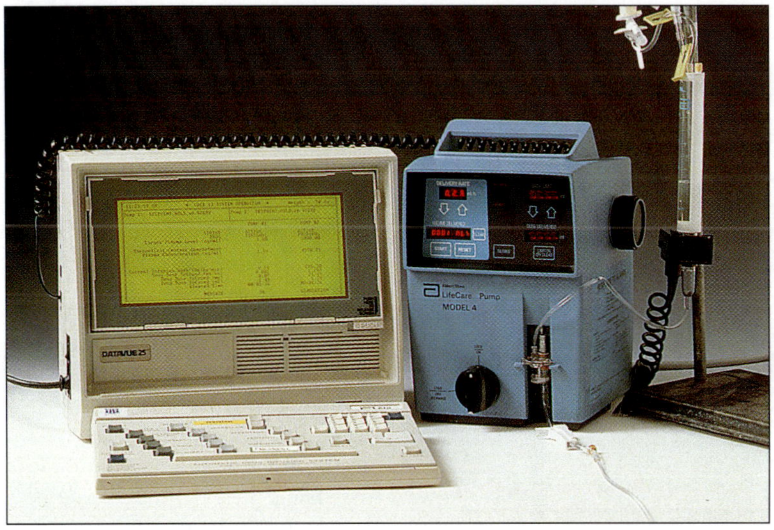

Figure 1-10. The present computer-assisted continuous infusion system (a target-controlled infusion device) used at Duke University Medical Center. It consists of a laptop computer electronically linked to an infusion pump. The desired drug plasma concentration is entered via the keyboard.

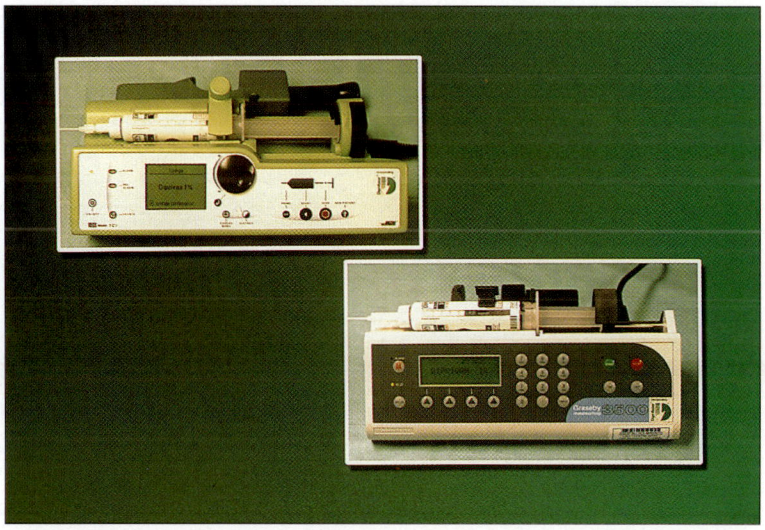

Figure 1-11. Illustrated is the first target-controlled infusion system that incorporates a diprifusor module (Zeneca Pharmaceuticals, Cheshire, England) into a Graesby 3500 (Graesby Medical Limited, Watford, UK) or Pilot Anesthesia (Fresenius Vial, Brezins, France) syringe pump. The diprifusor module contains the software that drives the pump. The diprifusor software is limited to the administration of propofol. It represents, however, the first commercially approved target-controlled infusion device.

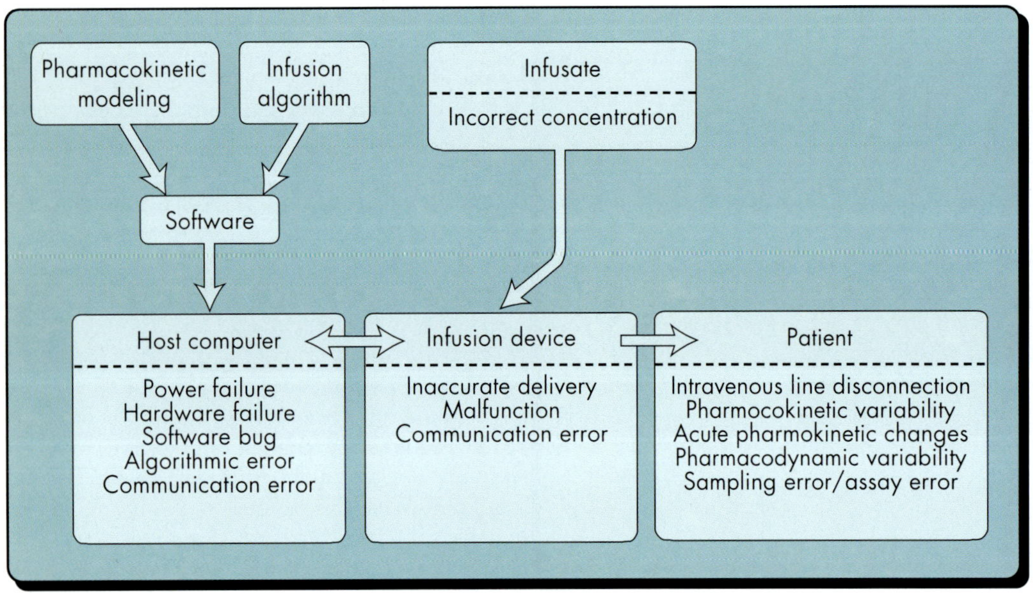

Figure 1-12. Sources of potential errors in pharmacokinetic model–driven drug delivery. In a commercial device, the computer functions would be incorporated into the infusion device itself. (*Adapted from* Glass and coworkers [3].)

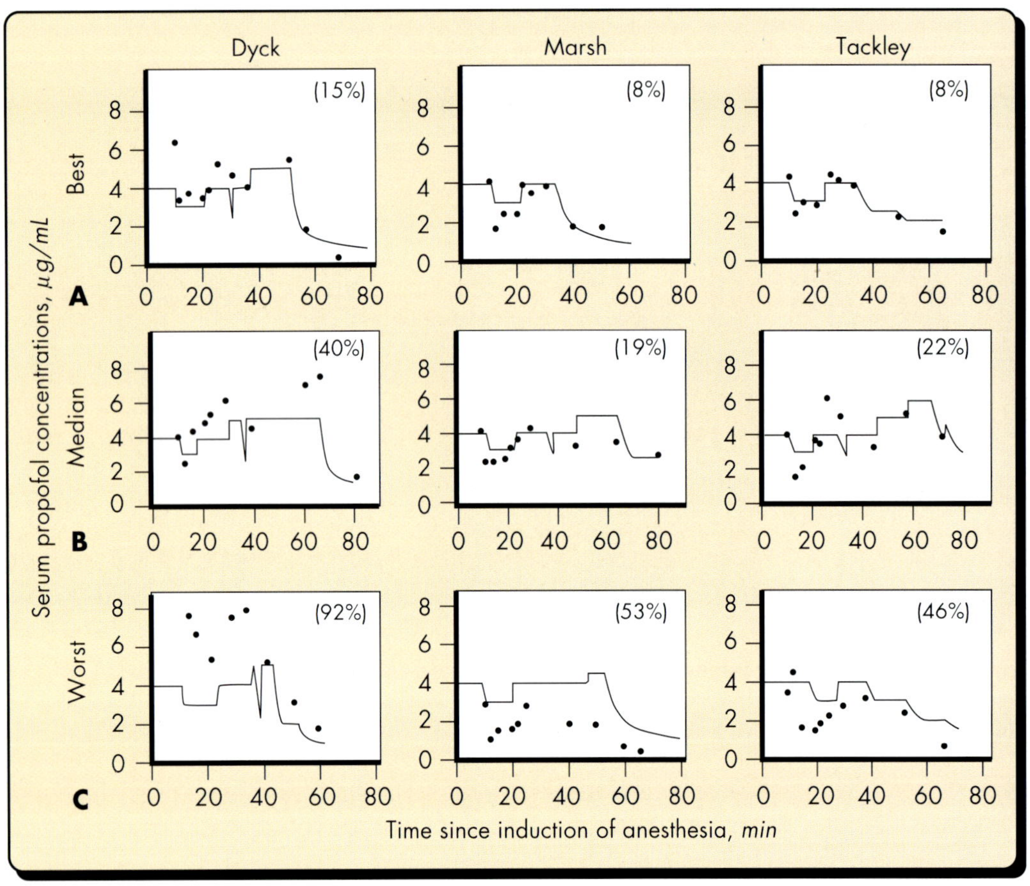

Figure 1-13. Plot of the measured to predicted concentration of propofol administered by means of a target-controlled infusion (TCI) device in patients using three different pharmacokinetic parameter sets. The *dots* are the actual measured arterial concentrations; the *solid line* represents the predicted concentration with the particular pharmacokinetic parameter set. Presented are the best (**A**), median (**B**), and worst (**C**) fit for an individual for that particular set of pharmacokinetic parameters. The numbers in parentheses indicate the median absolute performance error in that individual. The accuracy of any TCI device is primarily dependent on the set of pharmacokinetic parameters utilized within the device. In general, only a single set of parameters are used to represent the entire population. Thus it is highly unlikely in any given individual that the target concentration is the actual concentration present in that patient. A good set of pharmacokinetic parameters should result in there being no consistent over- or undershoot of the target to the measured concentration. This is represented by the bias, which should not be significantly different from 0. The target concentration should not stray far from the measured concentration within the population it is being used for. This is the absolute difference between the target and the measured concentration and is usually presented by the median absolute performance error (MAPE). This value should be less than 30% for a pharmacokinetic set considered to be adequate for use in clinical practice. The Marsh or Tackley pharmacokinetic parameters resulted in a bias of –09% and –2.8%, and a MAPE of 24% and 28%. Thus, either of these pharmacokinetic parameter sets would be suitable for use in an adult population. However, the Dyck parameters resulted in a bias of 43% and a MAPE of 47%, which would not be recommended for a similar population group. (*Adapted from* Coatzee [9].)

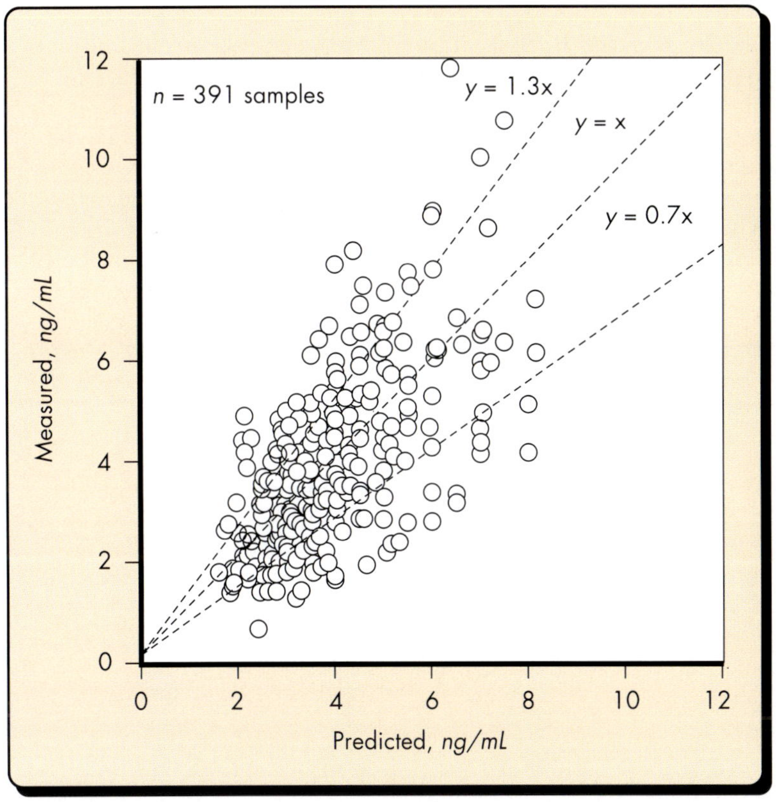

Figure 1-14. Plot of the measured to the predicted concentration of fentanyl administered via computed-assisted continuous infusion in 24 patients. In this study, the pharmacokinetic parameter set [7] resulted in excellent performance with minimal bias as seen by equal distribution around the line of identity and 70% of samples within ± 30% of predicted. (*Adapted from* Glass and coworkers [8].)

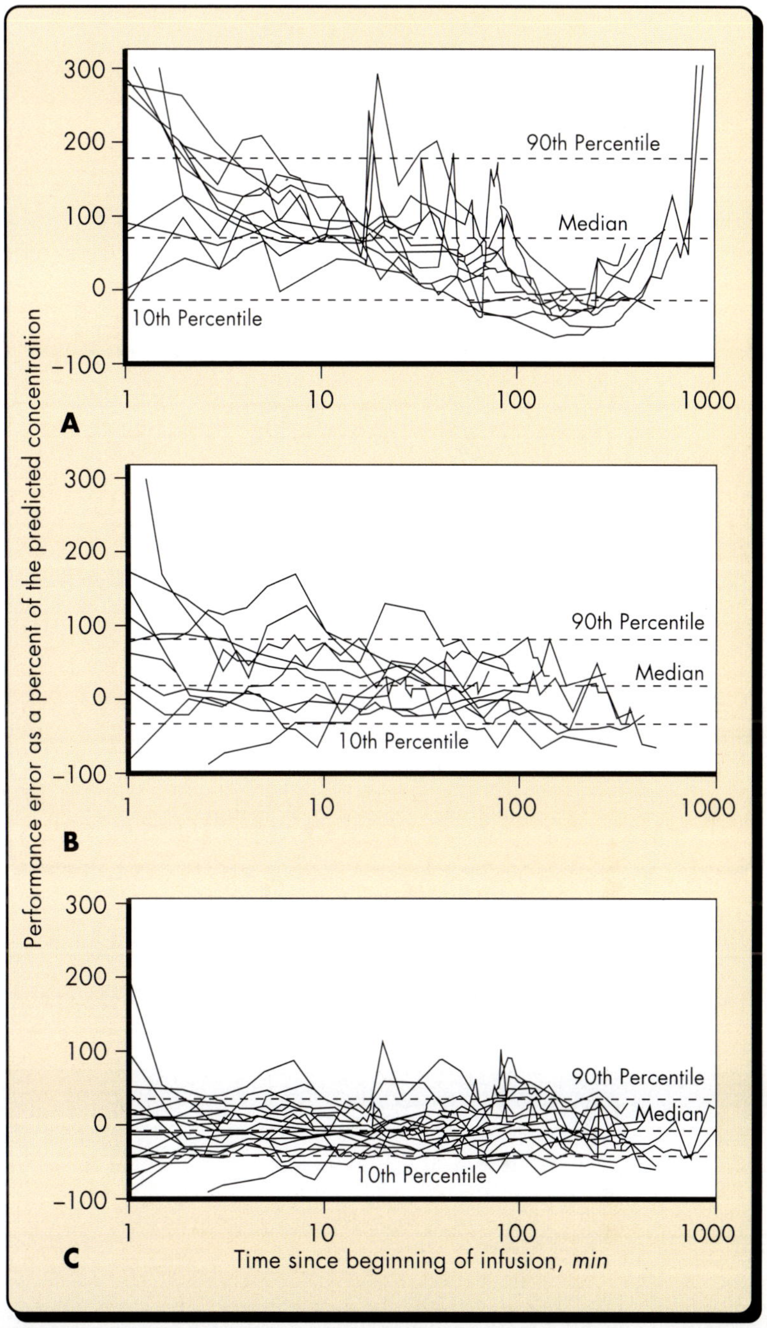

Figure 1-15. Performance error (measured and predicted) as a percent of the predicted concentration of fentanyl when administered via a target-controlled drug delivery system. Pharmacokinetic parameters shown include McLain and Hug (**A**), Scott and Stanski (**B**), and the pharmacokinetic parameters rederived from this population (**C**). Administration of intravenous anesthetics via a target-controlled drug delivery system both allows for the prospective testing of a set of pharmacokinetic parameters and allows a new set to be derived using tools such as NONMEM (nonlinear mixed effects model) that may provide greater accuracy for future use. (*Adapted from* Shafer and coworkers [10].)

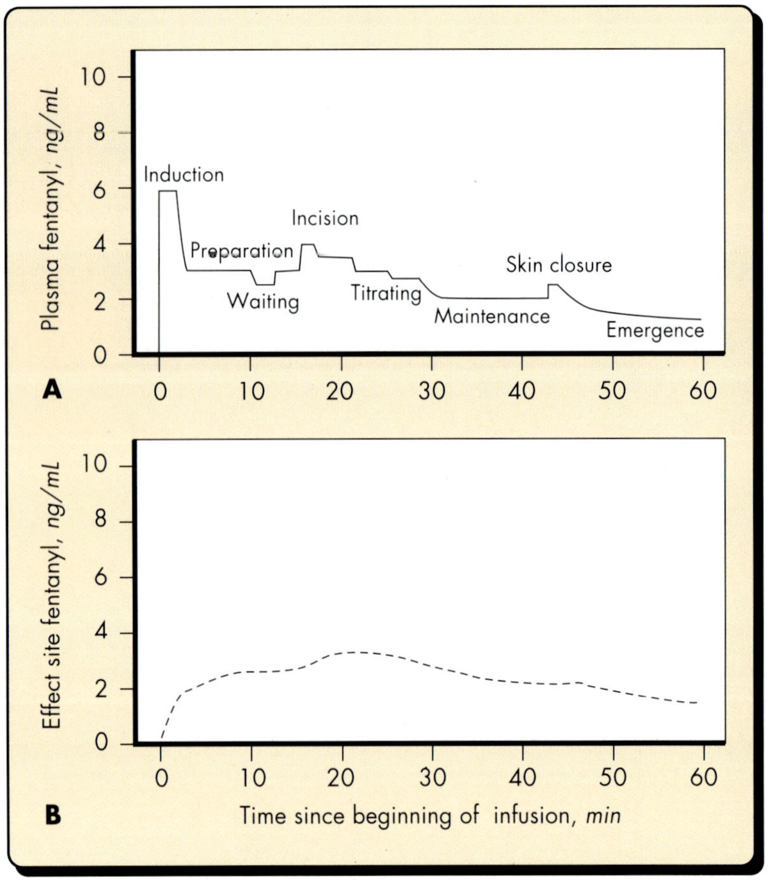

Figure 1-16. Targeted plasma concentration (**A**) and resultant simulated effect site (**B**) concentration. Most target-controlled infusion systems are programmed to target a plasma concentration. The plasma is not the site of drug effect. By measuring simultaneous drug concentration and dynamic effects, it is possible to determine the equilibration constant (k_{e0}) between plasma and the effect site (or biophase). As shown in this figure with a drug such as fentanyl, where the rate of equilibration between plasma and effect site is slow, targeting the plasma concentration provides a poor means of achieving the desired effect. Several prototype target-controlled infusion systems now allow the user to target the effect site concentration instead of the plasma concentration. This should make the titration of intravenous drugs even more precise. (*Adapted from* Shafer and Gregg [11].)

APPROXIMATE PLASMA DRUG CONCENTRATIONS REQUIRED FOR VARIOUS STIMULI

Drug	Skin incision	Major surgery	Minor surgery	Spontaneous ventilation	Awakening
Alfentanil, *ng/mL*	200–300	250–450	100–300	<200–250	—
Fentanyl, *ng/mL*	3–6	4–8	2–5	<2–3	—
Remifentanil	3–6	4–8	4–8	<2–3	
Sufentanil, *ng/mL*	1–3	2–5	1–3	<0.2–0.3	—
Propofol, *µg/mg*	2–6	2.5–7.5	2–6	—	0.8–1.8
Methohexital, *µg/mL*	5–10	5–15	5–10	—	1–3
Thiopental, *µg/mL*	7.5–12.5 (with N_2O) 35–45 (without N_2O)	10–20	10–20	—	4–8
Etomidate, *ng/mL*	400–600	500–1000	300–600	—	200–350
Midazolam, *ng/mL*	—	50–250 (when combined with an opiate)	50–250 (when combined with an opiate)	—	150–200 reduced to 20–70 in presence of an opiate
Ketamine, *mg/mL*	?	?	1–2	—	0.1–1.0

Figure 1-17. Approximate plasma drug concentrations required for various stimuli. These drug levels occur when combined with 65% to 70% nitrous oxide unless otherwise stated. Effective plasma concentrations may differ markedly depending on premedication and intraoperative drug combinations. (*Adapted from* Glass and coworkers [3].)

STEADY-STATE CONCENTRATIONS FOR PREDEFINED EFFECTS					
Drug	IC50 (±SD)	Cp50 incision or painful stimulus (±SD)	Cp50 LOC (±SD)	Cp50 spont vent (±SD)	Plasma blood concentration for a 50% reduction in isoflurane MAC
Alfentanil, *ng/mL*	50±123	241±16	500–1500	226±10	50
Fentanyl, *ng/mL*	6.9±1.9	4.2	(8–25)	(3–4)	1.67
Sufentanil, *ng/mL*	0.68±0.31	(0.3–0.4)	(0.7–2)	(0.3–0.4)	0.145
Remifentanil, *ng/mL*	14.7	(3–4)	25–75	(2–3)	1.27
Thiopental, *µg/mL*	17.9	39.8±3.3	15.6±1.1		
Propofol, *µg/mL*		15.8	3.4		

Figure 1-18. Steady-state concentrations for predefined effects. These values may provide a guide when intravenous drugs are administered by target-controlled infusions. IC50 is the steady-state serum concentration in equilibration with the effect compartment that causes a 50% slowing of the maximal electroencephalogram. Cp50 skin incision is the steady-state plasma concentration in equilibration with the effect compartment that will prevent a somatic or autonomic response in 50% of patients. Cp50 loss of consciousness (LOC) is the steady-state plasma concentration in equilibration with the effect compartment, which provides absence of a response to a verbal command in 50% of patients. For the opioids, a Cp50 LOC is provided. However, LOC is not consistently achieved with opioids, and the range is extremely large as compared with conventional hypnotics. Cp50 spontaneous ventilation is the steady-state concentration in equilibration with the effect compartment that is associated with adequate spontaneous ventilation in 50% of patients following surgery. This value is considerably higher than the opiate concentration, causing a 50% depression in minute ventilation in volunteers. MEAC is the minimum effective anesthetic concentration providing postoperative analgesia. Values in parentheses are estimated by scaling to the alfentanil Cp50 and where the potency of the opioid to alfentanil has been established. MAC—minimum alveolar concentration. (*Adapted from* Glass and coworkers [3].)

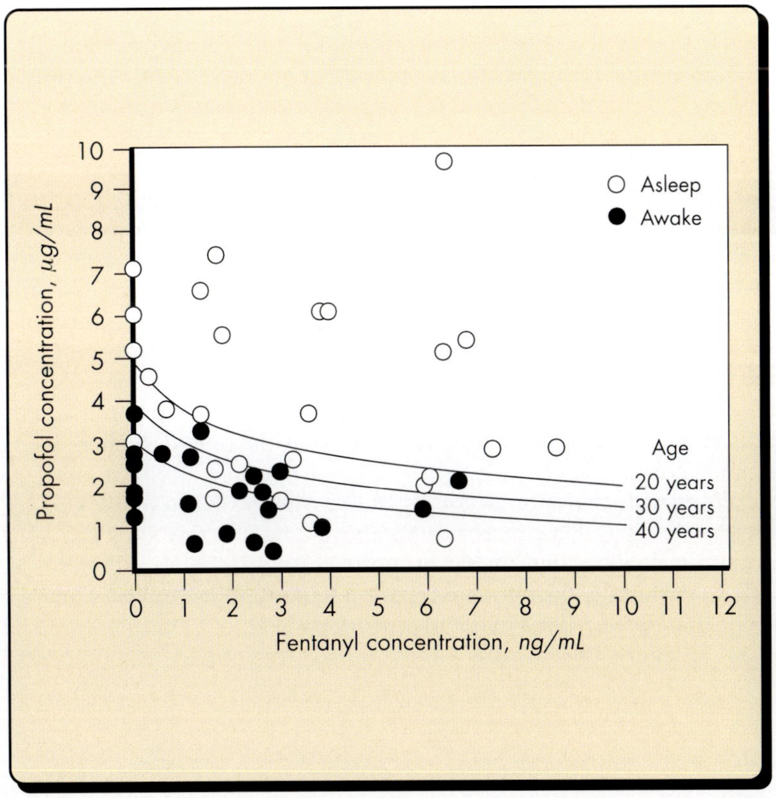

Figure 1-19. The interaction between fentanyl and propofol to provide loss of consciousness. The *solid lines* represent the concentration of propofol at a given concentration of fentanyl at which 50% of patients did not respond to a simple verbal command. It can be noted that both increasing age and increasing fentanyl concentration decrease the concentration of propofol required to produce loss of consciousness. Although fentanyl (and probably any other opioid) decreases the concentration of propofol required to produce loss of consciousness, this interaction is far less marked than that seen when these same two drugs are combined to prevent a response to a noxious stimulus, *ie*, skin incision (*see* Figs. 1-16 and 1-17). (*Adapted from* Smith and coworkers [12].)

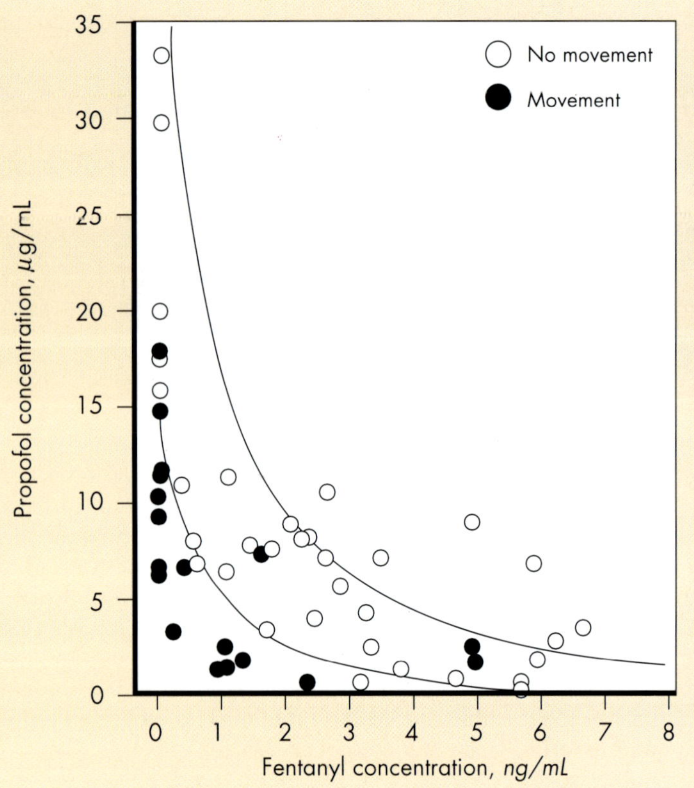

Figure 1-20. The interaction between propofol and fentanyl that results in lack of a somatic response to a noxious stimulus. The *solid line* represents the concentration of propofol at a given concentration of fentanyl at which 50% of patients did not respond to a surgical incision. For a noxious stimulus, analgesic concentrations of fentanyl (1 to 2 ng/mL) markedly reduce the concentration of propofol required to provide adequate anesthesia. Also, the ability of fentanyl (or any other opioid) to reduce the requirement of propofol to ensure absence of a response reaches a plateau. This plateau is close to the Cp50 for loss of consciousness with propofol (*ie*, 3 μg/mL). Thus, in using a total intravenous technique, a minimum concentration of propofol to provide loss of consciousness is required and there is little value in increasing the opioid much above an equivalent concentration of fentanyl of 4 to 6 ng/mL. A similar interaction occurs between the opioids and volatile anesthetics, and the same principles hold true. (*Adapted from* Smith and coworkers [12].)

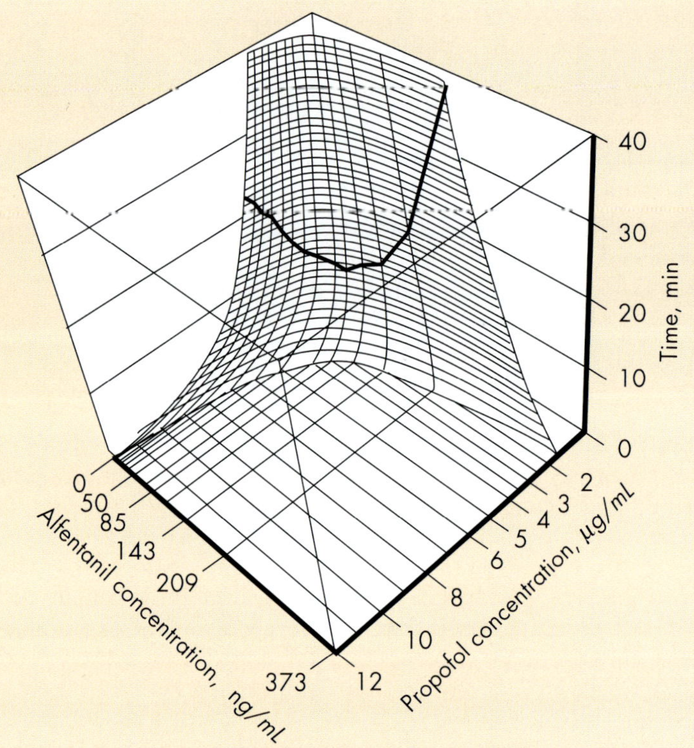

Figure 1-21. The interaction between propofol and alfentanil to prevent a somatic response to skin incision. The interaction is very similar to that illustrated between propofol and fentanyl (*see* Fig. 1-16) and confirms the principles outlined previously. The interaction between propofol and opioid is complex, and thus it is difficult to decide if it is better to administer more propofol or more opioid in obtaining an adequate state of anesthesia. Part of that decision should be based on the ability of the patient to awaken and breathe spontaneously at the end of the procedure. Illustrated on the z axis in this figure is the time required for adequate recovery to occur with each drug combination. For the most rapid recovery, a propofol concentration of 3.5 μ/mL combined with an alfentanil concentration of 80 ng/mL will provide adequate anesthesia in 50% of patients and the fastest recovery. Thus, the optimal drug combination depends on the drug interaction and the recovery characteristics of the individual drugs being used. If remifentanil was used as the opioid, higher opioid concentrations and slightly lower propofol concentrations would provide the optimal combination, whereas when fentanyl is used as the opioid, a concentration above 2 ng/mL may slow recovery substantially. Thus, higher propofol concentrations are preferable to ensure the fastest recovery for a fentanyl-plus-propofol anesthetic. (*Adapted from* Vuyk and coworkers [13].)

AUTOMATED CLOSED-LOOP DRUG DELIVERY SYSTEMS

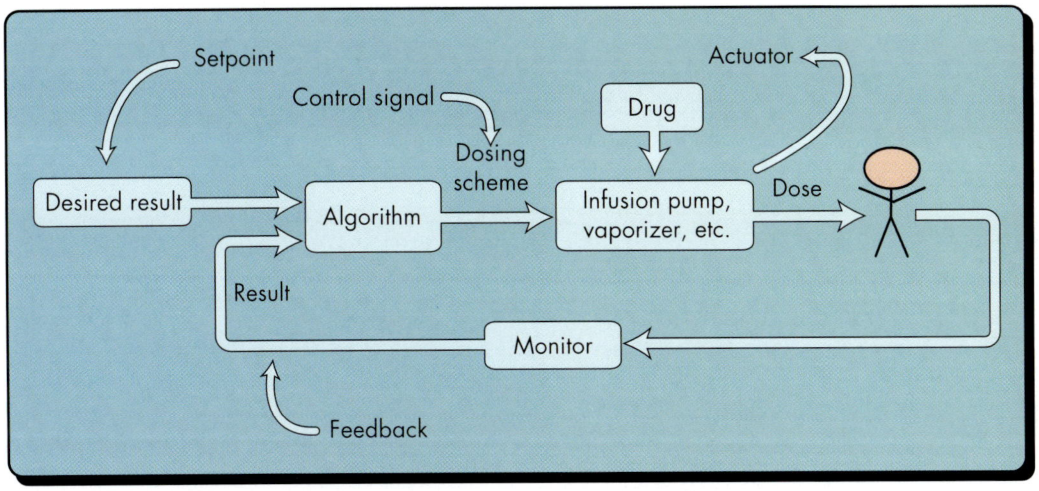

Figure 1-22. The components of a typical fully automated drug delivery system. This system differs from a target-controlled infusion device in that it contains a monitor of effect. In a closed-loop drug delivery system, the user inputs the desired result (*eg*, maintain neuromuscular blockade T_1 [the first twitch of the train-of-four] at 10% of control). The device automatically adjusts its dosing based on an algorithm (often incorporating pharmacokinetic parameters) to achieve the set effect. (*Adapted from* Jacobs and coworkers [5].)

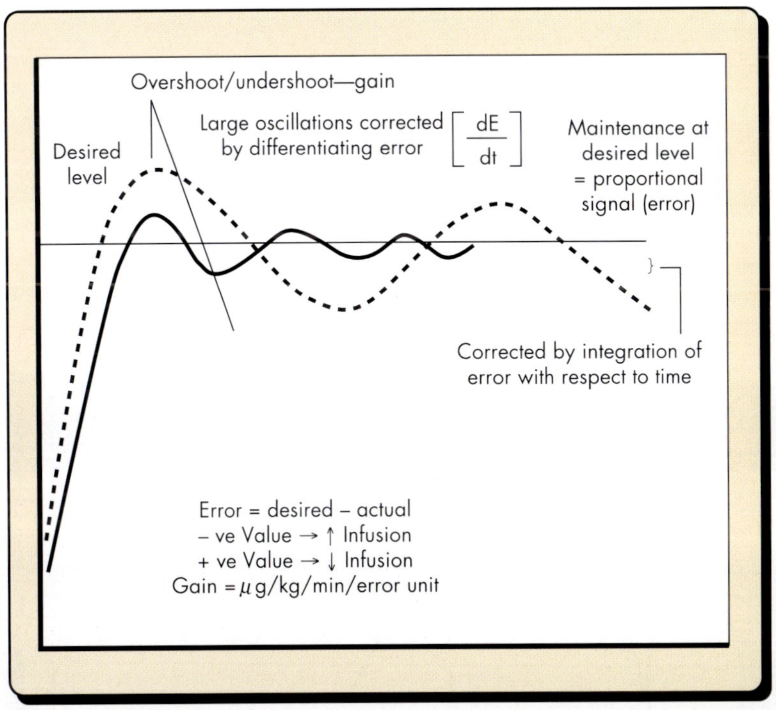

Figure 1-23. How the proportional, integral and derivative of the error is used to provide closed-loop control. A measured value of a parameter (the "output") is arithmetically subtracted from the desired value (the "setpoint"), producing a difference value (the "error"). This error signal is used to drive some device (the "prime mover") in such a way as to decrease the error (*ie*, "negative feedback"). Thus, the system tends toward an equilibrium where the setpoint is equal to the output, and the error signal is zero. If the setpoint or output is subsequently changed, the system automatically corrects the situation. Proportional controllers are simple in concept, but perform poorly where there is an appreciable delay in the response of the prime mover. Then they tend to overcorrect and oscillate. This limitation led to the development of the "proportional-derivative" (PD) controller, which generates an error to signal based not only on the difference between the setpoint and the output but the time rate of change of this difference as well. In principle, a PD controller will detect the condition where the error signal is rapidly approaching zero, and thus slow the corrective action of the prime mover. PD controllers perform well in mechanical servo applications, but a slight limitation exists whenever the output is biased by a constant factor such as a mechanical load. In this situation, the PD controller comes into equilibrium with a small constant error that exactly balances the effect of the load. Often the error is small enough to be negligible, but it can often be corrected by adding a third component consisting of the time integral of the error, forming a "proportional-integral-derivative" (PID) controller. The integral component corrects for the constant error and forces the output to be exactly equal to the setpoint.

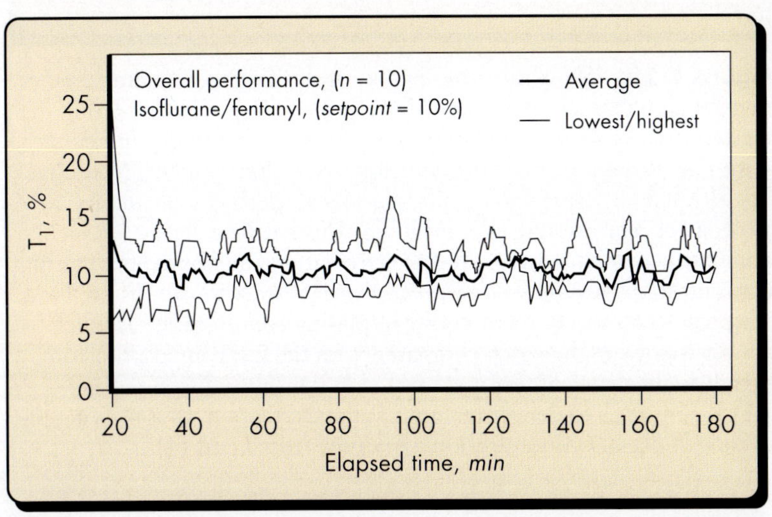

Figure 1-24. Typical performance of an automated closed-loop device for neuromuscular blockade when used to administer vecuronium to a setpoint of 10% of the original T_1 (the first twitch of the train-of-four) in the presence, of isoflurane and fentanyl. The *bold line* is the average performance in 10 patients; the *top* and *bottom lines* are the highest and lowest T_1 within the 10 patients at that time point. With an appropriate physiologic monitor, drugs can be delivered to provide very accurately the desired effect. (*Adapted from* Glass [4].)

ALTERNATE NOVEL DRUG DELIVERY SYSTEMS FOR INTRAVENOUS ANESTHETICS

Transdermal	Transmucosal
Passive patch	Oral
Iontophoretic patch	Nasal
	Rectal
	Inhaled

Figure 1-25. Alternate novel delivery systems for intravenous anesthetics.

ADVANTAGES AND DISADVANTAGES OF THE TRANSDERMAL FENTANYL PATCH

Advantages
- Provides a simple and convenient mode of drug delivery
- Allows a more precise control over plasma drug concentrations than intermittent dosing
- Reduces amount of drug needed daily to achieve a therapeutic effect by avoiding first-pass loss
- Avoids variability of gastrointestinal absorption
- Provides an alternative route when oral administration is not practical
- Provides a parenteral route without the inconvenience of intravenous infusions or intramuscular injections
- Allows delivery to be altered by changing patch size

Disadvantages
- Long lag time between placing patch and reaching therapeutic levels
- Cannot rapidly alter concentration
- Patients cannot interact with system to titrate themselves to their own effective plasma concentration
- If overdose occurs extremely long elimination of drug

Figure 1-26. Advantages and disadvantages of the transdermal fentanyl patch. (*Adapted from* Glass [4].)

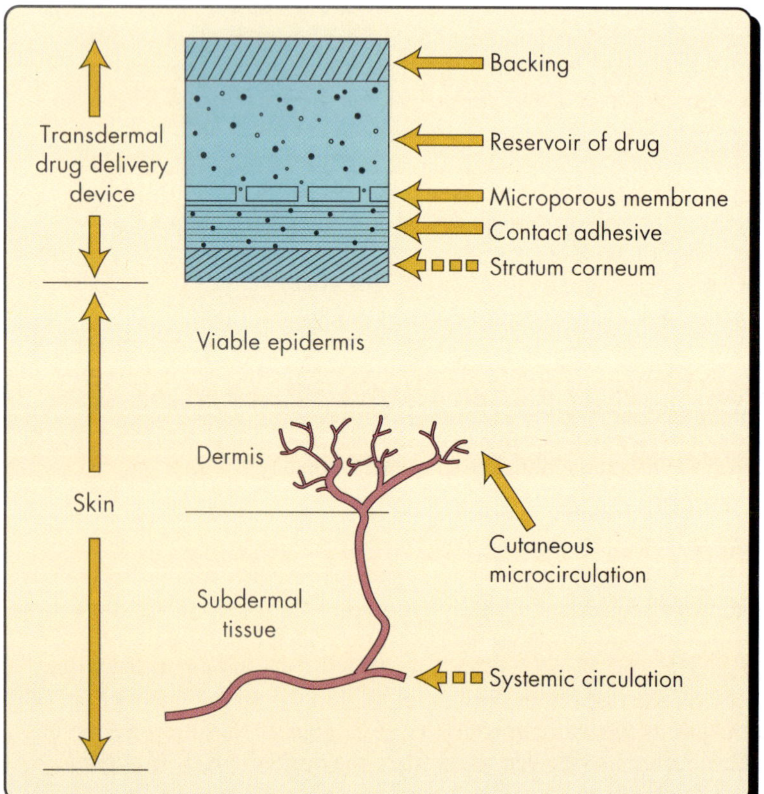

Figure 1-27. Transdermal drug delivery system. To provide absorption through the skin, a very high concentration gradient is necessary. To achieve this a drug reservoir is created. Absorption through the skin can also be very variable according to application site, state of the cutaneous microcirculation, and so on. To ensure consistent absorption, the device contains a rate-limiting membrane that thus minimizes the variability. To increase the delivery rate, a larger patch is applied. (*Adapted from* Varvel and coworkers [14].)

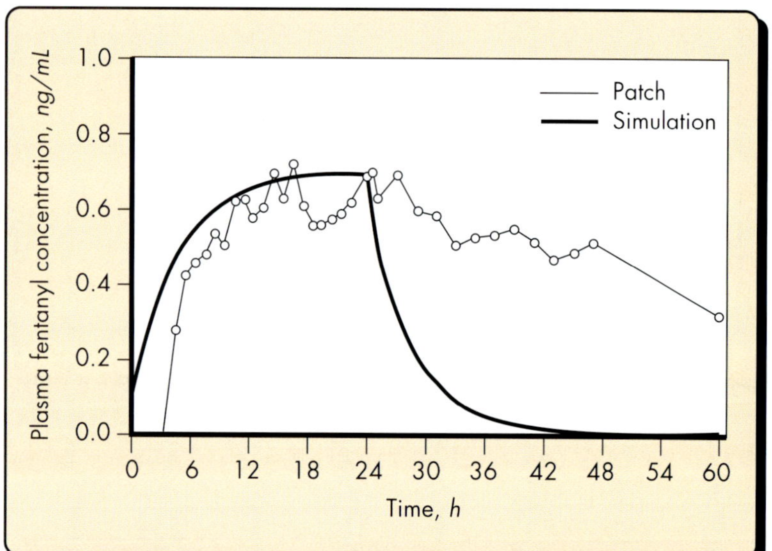

Figure 1-28. The absorption uptake and elimination characteristics of a 50-μg/h transdermal drug delivery patch. These data are contrasted to a computer simulation of the theoretical uptake and elimination of 50-μg/h intravenous infusion in the same patient. Note that initially, fentanyl is absorbed into the subcutaneous tissue and its plasma concentration rises very slowly. Ultimately, delivery between patch, subcutaneous tissue, and the circulation equilibrate and plasma concentrations reach those achieved by the intravenous infusion. Once the patch is removed, the decrease in plasma concentration is much slower following the patch compared with the intravenous infusion owing to the depot of fentanyl created in the subcutaneous tissue, which continues to deliver fentanyl to the circulation, thus slowing the decline in plasma concentration. (*Adapted from* Glass [4].)

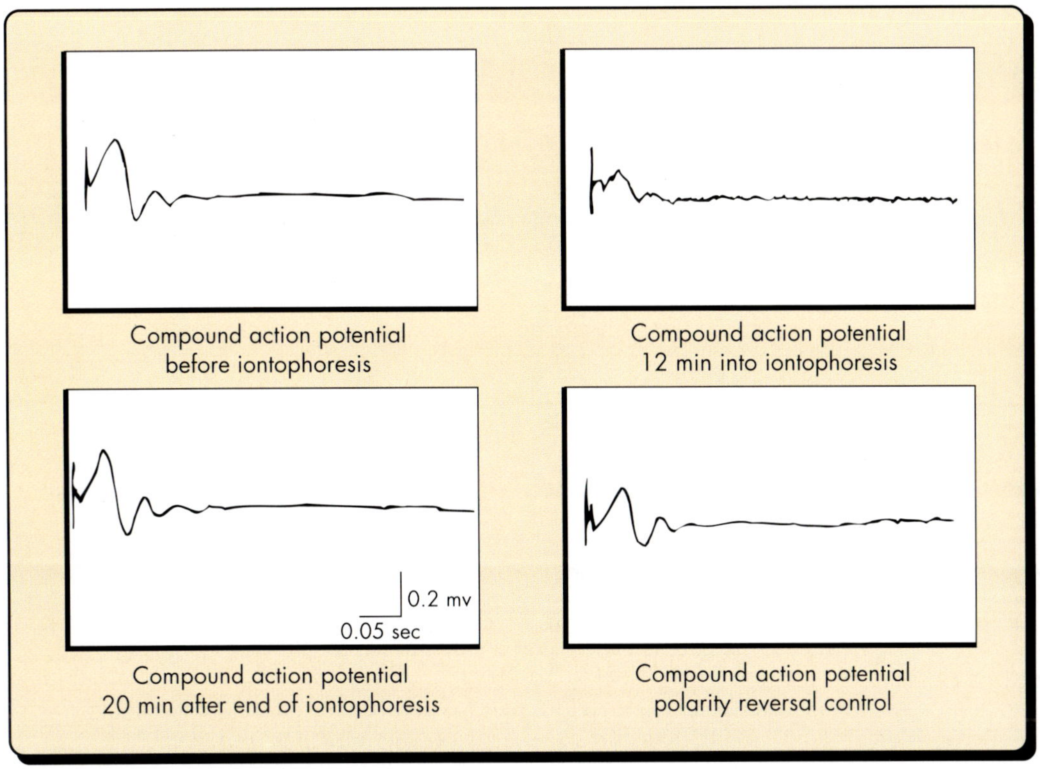

Figure 1-29. Iontophoresis provides active transfer of polar drugs across the skin by means of an electric current. Iontophoresis of lidocaine has been used to provide local anesthesia to the underlying skin. In very superficial nerves it is also possible, as shown in this figure, to actually cause neural blockade. This potential for local anesthetic iontophoresis has not yet been fully explored. Several opioids (morphine, fentanyl, and sufentanil) have also been administered via iontophoresis to reach therapeutic concentrations. These therapeutic concentrations are achieved more rapidly than is observed when a passive patch is applied.

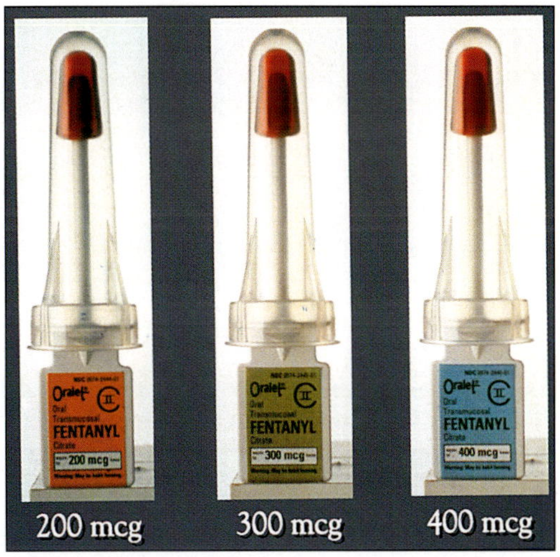

Figure 1-30. Different dosage strengths of oral transmucosal fentanyl citrate (OTFC). This form of fentanyl drug delivery is presently approved for premedication in children. Although OTFC is well accepted in this population group and enhances parental separation, it does result in occasional incidences of depressed ventilation, increased rigidity on induction of anesthesia, and an increased incidence of nausea and vomiting. The major utility of OTFC is probably for brief painful procedures in children done under sedation or for breakthrough pain in cancer patients.

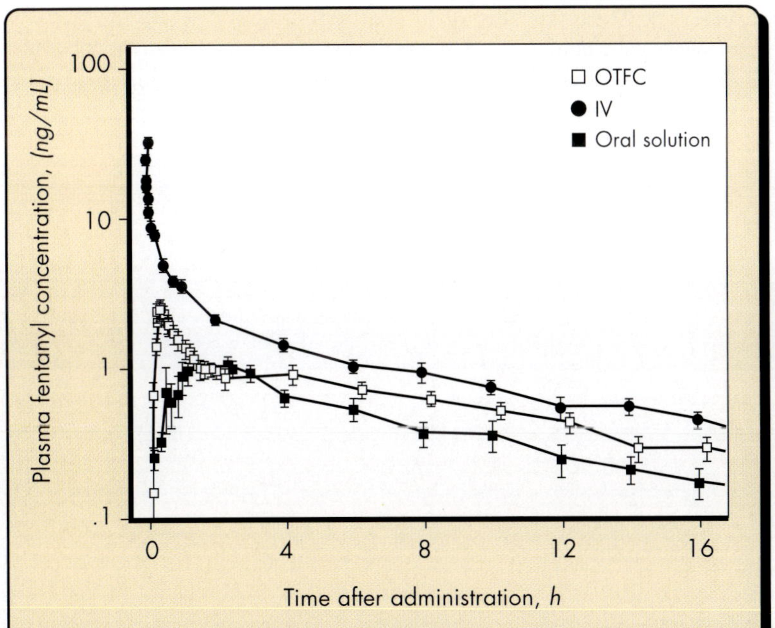

Figure 1-31. The plasma concentrations of fentanyl following a dose of 15 µg/kg (800 µg) administered either intravenously (IV), via an oral transmucosal fentanyl citrate (OTFC) delivery system, or orally. Approximately 30% of the OTFC is swallowed and some of this dose undergoes first-pass metabolism, resulting in a 90% bioavailability of the OTFC formulation of fentanyl. OTFC administration of fentanyl provides some unique advantages. The absorption of fentanyl into the systemic circulation from the OTFC is rapid. However, the OTFC is consumed over approximately 15 minutes. This results in a fairly rapid achievement of analgesic concentrations (peak effect, 15 to 20 min) but as redistribution is occurring continuously with absorption, the peak effect site concentration after a dose of 800 µg does not generally exceed that, causing significant respiratory depression. This is in contrast to an intravenous (IV) bolus of the same dose of fentanyl, which would produce significant respiratory depression. Also, as extensive redistribution has occurred during consumption of the OTFC, the subsequent decrease in fentanyl concentration is primarily dependent on its elimination (rather than redistribution), thus providing a fairly long duration of analgesic action. (*Adapted from* Streisand and coworkers [15].)

DOSING AND ONSET WITH TRANSMUCOSAL ADMINISTRATION OF HYPNOTICS AND OPIOIDS				
Drug	Route	Time to peak effect, *min*	Bioavailibility, %	Dose, *μg/kg*
Midazolam	Intranasal	5–15	50	200
Midazolam	Oral	10–15	20–30	500
Fentanyl	Oral	20–30	90	10
Fentanyl	Intranasal	10–20	Approximately 70–80	0.3–2
Sufentanil	Intranasal	10–20	70–80	0.05–0.2

Figure 1-32. Dosing and onset with transmucosal administration of hypnotics and opioids.

REFERENCES

1. Major DJ: *Chirurgia Infusoria placidis CL: Virorium Dubiis impugnata, cum modesta, ad Eadem, Responsione*. Kiloni: 1667.
2. Dundee JW, Wyant GM: *Intravenous Anaesthesia*, edn 2. London: Churchill Livingstone; 1988.
3. Glass PSA, Shafer SL, Jacobs JR, Reves JG: *Intravenous Drug Delivery Systems*. In *Anesthesia*, edn 4. Edited by Miller R. New York: Churchill Livingstone; 1994:389–416.
4. Glass P: Intravenous Drug Delivery Systems. In *Drug Infusions in Anesthesiology*, edn 2. Edited by Fragen RJ. Lippincott-Raven Press; 1996:25–70.
5. Reves JG, Jacobs JR, Glass PSA: Automated Drug Delivery in Anesthesia. In American Society of Anesthesiologists *Refresher Course in Anesthesiology*. 1991, 19:127–137.
6. Jacobs JR, Glass PSA, Reves JG: Opioid administration by continuous infusion. In *Opioids in Anesthesia*, edn2. Edited by Estafanous FG. Boston: Butterworth Heinemann; 1990:241–253.
7. McClain DA, Hug CC Jr: Intravenous fentanyl kinetics. *Clin Pharmacol Ther* 1980, 28:106–114.
8. Glass PSA, Jacobs JR, Smith RL, *et al.*: Pharmacokinetic model-driven infusion of fentanyl: assessment of accuracy. *Anesthesiology* 1990, 73:1082–1090.
9. Coetzee JF, Glen JB, Wuim CA, Boshoffl: Pharmacokinetic model selection for target-controlled infusions of propofol. *Anesthesiology* 1995, 82:1328–1345.
10. Shafer SL, Varvel JR, Aziz N, Scott JC: The pharmacokinetics of fentanyl administered by computer controlled infusion pump. *Anesthesiology* 1990, 73:1091–1102.
11. Shafer SL, Gregg K: Algorithms to rapidly achieve and maintain stable drug concentrations at the site of drug effect with a computer controlled infusion pump. *J Pharmacokinetic Biopharm* 1992, 20:147–169.
12. Smith C, McEwan AI, Jhaveri R, *et al.*: The interaction of fentanyl on the Cp_{50} of propofol for loss of consciousness and skin incision. *Anesthesiology* 1994, 81:820–828.
13. Vuyk J, Lim T, Engbers FHM, *et al.*: The pharmacodynamic interaction of propofol and alfentanil during lower abdominal surgery in female patients. *Anesthesiology* 1995, 83:8–22.
14. Varvel JR, Shafer SL, Hwang SS, *et al.*: Absorption characteristics of transdermally administered fentanyl. *Anesthesiology* 1989, 70:928–934.
15. Streisand JB, Varvel JR, Stanski DR, *et al.*: Absorption and bioavailability of oral transmucosal fentanyl citrate. *Anesthesiology* 1991, 75:223–229.

2

Inhaled Anesthetic Delivery Systems

James F. Szocik

This chapter is divided into three parts. The first deals with the principles of inhaled anesthesia delivery systems, that is, the chemistry and physics of gas and vapor storage, delivery, and elimination. The second delves into the equipment used to anesthetize patients and support their physiology, including some aspects of manufacture, storage, and delivery of anesthetic gases and vapors. A historical perspective is used for vaporizers and anesthesia machines to illustrate the changes that have been made to these devices as understanding of the underlying principles has evolved. The third portion enumerates some of the complications associated with use of the equipment described previously.

After viewing this material, the reader should have a greater understanding of how anesthesia equipment works, of the limitations imposed by physics and physiology, and of the complications that can arise through use and misuse of anesthesia equipment. Understanding these principles will also allow the reader to interpret future directions in anesthesia machine development. Modern anesthesia equipment is well-designed, safe, and reliable; however, a significant portion of the safety and reliability is in the hands of the person administering the anesthetic, just as in the days of open-drop ether.

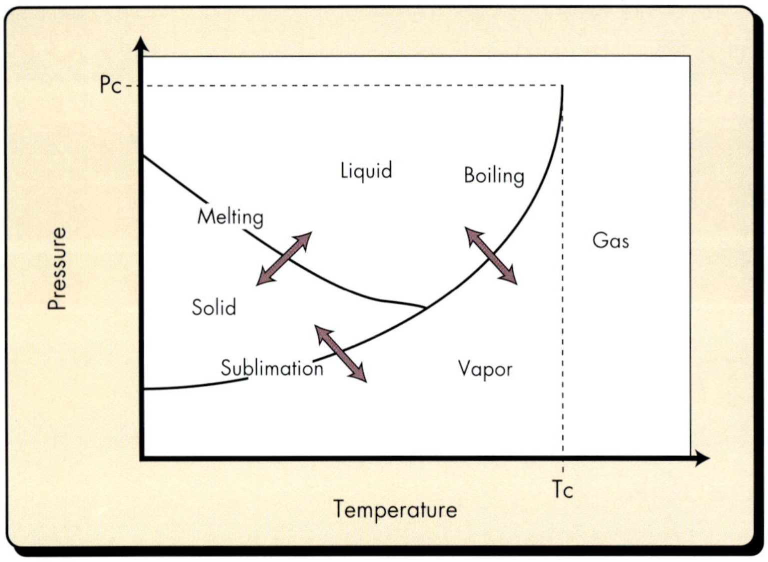

Figure 2-1. Solids, liquids, fluids, vapors, or gases? Matter can exist in several states, depending on temperature and pressure [1,2]. A familiar example is water, which is solid at temperatures below 0°C (and 1 atm pressure), becomes liquid at temperatures greater than 0°C, with a vapor pressure dependent on temperature. At 100°C the vapor pressure equals atmospheric pressure, and water becomes a vapor and "boils." The boiling point of a liquid is simply that temperature at which the vapor pressure equals the atmospheric pressure. As altitude increases above sea level, water boils at a lower temperature because the atmospheric pressure is lower. Vapors are the "gaseous" phase of a material that exist in equilibrium with liquid at that temperature and pressure. Above its critical temperature, a substance can only exist as a gas. Critical temperature (T_c) is that temperature above which a gas cannot be liquefied by pressure. Critical pressure (P_c) is the pressure required to liquefy a gas at its critical temperature. To further confuse things, the terms *fluid* and *liquid* are commonly used interchangeably, when indeed they are not synonymous. Vapors and gases are compressible fluids, whereas liquids are incompressible fluids.

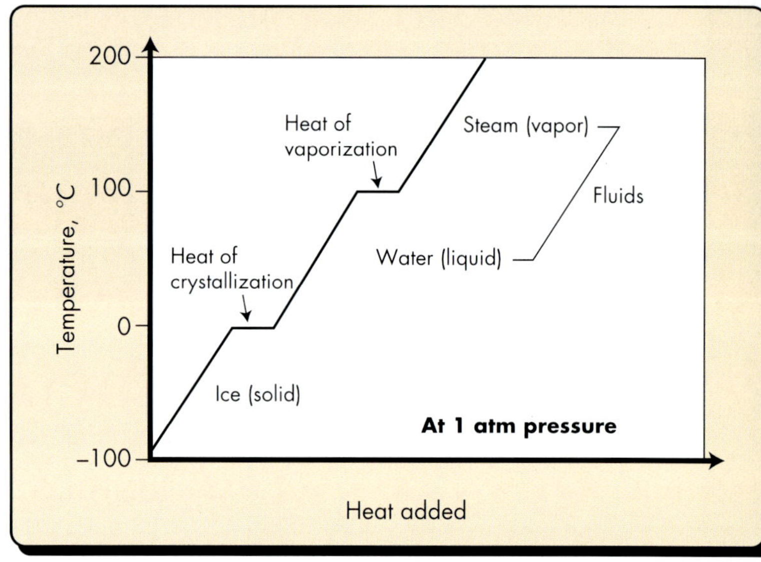

Figure 2-2. Heat of vaporization. When solids melt or liquids vaporize, these state transitions require extra energy (heat of crystallization and heat of vaporization). Anesthetic equipment that involves vaporizing liquids must be constructed to deliver this energy in some form. (*Modified from* Mushin and Jones [3].)

IDEAL GAS LAWS

Eponym	Mathematical expression	Extrapolation
Boyle's law	PV=k	For a constant quantity of gas, as volume decreases, pressure increases (and vice versa)
Charles' law	$V \propto T°C + 273$ $V \propto T°K$	Gases expand and contract with temperature (if pressure remains constant)
Gay-Lussac's law	$P \propto T°C + 273$ $P \propto T°K$	Gases increase or decrease in pressure as the temperature increases or decreases (if the volume remains constant)
Dalton's law	$PV \propto (N1+N2)kT$	Total pressure of a mixture of gases is the sum of individual pressures in proportion to the number of molecules of each gas
Definitions	P—pressure V—volume T—temperature k—a constant N—number of moles	*Notes.* The constants here are not identical to each other. T°K = T°C+273

Figure 2-3. Ideal gas laws and their design implications. For *ideal gases* (those with theoretically no molecular interaction between their particles), the ideal gas laws describe the interrelationship between pressure, volume, and temperature. As compressed gases expand, pressure and temperature decrease. For this reason, compressed gases must be dry to prevent condensation or freezing of water vapor inside the apparatus. In addition, in the cylinder yoke, trapped gases can be compressed when the cylinder valve is opened, with a resultant increase in temperature. For this reason, no grease or oil is used on gas valve fittings because the temperature increase could ignite any flammable material [3]. These laws form some of the basis of anesthesia machine design and will be referred to in subsequent illustrations.

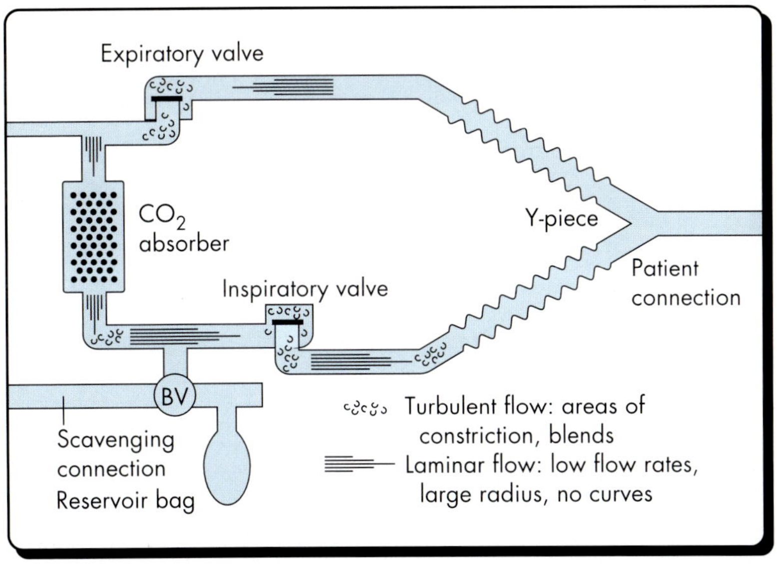

Figure 2-4. Moving gases: flows and resistance. Gases and liquids flow down pressure gradients in an attempt to lower their energy and increase their entropy. At low flow rates (below the critical velocity), flow is laminar and resistance is related to viscosity and flow rate. The Hagen-Pouiseuille equation ($p=8\eta V/\pi r^4 t$ or $Q=V/t=\pi r^4 p/8\eta$) describes the pressure decrease (p) and flow (Q=volume(V)/time(t)) given the viscosity of the fluid (η) and the length (l) and radius (r) of the tube [3]. This is the familiar r to the fourth power rule for flow through a tube, *ie*, a catheter. As flows exceed the Reynold's number ($Re=\rho Ul/\mu$), flow becomes turbulent, and resistance increases and is affected by density (ρ) (U=mean flow velocity) [2]. Flow in turbulent systems is not truly predictable but may follow some empirically derived formulas. Anesthetic circuits have areas of both laminar and turbulent flow. Turbulent flow occurs at high flow rates, with fluids of high viscosities, and at areas of constriction or bends in tubing. BV—bag ventilator selector switch; CO_2—carbon dioxide. (*Modified from* Dorsch and Dorsch [4].

A. CHARACTERISTICS OF COMMONLY USED GASES AND VAPORS

Chemical Name	Formula, Molecular Mass	Boiling Point, °C	Vapor Pressure at 20°C, *mm Hg*	Heat of Vaporization, *kJ/g*	Critical Temperature, °C	Critical Pressure, *atm*
Water	H_2O, 18.0	100	17	2.45	374	215
Ethyl alcohol	CH_3•CH_2OH, 46.1	78.3	44	0.92	243	62
Diethyl ether	C_2H_5•O•C_2H_5, 74.1	34.6	441	0.37	194	350
Chloroform	$CHCl_3$, 119	61.2	160	0.28	263	53
Trichloroethylene	CHCl: CCl_2, 131	87	65	0.24	271	49
Halothane	CF_3•CHClBr, 197	50.2	242	0.15	296	38
Methoxyflurane	CH_3•O•CCl_2•CHF_2, 165	105	23	0.21	—	—
Enflurane	CHF_2•O•CF_2CHClF, 185	56.5	173	0.16	—	—
Isoflurane	CHF_2•O•$CHClCF_3$, 185	48.5	240	0.15	—	—
Carbon dioxide	CO_2, 44	-78	428	0.15	31	73
Nitrous oxide	N_20, 44	-88.6	390	0.37	36.4	72
Cyclopropane	CH_2•CH_2•CH_2, 42.1	-33	56	0.47	125	54
Oxygen	0_2, 32	-183	—	0.21	-118	50
Nitrogen	N_2, 28	-196	—	0.20	-147	34
Air	29	-194	—	0.21	-141	37
Hydrogen	H_2, 2.02	-253	—	0.45	-240	13
Helium	He, 4	-269	—	0.025	-268	2
Xenon	Xe, 131	-108	—	0.096	16.5	58
Desflurane	CHF_2•O•$CHFCF_3$, 168.04	22.8	669			
Sevoflurane	CH_2F•O•$CH(CF_3)_2$, 200.05	58.6	157			

Figure 2-5. Commonly used gases and vapors. Many of these properties are interrelated. For example, one cannot define the boiling point without specifying the pressure, because the true definition of boiling point is the temperature at which the vapor pressure equals the ambient or atmospheric pressure (**A**).

(*Continued on next page*)

B. OSTWALD PARTITION COEFFICIENT FOR COMMONLY USED GASES AND VAPORS (AT 37°C)

Chemical Name	Water/Gas	Oil/Gas	Blood/Gas	Muscle/Gas	Fat/Gas	Brain/Blood	Muscle/Blood	Fat/Blood	MAC, *vol %*
Water	—	—	—	—	—				—
Ethyl alcohol	—	—	—	—	—				—
Diethyl ether	13	65	12	10	50	1.1	0.9	5	1.92
Chloroform	4.00	400	8	12	280				0.77 (dog)
Trichloroethylene	1.70	900	9	12	600				0.6 (rat)
Halothane	0.80	220	2.4	6.0	155	2.6	2.5	60	0.8
Methoxyflurane	4.50	950	11	20	670				0.16
Enflurane	0.80	98	1.9	3	70	2.6	1.7	105	1.68
Isoflurane	0.62	97	1.4	5.6	68	3.7	4	45	1.15
Carbon dioxide	0.64	1.0	40	—	—				
Nitrous oxide	0.47	1.4	0.47	0.4	1.1	1.1	1.2	3	101
Cyclopropane	0.2	11.5	0.55	0.4	8				9.2
Oxygen	0.03	—	—	—	—				
Nitrogen	0.024	—	0.015	—	0.054				>1 atm
Air	—	—	—	—	—				—
Hydrogen	—	—	—	—	—				—
Helium	—	—	—	—	—				—
Xenon	0.09	1.8	0.14	0.10	1.3				0.71 atm
Desflurane		18.7	0.424						6.00
Sevoflurane	0.36	47–54	0.63						2.60

Figure 2-5. (*Continued*) Note the Ostwald partition coefficients (**B**) that parallel the anesthetic potency as part of the Meyer-Overton hypothesis. Some of the agents are included for historical perspective. Note that the concept of minimum alveolar concentration (*MAC*), an ED_{50} dose of anesthetic, did not exist before the 1960s. Hence, no MAC values are available for humans in these older agents. (Chloroform is now listed as a carcinogen and is not used). (*Modified from* Mushin and Jones [3].)

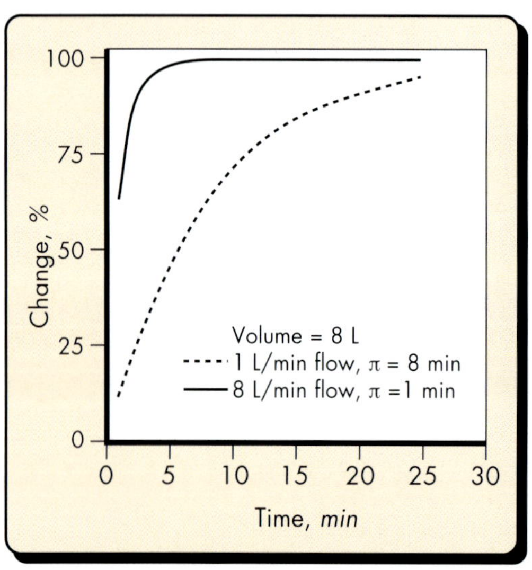

Figure 2-6. Time constants. As gases flow into a circuit or reservoir bag, they mix. The composition of the gas in the circuit can be predicted by mathematical principles. The time constant is defined as the volume divided by the flow rate and has units of time. Imagine trying to change the concentration in an anesthetic circuit. As new gas enters and mixes, the mixture will exit via the pop-off valve to the scavenging system. If the circuit holds 8 liters and the flow rate is 1 L/min, the time constant is 8 minutes (8 L/1 L per minute). If the flow rate increases to 8 L/min, the time constant decreases to 1 minute. The following formula allows one to predict the new concentration at time t. $C_{(t)} = C \times (1-e^{(-t/\tau)})$. At one time constant, the gas concentration is 68% toward the new equilibrium; at two time constants, 86%; and at three time constants, 95%.

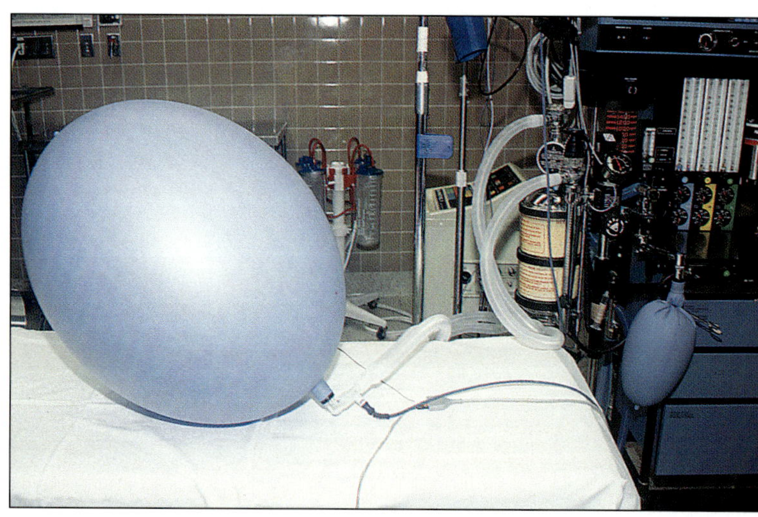

Figure 2-7. Compliance. The definition of *compliance* is change in volume for a change in pressure. Inverse compliance is termed *elastance*. Anesthetic circuits have compliance in that a given change in pressure during the respiratory cycle is accompanied by a change in volume. The reservoir bag is designed to be highly compliant to limit the chance of patient injury owing to high pressure.

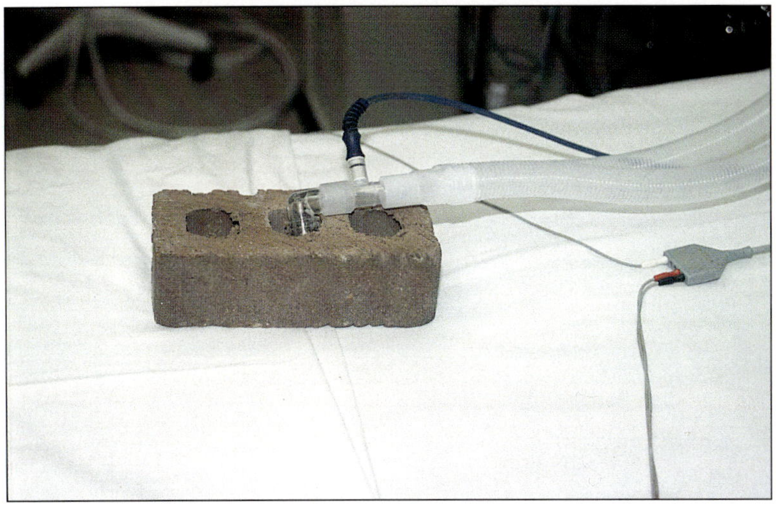

Figure 2-8. Noncompliant. Some patient's lungs may become noncompliant or "stiff" owing to pulmonary edema or other pathologic processes.

Carbon dioxide absorption

Initial reaction

$CO_2 + H_2O \rightarrow H_2CO_3$

Soda lime

$2NaOH + 2H_2CO_3 + Ca(OH)_2 \rightarrow CaCO_3 + Na_2CO_3 + 4H_2O$

Baralyme

$Ba(OH)_2 \bullet 8H_2CO + CO_2 \rightarrow BaCO_3 + 9H_2O$

Figure 2-9. Carbon dioxide (CO_2) absorption. CO_2 formed by the body is eliminated by respiratory exchange with an atmospheric pool much larger than our lungs. When the pool is decreased in size (such as when breathing into a paper bag or an anesthetic circuit), oxygen content is decreased and CO_2 is then increased, leading to rebreathing. Therefore, anesthesia circuits need to either have flows greater than minute ventilation or a means of eliminating the CO_2. Two chemicals are commonly used for this purpose, soda lime and baralyme. The size of the granules at 4 to 8 mesh is an empiric balance between the surface area for absorption of CO_2 and the resistance to gas flow.

EQUIPMENT USED TO DELIVER INHALED ANESTHETICS

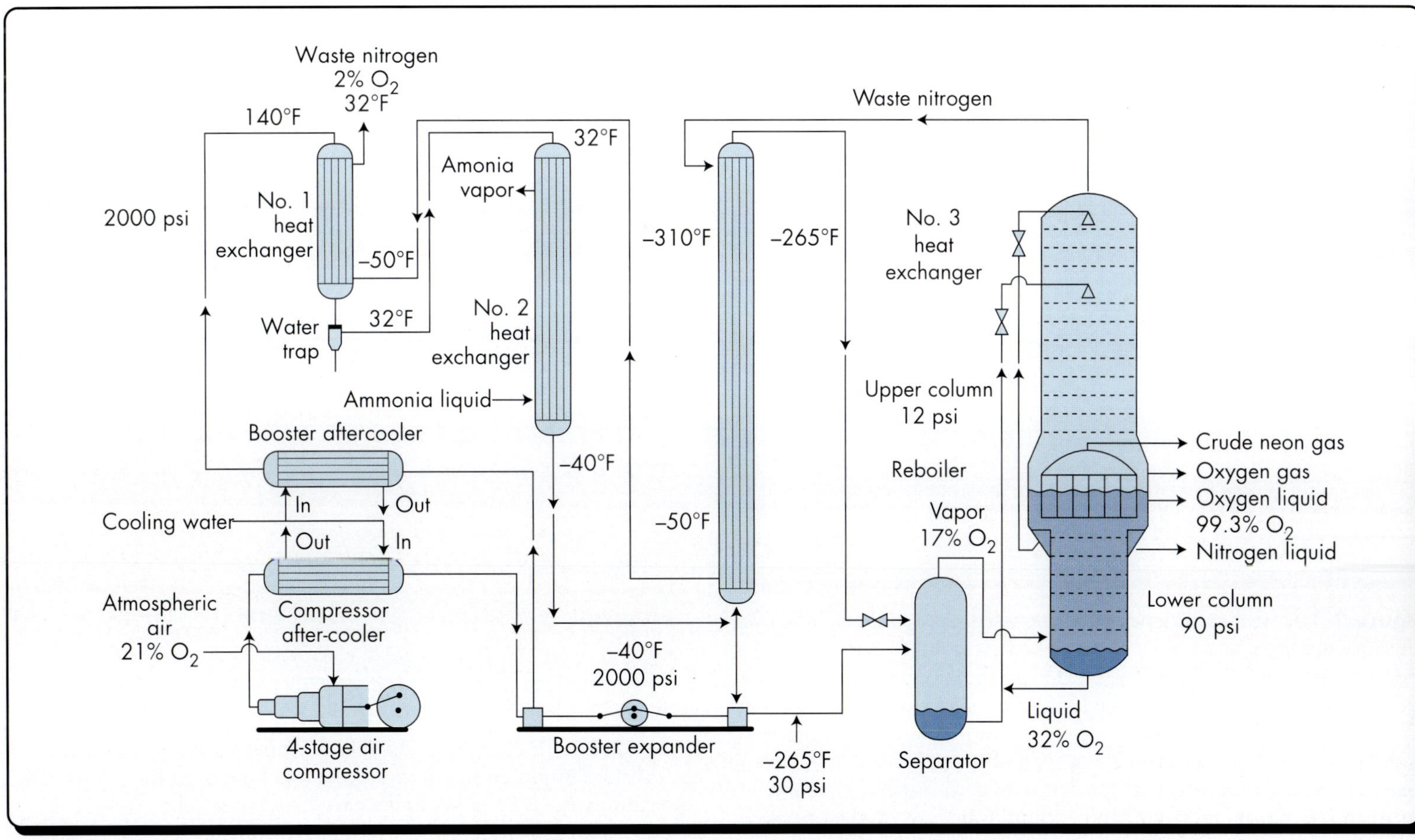

Figure 2-10. Manufacture of gases. Oxygen is purified from the atmosphere by fractional distillation of air [5]. Nitrous oxide (N_2O) is created from the decomposition of ammonium nitrate (NH_4NO_3) by heat. ($NH_4NO_3 \rightarrow N_2O + 2H_2O$) and further purified to eliminate the toxic higher oxides of nitrogen [3]. "Gases" can be stored either as liquids or compressed gases, depending on their critical temperature. (*Adapted from* Kacmarek [5]; with permission.)

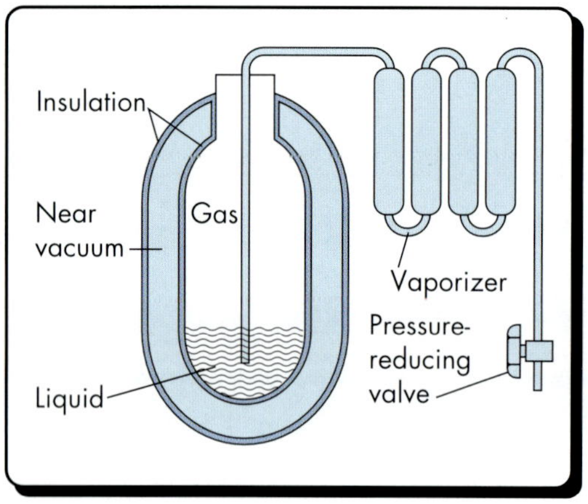

Figure 2-11. Oxygen storage. To physicists, a compressed gas is any material above its critical temperature and above atmospheric pressure. The Compressed Gas Association [6] defines a compressed gas to be any material or mixture having in the container an absolute pressure exceeding 40 psi at 70°F, or, regardless of pressure at 70°F, having an absolute pressure exceeding 104 psi at 130°F, or any liquid having a vapor pressure exceeding 40 psi absolute at 100°F. A nonliquefied compressed gas is a gas that does not liquefy at ordinary terrestrial temperatures and under pressures that range from 2000 to 2500 psig. A liquefied compressed "gas" is a "gas" that becomes liquid to a very large extent in containers at ordinary temperatures and at pressures from 25 to 2500 psig. Oxygen can be stored at very high pressures as a gas, or cooled (kept cool) and stored as liquid at a reasonable pressure. Liquid oxygen cannot be stored at room temperature, because room temperature (20°C) is well above the critical temperature of oxygen (-118°C). Any container filled with liquid oxygen and allowed to warm is at tremendous pressure and is likely to rupture and explode. (*From* McPherson and Spearman [7].)

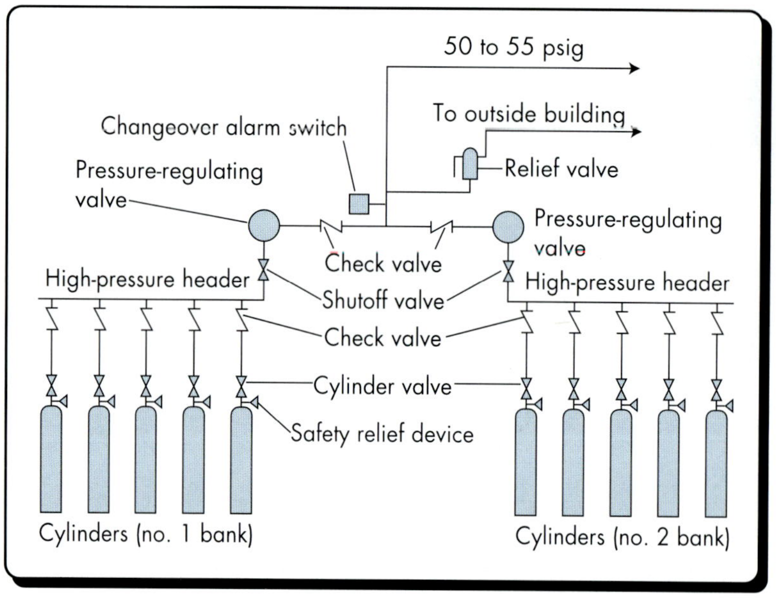

Figure 2-12. Compressed gas storage. For nitrous oxide, the critical temperature and pressure are within practical ranges. Nitrous oxide is stored as a liquid in compressed "gas" tanks, more properly termed liquefied compressed vapor tanks. (*From* McPherson and Spearman [7].)

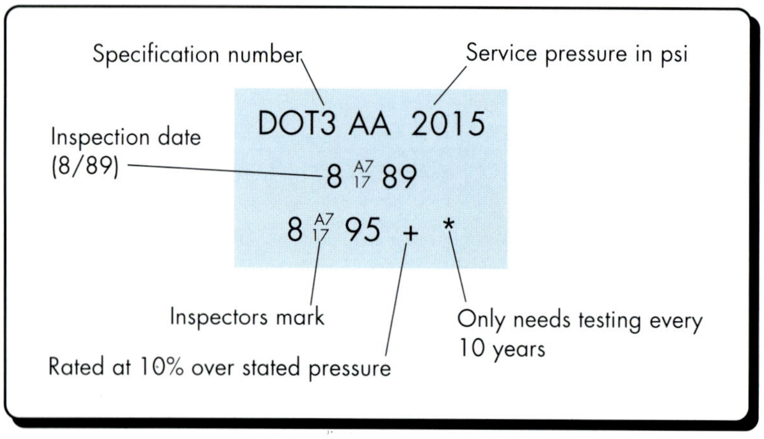

Figure 2-13. Characteristics of compressed gas cylinders. What do all those numbers and colors mean? The first number is a Department of Transportation (DOT) specification number, which indicates the type of material used in the construction of the cylinder. The second number is the service pressure in psi. The third number is the serial number and identifying symbol for either the user, purchaser, or manufacturer. Finally, a test date with inspector's mark between the month and year can be found fourth or on the opposite shoulder of the cylinder [4].

CYLINDER COLOR AND E-CYLINDER SPECIFICS

Gas	Cylinder Color	Contents at 1 atm, *L*	Pressure, *psi*
Oxygen	Green (U.S.)	660	1900
	White (Canada)		
Nitrous oxide	Blue	1590	745
Air	Yellow (U.S.)	625	1900
	Black and white (Canada)		
Helium	Brown	500	1600
Nitrogen	Black	610	1900
Carbon dioxide	Gray	1590	838

Figure 2-14. E cylinders. The most common size of a compressed gas cylinder mounted to an anesthesia machine is an E cylinder. The color and content of full cylinders are listed here. The internal volume of an E cylinder is approximately 5 liters.

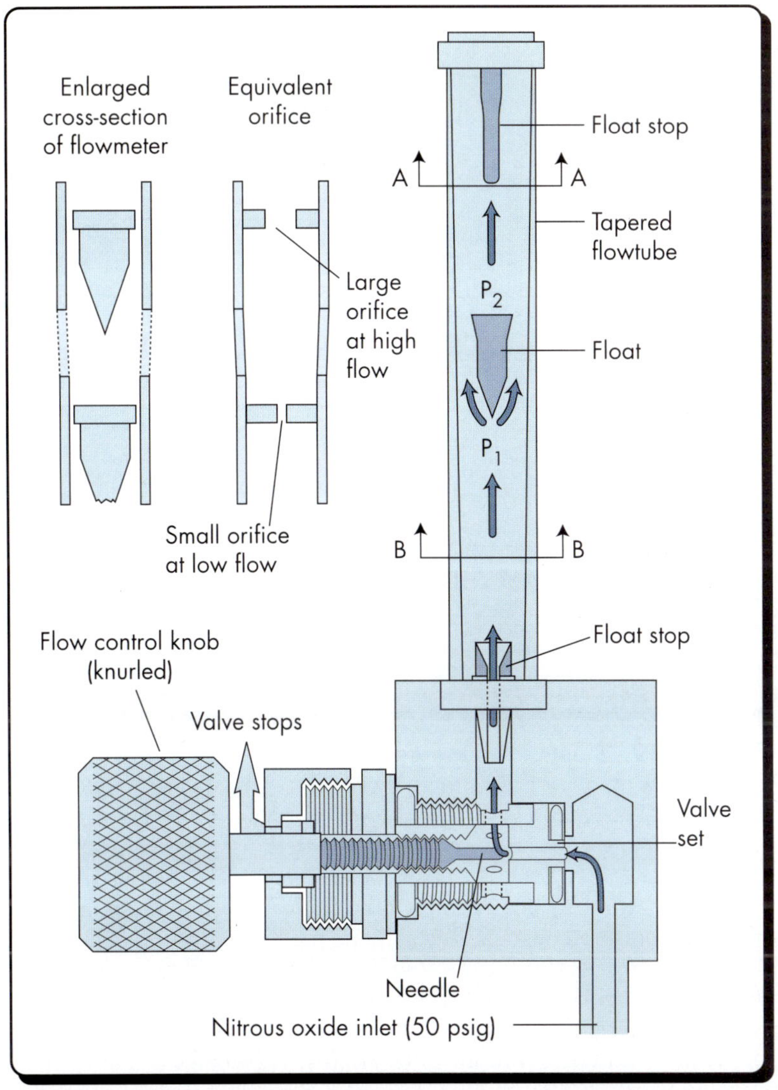

Figure 2-15. Thorpe tube. Two physical principles are used to measure gas flow: a variable orifice and fixed pressure, or variable pressure and fixed orifice. Historically, several methods based on these principles have been tried. The Thorpe tube is the final evolution of the variable orifice design, which began with perforated tubes providing the orifice. The Thorpe tube depends on the balance of the pressure above and below the float and gravity. (*Modified from* Bowie and Huffman [8], Mushin and Jones [3], and Cicman and coworkers [9].)

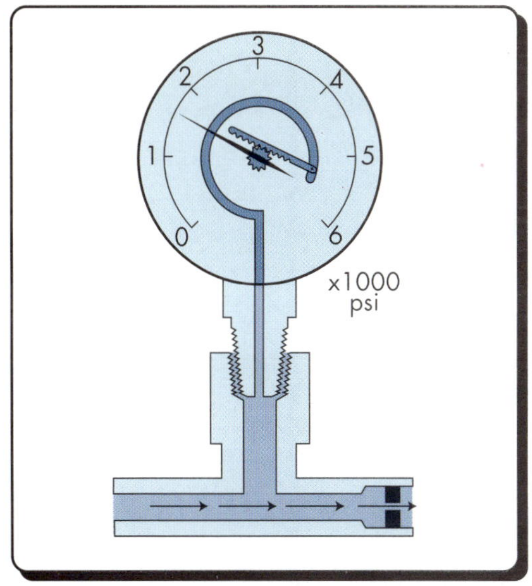

Figure 2-16. Bourdon tube. The Bourdon tube uses the pressure decrease to mechanically move a dial and measure the pressure. An excessively large orifice results in underreading of the actual flow, whereas a small orifice (often resulting from dirt accumulation) results in an overestimation of flow. (*Modified from* Mushin and Jones [3] and Cicman and coworkers [9].)

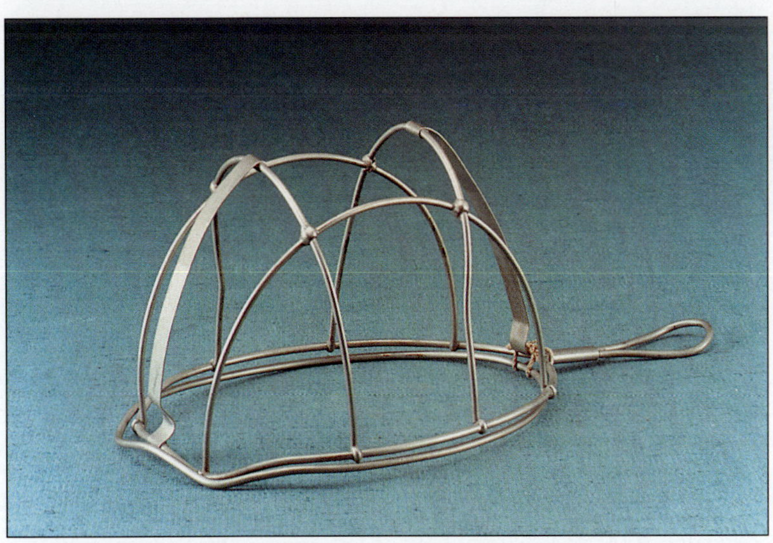

Figure 2-17. An early vaporizer. As illustrated in Figure 2-1, extra energy is required to convert matter from a liquid form to a vapor, which results in cooling of the liquid and decreased vaporization. Because the vapor pressure is dependent on temperature, this also results in a decrease in the amount of vapor formed. Vaporizer design has been determined by these two principles to deliver known concentrations of anesthetic agents. Simple mask vaporization results in delivery of an agent at an unknown concentration, depending on the ambient temperature, rate of breathing, which determines vaporization and cooling, and so on. Some of these protect against overdose, that is, as gas flow through the mask increases, cooling increases and then vaporization decreases. Additionally, supplemental oxygen dilutes the anesthetic. Some of these problems were addressed in the next generation of vaporizer. (*From* Reeves [10].)

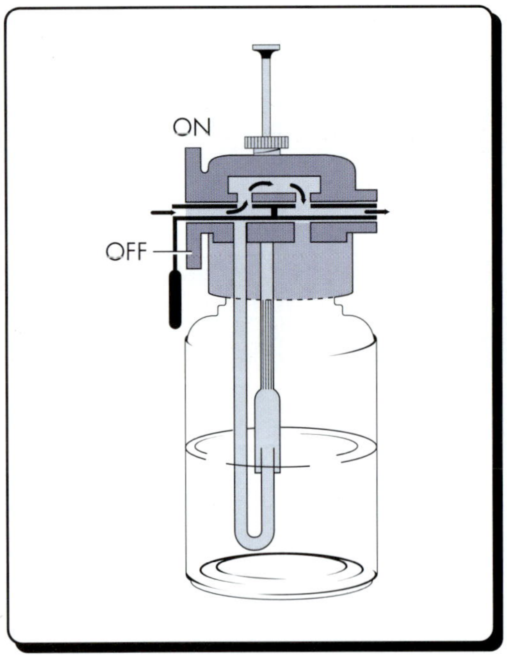

Figure 2-18. Boyle's bottle. This "second-generation" vaporizer allows for higher and somewhat controlled concentration of agent to be delivered. The surface area for equilibration is limited, because it varies between the surface of liquid in the chamber and that of a stream of bubbles under the surface. In addition, as the liquid vaporizes, the temperature decreases, resulting in decreased vaporization. These problems were addressed in the design of the copper kettle. (*From* Mushin and Jones [3].)

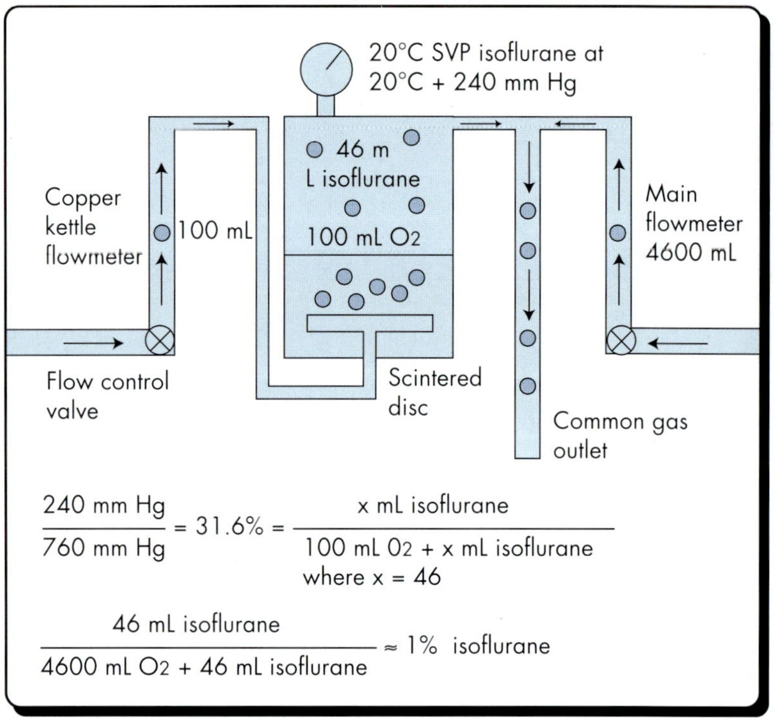

Figure 2-19. Copper Kettle/Vernitrol. A copper kettle vaporizer incorporates many of the features found in its descendant, modern vaporizers. The carrier gas flows through a device to increase the surface area and allow equilibration (scintered disc). The vaporizer is made of a metal with a high specific heat–thermal conductivity so that it can readily absorb heat from the environment and remain relatively temperature-constant. To calculate the concentration delivered from the vaporizer, one must know the temperature, flow of gas through the vaporizer, bypass flow, and vapor pressure of the agent at that temperature. For example: 100 mL of oxygen flowing through a copper kettle full of isoflurane (SVP at 20°C = 240 mm Hg, atmospheric pressure = 760 mm Hg, 240/760 = 31.6%, or 0.316 of the output, which must be x/100 + x = 0.316 or amount delivered = (SVP/atm * copper kettle flows)/(1-SVP/atm) = 46 mL such that 46/146 = 31.6% This must be diluted with extra gas (4600 ml in the example) to decrease the concentration to a nonfatal level (1% vol/vol). *Asterisk* denotes multiplication. (*Modified from* Hill [11].)

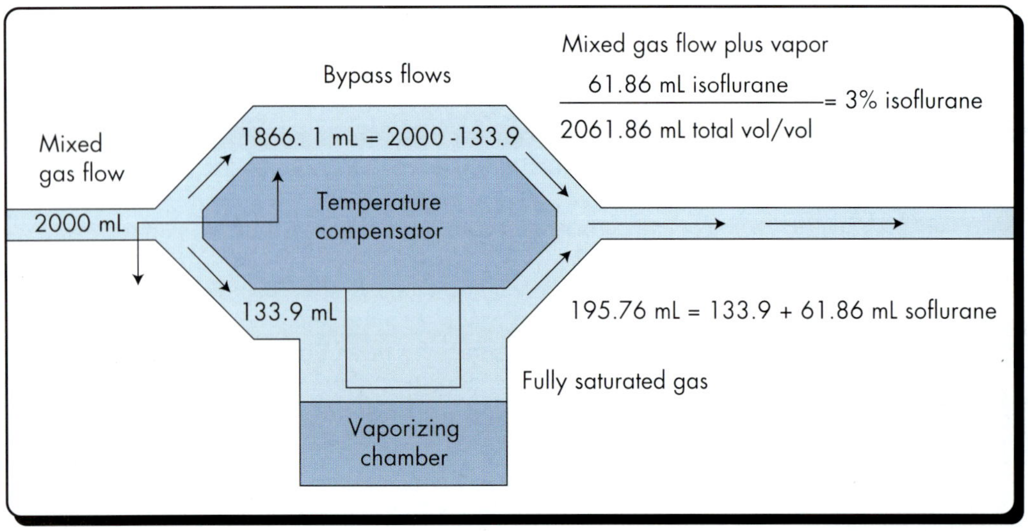

Figure 2-20. Temperature compensated, flow over vaporizer, out of circuit. Using the equations from the copper kettle illustration, it is possible to calculate the amount passing through the vaporizing chamber and the bypass area. For example, if the flowmeters are delivering 2000 mL/min to the isoflurane vaporizer, which is set at 3% (vol/vol), how much of the flows are going through the bypass and how much are going through the vaporizing chamber and being saturated with isoflurane? First, a certain amount of isoflurane must be *added* to the 2000 mL to make a 3% vol/vol mixture. The formula to determine this is x% * flows/(100-x%). In this case, 3%, * 2000/(100-3%) = 61.86 mL of isoflurane vapor is added to 2000 such that 61.86/2061.86 = 3%. To create this 61.86 mL of pure isoflurane vapor, some amount of flow must go through the vaporizing chamber and become completely saturated with isoflurane (dependent on the temperature). At 20°C, the saturated vapor pressure of isoflurane is 240 mm Hg, with an atmospheric pressure of 760 mm Hg (at sea level), 240/760 or 31.6% of the mix is isoflurane vapor. Therefore, the question becomes, how much flow needs to go through the vaporizing chamber to result in 61.86 mL isoflurane vapor. The flow needed to provide 61.86 mL of isoflurane vapor at 20°C equals (61.86 mL) * (100-31.6)/31.6, or 133.9 mL of fresh gas entering the vaporizing chamber. A total flow of 195.76 mL exits the vaporizing chamber, of which 31.6% (61.86 mL) is isoflurane. *Asterisk* denotes multiplication. (*Modified from* Cicman and coworkers [9].)

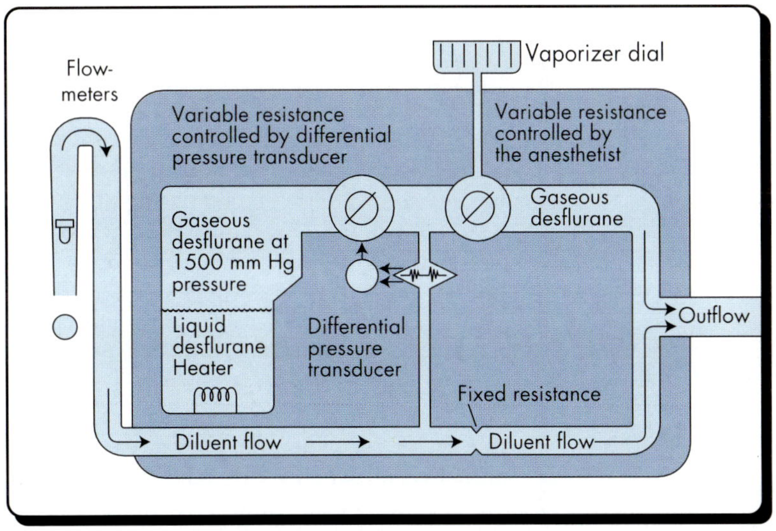

Figure 2-21. Postmodern vaporizer (desflurane). This design is unique in that no fresh gas enters the vaporizer. This is possible because the high vapor pressure of desflurane is increased even further by heating so that pure vapor is added to the main flows. Note the absence of wicks or any device to saturate a gas flow because pure vapor is added to the fresh gas flows. (*From* Egar [12]; with permission.)

ANESTHETIC CIRCUIT COMPONENTS	
Connective Tubing	Links components together
Fresh gas inlet	Determines where fresh gas enters the circuit
Pop-off valve	Determines where excess gas leaves the circuit
Patient connection	Where the mask or endotracheal tube connects the patient to the circuit
Carbon dioxide absorber	Where respiratory carbon dioxide is converted from gas to a solid compound and removed from the gas mixture
Inspiratory valve	One-way valve that prevents exhaled gases from entering the inspiratory limb
Expiratory valve	One-way valve that prevents inhalation of exhaled gases
Y-piece	Connects the inspiratory and expiratory limbs of a circle system
Reservoir bag	Serves as a reservoir for anesthetic gases, mixing place, and counterlung for assisted-controlled ventilation

Figure 2-22. Anesthetic circuits. The purpose of an anesthetic circuit is to deliver a desired quantity and content of gases from the anesthesia machine proper to the patient. Numerous designs have evolved over time, with various advantages and disadvantages. The nomenclature has been a confusing eponymic alphabet soup. To complicate this even further, the functional characteristics of an anesthetic circuit can change depending on the flow rate of the fresh gas and the nature of respiration (spontaneous or controlled). However, a description of the components and their arrangement will describe the static circuit. The functional analysis then depends on variables such as mode of ventilation and fresh gas flows, which are dynamic.

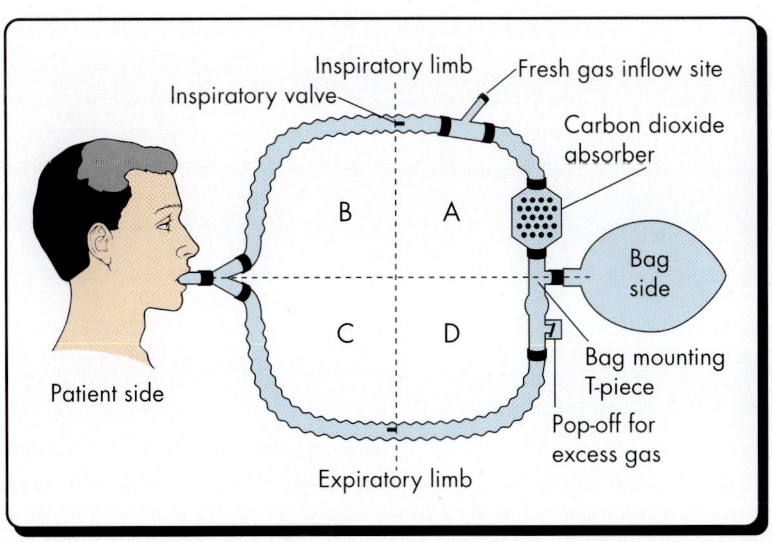

Figure 2-23. Circle circuit. The components of a circle system may be arranged in various configurations. A common one is illustrated. Rebreathing is determined by fresh gas flow (*quadrant A*). A circle system can be made nonrebreathing by increasing the fresh gas flow. Complete rebreathing can be achieved by decreasing the fresh gas flows to just meet the demands of uptake and use. (*Modified from* Smith [13].)

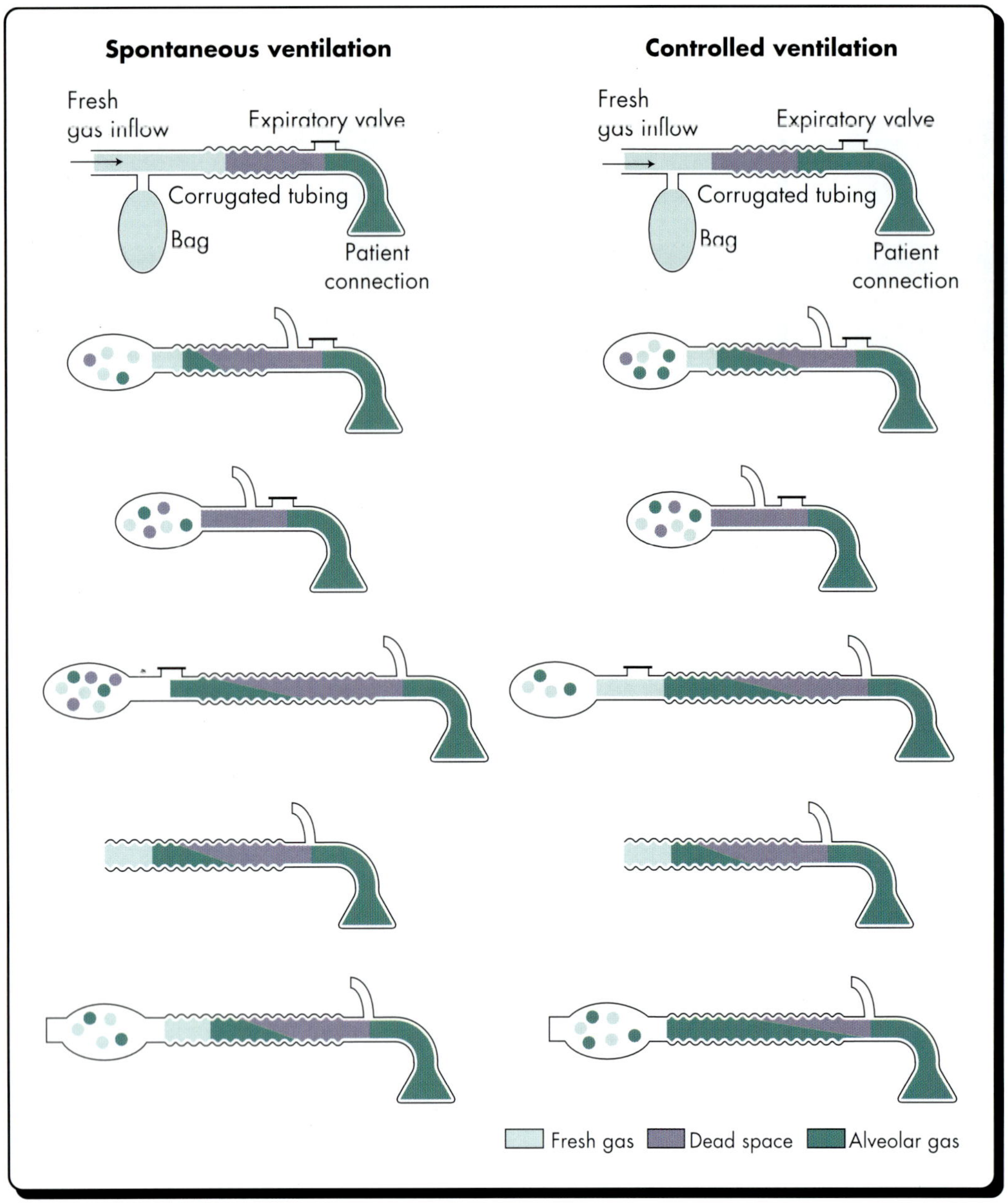

Figure 2-24. Mapleson circuits. *A* through *F* in controlled and spontaneous ventilation. Rebreathing is determined by fresh gas flow. The most commonly used Mapleson circuit in the United States probably is the Mapleson *D* and its co-axial variation, the Bain circuit. Of note in comparing the Mapleson *A* and *D* is that the single limb can be thought of as both an inspiratory limb or expiratory limb, depending on the location of the fresh gas flow and reservoir bag. Rebreathing in a circuit is determined by a number of factors, some of which are static (location of fresh gas inflow, expiratory valve, reservoir bag, length of tubing), and some of which are dynamic (tidal volume, dead space ratio, fresh gas flow, spontaneous or controlled ventilation, expiratory pause). In the circuit gases flow along the path of least resistance. For example, during a spontaneous ventilation in a Mapleson *D*, at the beginning of inspiration the inspiratory flow exceeds the fresh gas flow and the patient also inspires gases from the volume of the circuit and reservoir bag. (*Modified from* Sykes [14].)

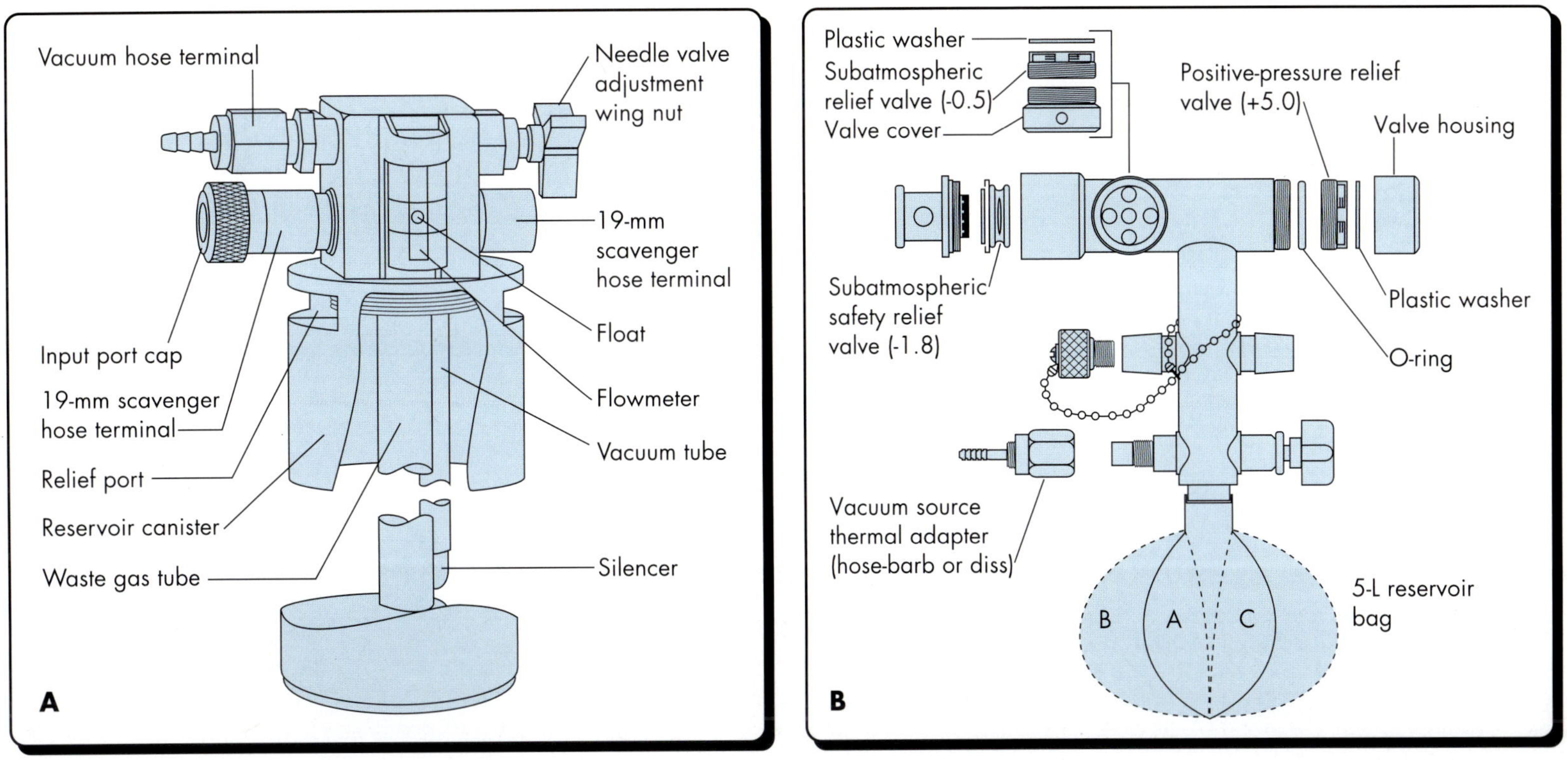

Figure 2-25. Scavenging systems. Scavenging systems serve to remove excess gases from the circuit and decrease operating room pollution. There are two major types of scavenging arrangements, open (**A**) and closed (**B**). An open system has no relief valves and uses flows of approximately 25 L/min to remove the waste gases. Closed scavenging systems may use an air-conditioning exhaust or a vacuum system. Low-pressure passive systems may only have a positive-pressure relief valve, whereas high pressure must have both positive-pressure and negative-pressure relief valves. Reservoir bags may be incorporated to accommodate momentary increases in flows without venting to the atmosphere. *Panel B* shows a 5-L reservoir bag overinflated (*B*), completely deflated (*C*), and slightly inflated (*A*). (*Modified from* Cicman and coworkers [9].)

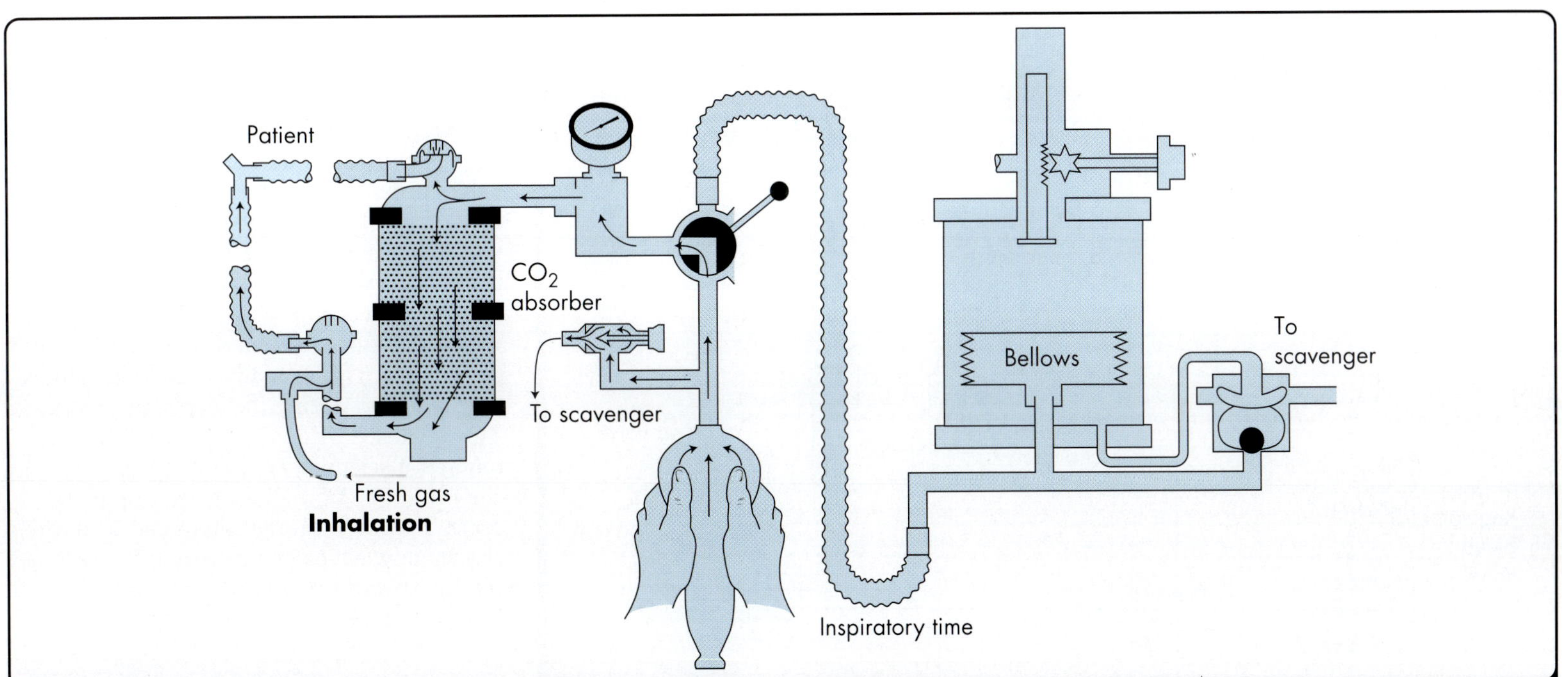

Figure 2-26. Classification of ventilators: the ultimate anesthetic ventilator. Manual ventilation is achieved through the use of the reservoir bag as a counter lung to provide positive-pressure inflation of the patient's lungs. Most anesthesia ventilators can be understood as a bag in a bottle with pressurized gas flows providing the force instead of an anesthesiologist's hand. During inspiration, a pressure-operated switch closes the pressure relief valve, resulting in a potential for barotrauma if the oxygen flush is activated during this time. The commonly used parameters of respiratory rate, tidal volume, and inspiration-to-expiration ratio are more properly thought of as a combination of inspiratory time, expiratory pause, and gas flow rate. Anesthesia ventilators use these later variables to control ventilation. Anesthetic ventilators are classified by the bellows motion during expiration. Current ventilators use an ascending bellows design. During a circuit disconnect, an ascending bellows fails to fill with expiratory gases, resulting in a quick detection of a dangerous situation. With a descending bellows, the ventilator draws in room air and continues to function, apparently normally, with great potential for hypoventilation of the patient. Because of the nature of ascending bellows, an obligatory positive end-expiratory pressure is required to raise the bellows against gravity. (*Modified from* Cicman and coworkers [9].)

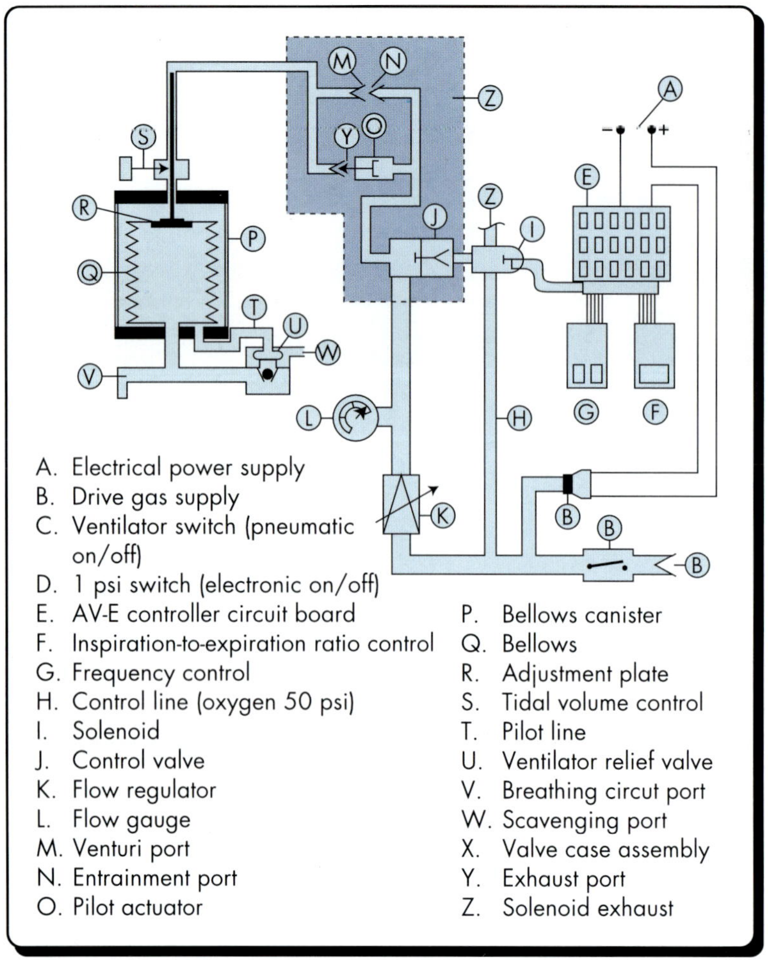

Figure 2-27. Dräger ventilator (Telford, PA). As in most anesthetic ventilators the drive gas is separate from the patient circuit. The Dräger ventilator uses the Venturi effect to entrain air as part of the driving gas. This has the potential to lower inspired oxygen and increase inspired nitrogen if a leak in the bellows is present. When the bellows are fully compressed and the set tidal volume delivered, the excess drive gas is vented through a Venturi port. (*From* Cicman and coworkers [9].)

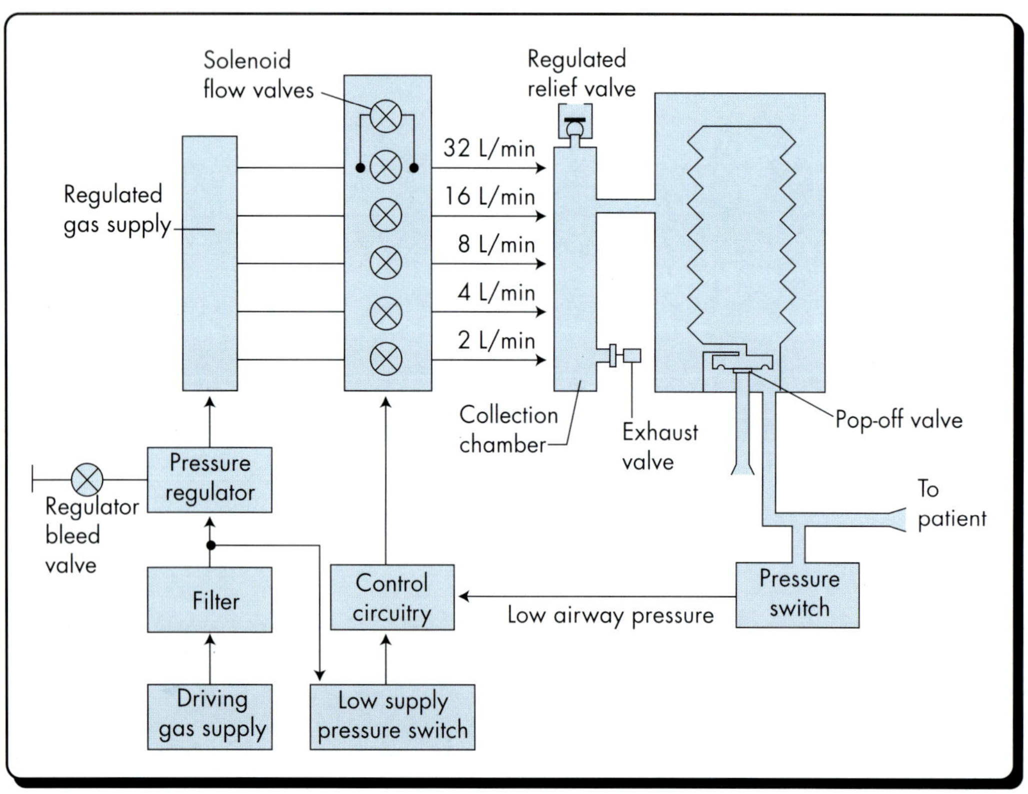

Figure 2-28. Ohmeda ventilator (Ohmeda/Anaquest, Madison, OH). Like most anesthetic ventilators, the drive gas and patient gas are kept separate. Compressed oxygen controlled by a series of selenoid valves provides the drive gas. Therefore, in case of a bellows leak, the patient circuit will receive an influx of 100% oxygen. The bellows in the Ohmeda 7000 ventilator do not completely empty as in the Dräger ventilator. Tidal volume is set by the driving gas volume. Occasionally, a clicking sound may be heard during the inspiratory cycle. This is caused by a volume setting that requires a selenoid to rapidly open and close multiple times during the respiratory cycle. The noise can be eliminated by a tiny change upward or downward in the volume setting. (*Courtesy of* Ohmeda/Anaquest, Madison, OH).

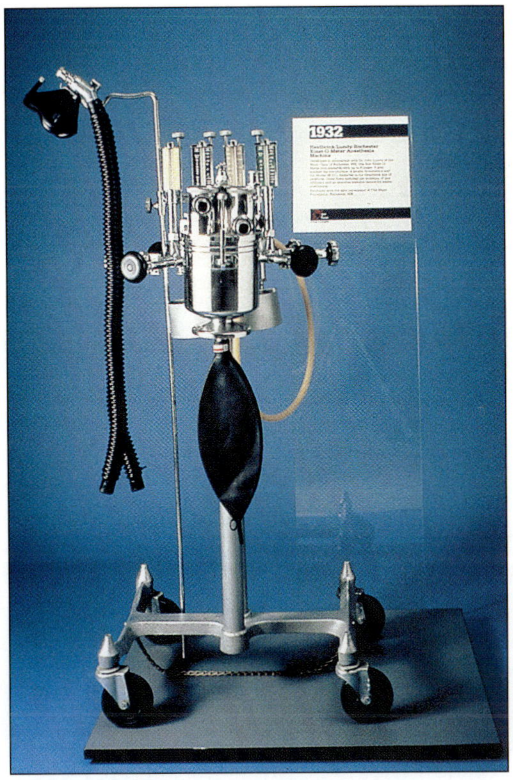

Figure 2-29. The anesthesia machine. When all the components, gas supply, flowmeters, vaporizers, circuits, and ventilator are put together, we have created a modern anesthesia machine. An early example of a Heidbrink/Lundy-Rochester Kinet-O-Meter Anesthesia Machine is shown. This device allowed the use of up to four gases, incorporating a carbon dioxide absorber and pin-indexing of gas cylinders. (*Courtesy of* Ohmeda/Anaquest, Madison, OH.)

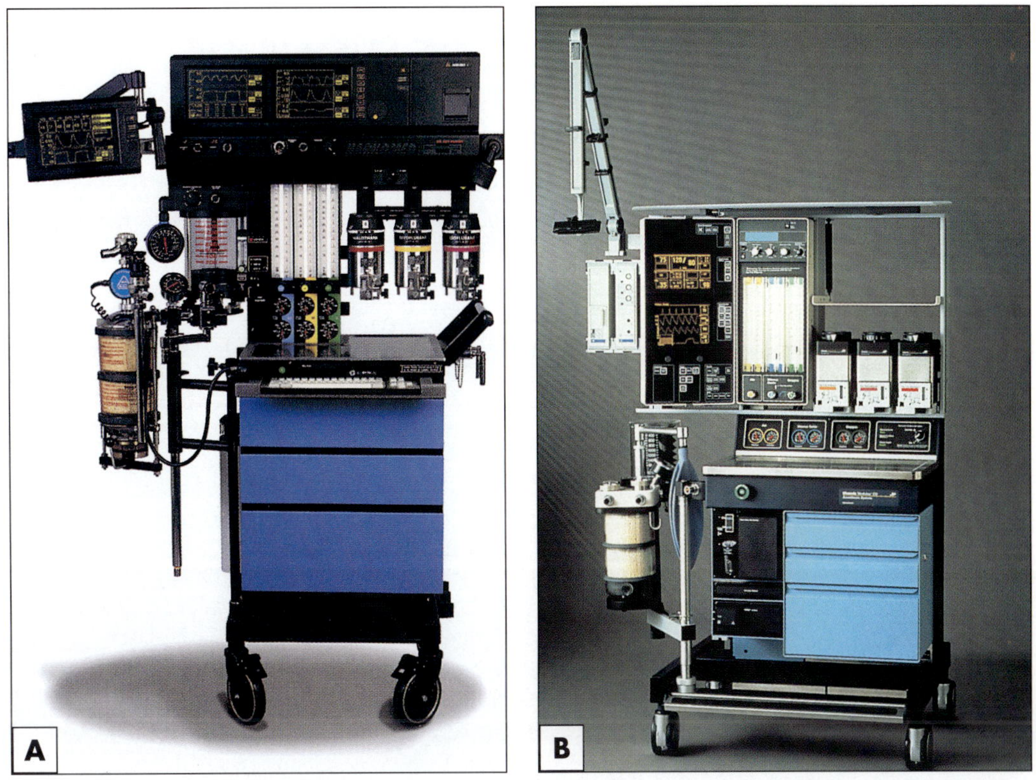

Figure 2-30. Current anesthesia machines. In the United States, there are two primary manufacturers of anesthesia machines: North American Dräger and Ohmeda. Their current models are the Dräger Narkomed 4 (**A**) and the Ohmeda Modulus CD (**B**). Both incorporate many safety devices, although these differ in their specifics. Modern anesthesia machines include integrated vaporizers, ventilators, and alarms. The American Society for Testing and Materials (ASTM) has established minimum performance and safety requirements for components and systems of anesthesia gas machines known as ASTM F1161-88. These new standards include automatic activation of an oxygen analyzer, a breathing pressure monitor, and either a carbon dioxide monitor or exhaled volume monitor. (Part A courtesy of North American Dräger, Telford, PA; part B *courtesy of* Ohmeda/Anaquest, Madison, OH.)

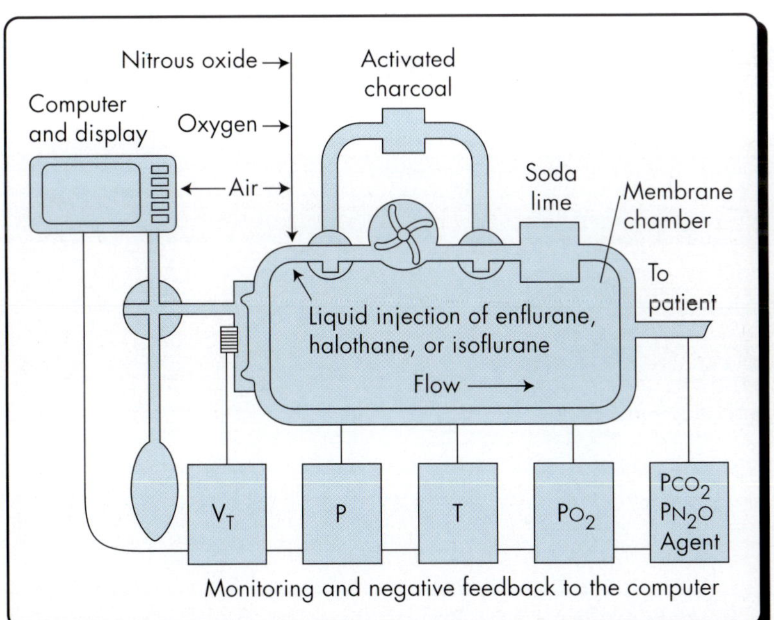

Figure 2-31. Future anesthesia machines. The future of anesthesia machines is uncertain. Two concepts persist, that of a modular machine, with the advantages of interchangeable units that can be expanded or upgraded as advancements are made. The other concept, that of a combined machine, incorporates an "all-in-one" concept with the advantage of unified monitors and standardized alarms. Newer advances in communications technology may allow a blending of these two, wherein disparate components can be unified into a standard interface. A final approach uses feedback loops so that the anesthesiologist no longer adjusts individual variables, but decides on a state to achieve, and the machine through negative feedback loops adjusts infusions to maintain homeostasis, relegating the anesthesiologist to an active bystander in the process. P—pressure; PCO_2—partial pressure of carbon dioxide; P_{N2O}—partial pressure of nitrous oxide; PO_2—partial pressure of oxygen; T—temperature; V_T—tidal volume. (*Modified from* Grogono and Travis [15]; with permission.)

APPLICATIONS AND COMPLICATIONS OF INHALED ANESTHESIA DELIVERY SYSTEMS

COMPRESSED GAS HAZARDS AND SAFEGUARDS

Hazards	Safety Features
Adiabatic heating resulting in ignition in valve area	Small valve so heat content is less; no grease or oil in valve seat
Fracture of valve stem when tank falls over	Hospital rules state that all gas cylinders must be supported
Mismatch of tank and yoke	Pin index system to prevent wrong gas being administered
Changeover of gas in wall supplies resulting in hypoxic gas mixture	Gas analyzer and sensor in circuit
Loss of wall pressure	Food and Drug Administration machine check-out requiring reserve of 1000 psi oxygen
Valve leak	Machine checkout
Loss of oxygen pressure	Oxygen pressure alarms
Exposure of tank to excessive heat leads to increased pressure, rupture, and explosion	Specific regulations as to storage; pressure relief valves built into tank valve

Figure 2-32. Compressed gas hazards and safeguards. Physical hazards. Compressed gas cylinders must be stored properly. If an unsupported tank falls over and the valve assembly is damaged, an E cylinder can become a 2000 psi torpedo, weighing over 7 kg (14 lbs when empty) and generating a force of 2000 psi = 1.379×10^7 N/m^2 . If the valve area is 1 cm^2, then the force is 1.379×10^4 N. If the "burn time" of this compressed gas rocket were 1 second, it would accelerate a 7-kg tank at 197 m/s^2, or 20 times the acceleration owing to gravity. At 1 second, the speed would be 197 m/s or 440 mph. (In reality, the acceleration would slow down as the pressure decreased and the speed would be less, only 83 m/s. The compression of gas in the valve assembly can result in heating and ignition of flammable materials. For this reason valves are made small and are not lubricated with any grease or oil. The wrong tank can be mounted, resulting in errors in gas delivery.

FLOWMETER HAZARDS AND SAFEGUARDS

Hazards	Safety Features
Leak in flowmeter	Machine checkout
Oxygen flowmeter misadjusted	Color coding, physical fluting, and size of knob
Flowmeters unintentionally changed	Knobs above workspace or protected by a bar
Wrong flowmeter replaced during service	Index system for flowmeters
Low-flow flowmeter adjusted versus high flow	Elimination of separate flowmeters for one double taper Thorpe tube or two tubes in series
Hypoxia due to loss of oxygen	Oxygen flowmeter last in series
Inadvertent flowmeter reading due to sticking indicator	Antistatic coating on tubes; rotameter design to confirm gas flow; tube design so that float cannot become stuck at the top
Hypoxic mixture set	Oxygen ratio monitor controller or Link25 proportioning system oxygen sensor in circuit
Flowmeter misread due to confusing scale	Scale standardized to right of tube or, preferably, permanently marked directly onto the tube

Figure 2-33. Flowmeter hazards and safeguards. Many design features have been incorporated into the flowmeters on anesthesia machines, including color coding, order, and arrangement. None of these will absolutely prevent operator error.

VAPORIZER HAZARDS AND SAFEGUARDS

Hazards	Safety Features
Wrong agent in vaporizer resulting in error in dosing	Key index filling system
Back pressure causing pumping effect and increased agent delivered	Check valve in anesthesia machine or vaporizer design with baffles
More than one vaporizer turned on resulting in overdose to patient and formation of azeotropic mixture in downstream vaporizer	Interlock system
Leak in vaporizer	Machine check with vaporizer on
Empty vaporizer resulting in inadequate anesthesia	Agent analyzer in circuit; sight glass
Excess dosing caused by tipping and liquid anesthetic in fresh gas pathway	Agent analyzer; tip proof systems

Figure 2-34. Vaporizer hazards and safeguards. Despite safeguards, hazardous conditions can exist owing to operator error. Interlock systems have been forced and index specific filling systems bypassed, among others things. With the advent of routine agent monitoring, most of the hazards of inadequate, excessive, or inadvertent agent administration may be avoided.

CIRCUIT HAZARDS AND SAFEGUARDS

Hazards	Safety Features
Circuit obstruction	Machine check out for proper function; clear tubing to visualize obstruction
Valve malfunction	Clear housing to visualize valve; carbon dioxide analyzer to detect rebreathing
Fresh gas flow disconnect	Locking design for fresh gas flow
Circuit leak	Machine checkout; use of low flows

Figure 2-35. Circuit hazards and safeguards. The circuit is the weakest link in the delivery of anesthetic to the patient, filled with multiple connections and hazards. A thorough machine checkout using a reservoir bag as an artificial lung, allows the anesthesiologist to observe the proper operation of all the components. Additionally, the intrinsic volume and pressure monitors incorporated into the anesthesia machine help verify the proper integrity and function of the anesthesia circuit.

VENTILATOR HAZARDS AND SAFEGUARDS

Hazards	Safety Features
Excessive pressure resulting in barotrauma	Pressure limiting capabilities of ventilator
Leak or disconnect resulting in hypoventilation	Integral pressure alarm/minute volume alarm; ascending bellows design
Ventilator failure (power)	Backup power; ability to hand ventilate
Bellows leaks	Use of life-sustaining driving gas; monitoring of pressures; forced inspiratory oxygen (FIO_2)
Failure of ventilator scavenger	Excessive pressures delivered

Figure 2-36. Ventilator hazards and safeguards. Modern ascending bellows ventilators fail to operate during a disconnect, alerting the anesthesiologist of one potential problem. An additional degree of safety is obtained by carefully setting the ventilator alarm limits (pressure and minute volume) so as to decrease the number of false alarms, while retaining enough sensitivity to detect partial disconnections.

SCAVENGER HAZARDS AND SAFEGUARDS

Hazards	Safety Features
Excessive positive pressure resulting in barotrauma	Positive-pressure relief valve
Excessive negative pressure	Negative-pressure relief valve
Operating room contamination	Proper checkout before case begins

Figure 2-37. Scavenging hazards and safeguards. The scavenging system is often overlooked during machine checkout, yet serious patient injury can occur owing to excess positive or negative pressure administered to the patient because of faults in the system.

REFERENCES

1. *The International Dictionary of Physics and Electronics*. edn 2. Princeton, NJ: Van Nostrand Company; 1961.
2. Barker S, Tremper K: Physics applied to anesthesia. In *Clinical Anesthesia*. Edited by Barash P, Cullen B, Stoelting R. Philadelphia, PA: JB Lippincott; 1992:141–181.
3. Mushin W, Jones P, eds: *Physics for the Anaesthetist*. edn 4. 1987, Chicago: Year Book Medical Publishers; 1987:561–562.
4. Dorsch J, Dorsch S: *Understanding Anesthesia Equipment: Construction, Care and Complications*. edn 3. Baltimore: Williams & Wilkins; 1994:149–165.
5. Kacmarek R: Supplemental oxygen and other medical gas therapy. In *Foundations of Respiratory Care*. Edited by Pierson D, Kacmarek R. New York: Churchill Livingstone; 1992:859–889.
6. Compressed Gas Association: *Handbook of Compressed Gases*. edn 3. New York: Van Nostrand, Reinhold; 1990.
7. McPheson SP, Spearman CB: *Respiratory Therapy Equipment*, edn. 3. St. Louis: CV Mosby; 1985.
8. Bowie E, Huffman L: *The Anesthesia Machine: Essentials for Understanding*. Madison, OH: Ohmeda; 1985.
9. Cicman J, Himmelwright C, Skibo V, Yoder J, *et al.*: *Operating Principles of Narkomed Anesthesia Systems*. Telford, PA: North American Dräger; 1993.
10. Reeves C: *Julliard Ether Mask*. Color slide. Association of Anaesthetists of Great Britain and Ireland.
11. Hill D: The design and calibration of vaporizers for volatile anesthetic agents. *Br J Anaesth* 1968, 40:648–659.
12. Egar EL, II: *Desfluran (Suprane): A compendium and reference*. Rutherford, NJ: The Healthpress Publishing Group, Inc.; 1993:82.
13. Smith T: Anesthesia breathing systems. In *Anesthesia Equipment Principles and Applications*. Edited by Ehrenwerth J, Eisenkraft J. Mosby: St Louis; 1993:89–113.
14. Sykes M: Rebreathing circuits: a review. *Br J Anaesth* 1968, 40:666–674.
15. Grogono G, Travis J: Anesthesia ventilators. In *Anesthesia Equipment Principles and Applications*. Edited by Ehrenwerth J, Eisenkraft J. St. Louis: Mosby; 1993:140–147.

3

Principles of Monitoring Instrumentation

Steven J. Barker

Developments in patient monitoring within the past 20 years have had a major impact on anesthesiology, in terms of both how we practice our specialty and patient safety or outcome. Twenty years ago we routinely monitored patient oxygenation only at the level of the inspired gas oxygen fraction (F_{IO_2}). Today we routinely monitor arterial oxygenation via pulse oximetry, and we are beginning to determine organ-specific oxygen delivery by a variety of methods. We monitor cardiac output, brain function, inspired and expired anesthetic agents, and a host of other variables never routinely measured in the recent past. To use these devices intelligently, we as clinicians must possess and apply a basic fund of knowledge of both the physiology and engineering of monitoring.

First, the clinician must understand the general principles of the monitor itself: how does it measure the variable on the display? Each monitor begins with some sort of "transducer," which converts the quantity being measured (*eg*, pressure) into another form of energy, usually electrical. If the monitor is "direct," then the variable measured by the transducer is in fact the variable displayed as final output. An example would be an arterial blood pressure monitoring system. If the monitor is "indirect," then the variable measured by the transducer is used to calculate some other quantity, which is then displayed as output. An example of an indirect monitor is the pulse oximeter, in which the photodetector transducer measures light transmitted through perfused tissue, and the instrument uses this measurement to calculate arterial hemoglobin saturation. This calculation invokes several assumptions, and even uses empiric data from human volunteers in the case of pulse oximetry. As shown in the following figures, an indirect monitor usually has more potential sources of error. In addition to possible measurement error of the primary variable, changing patient conditions may invalidate the mathematical model used to calculate the derived variable. The user must understand the derivation of the indirect variable well enough to be able to anticipate conditions under which the computation is not likely to be valid.

In addition to the above, the clinician user must have a thorough understanding of the displayed variable and its physiologic implications. For example, what is the bispectral index and how is it calculated? What clinical conditions can be detected by monitoring of arterial hemoglobin saturation? As an illustration, the pulse oximeter will not reliably detect endobronchial intubation in the operating room (at F_{IO_2} > 0.30), whereas transcutaneous oxygen tension monitoring will (*see* Fig. 3-11). The integration and interpretation of monitored data is a crucial function of the anesthesiologist, one that distinguishes him or her from other care providers. One aspect of interpretation is "pattern recognition," or the ability of the trained user to rapidly distinguish normal from abnormal signal patterns simply by their appearance. The exact manner in which the output of a monitor is displayed plays an important role in this process. This chapter explores several examples of how instrument designers have met the challenge of displaying complex three-dimensional data in a simple two-dimensional format.

Finally, all of these figures illustrate one common principle: even the most sophisticated monitoring instrumentation is only a conduit of data to the clinician user. Monitors used intelligently can save lives; monitors used in ignorance can do more harm than good.

THE COMPONENTS OF A MONITOR

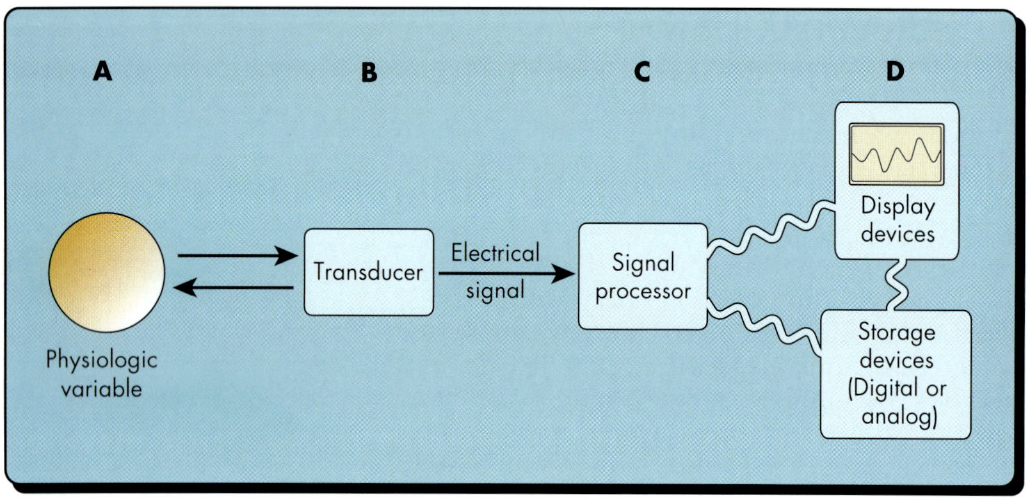

Figure 3-1. The basic building blocks of a monitor. First, the physiologic variable (**A**) to be monitored (*eg*, blood pressure) must affect the state or configuration of a transducer (**B**) (*eg*, variable capacitance pressure transducer). This change in the transducer state is converted to another form of energy, usually electrical. The resulting electrical energy is then amplified and processed (**C**) to yield a signal that is proportional to the physiologic variable being measured. Finally, the processed signal is displayed (**D**) in an analog or digital fashion that should be conducive to rapid and easy interpretation. The final data may also be stored in complete or edited form. (*Adapted from* Tremper and Barker [1].)

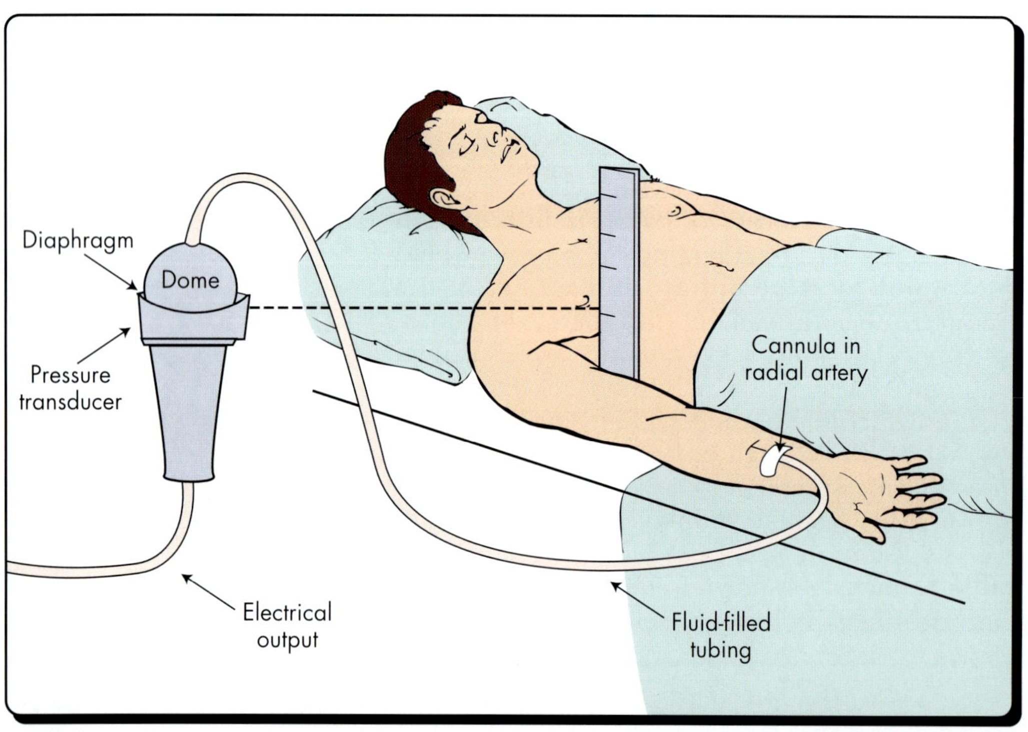

Figure 3-2. Intra-arterial blood pressure. An intra-arterial blood pressure monitor, illustrating the components of a monitor as described in Figure 3-1. The blood pressure in the radial artery is transmitted to the pressure transducer by means of fluid-filled tubing. The pressure transducer, which is at the level of the heart (*dotted line*), converts the blood pressure to an electrical signal—in this case a voltage that is related to pressure. The signal is then amplified, processed, and displayed, both as digital values of systolic and diastolic pressures and as a continuous waveform of pressure versus time. Errors can occur in any stage of this process, as illustrated in Figure 3-3. The intra-arterial blood pressure monitor is a "direct" monitor, in that the transducer directly senses the variable that is being measured (pressure). See Figure 3-6 to contrast this with an "indirect" monitor. (*Adapted from* Tremper and Barker [1].)

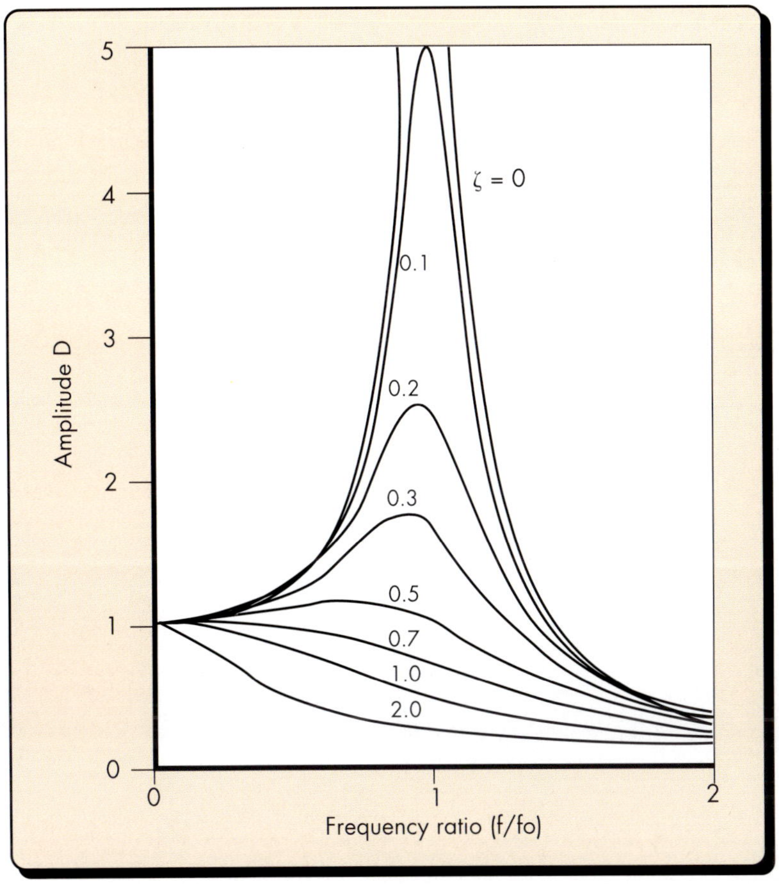

Figure 3-3. Resonance in a fluid-coupled system. The phenomenon of resonance is the most serious limitation of the fluid-coupled pressure monitor (*see* Fig. 3-2). The liquid in the tubing connecting the radial artery cannula to the transducer combines with the compliance of the transducer and tubing to form a harmonic oscillator. Any such oscillator will exhibit resonance, as illustrated in this figure, which plots the amplitude of the system response (*ie*, the transducer output) as a function of frequency. The various curves are for different amounts of friction in the system: higher values of the damping coefficient ζ (zeta) imply more friction. Frequency (f_o) is the resonant frequency, which depends on the compliance, the mass, and the friction in the system. Note that as the driving frequency (in this case the pulse rate) approaches the resonant frequency, amplification of the signal occurs. Typical transducer and tubing systems have a ζ value of 0.2 to 0.3, which results in a maximum pressure amplification factor of 2 to 2.5. This amplification of frequencies near resonance will distort the shape of the pressure waveform and result in erroneous pressure values [2]. (*Adapted from* Tremper and Barker [1].)

CATHETER–TUBING–TRANSDUCER SYSTEM CHARACTERISTICS*

Number	Description	Natural Frequency (Hz), f_0	Damping Coefficient ζ
1	5-Fr two-lumen pulmonary artery HP transducer; dyne diaphragm dome	9.5	0.32
2	5-Fr two-lumen pulmonary artery HP transducer; HP diaphragm dome	10.0	0.30
3	4-Fr two-lumen pulmonary artery (47 cm); Bell & Howell transducer and diaphragm dome	12.0	0.30
4	6-Fr two-lumen pulmonary artery HP transducer; no diaphragm dome	13.0	0.15
5	5-Fr two-lumen pulmonary artery HP transducer; no diaphragm dome	14.0	0.25
6	7-Fr four-lumen thermodilution pulmonary artery (#1)	14.5	0.20
7	CAP 18-gauge with 24-in pressure tubing	15.0	0.72
8	7-Fr pulmonary artery (#2) (*see* #6)	15.5	0.20
9	7-Fr pulmonary artery (#3) (*see* #6)	14.0	0.32
10	Vinca + 84-in pressure tube (#1)	16.0	0.10
11	Vinca + 84-in pressure tube (#2) (*see* #10)	16.0	0.20
12	CAP 18-gauge direct	20.0	0.30
13	48-in pressure tubing direct	24.0	0.28
14	7-Fr pulmonary artery	25.0	0.15
15	Vinca + 24-in PVC pressure tubing	38.0	0.10
16	Vinca + 48-in PVC pressure tubing	45.0	0.13
17	Vinca + 24-in polyethylene pressure tubing	48.0	0.14

*Unless otherwise specified, runs were made with Bentley Model 800 transducer without a diaphragm dome.
CAP—18-gauge CAP catheter-Sorenson; HP—Hewlett-Packard; PVC—polyvinyl chloride; Vinca—2-in, 18-gauge over-the-needle arterial catheter.

Figure 3-4. Catheter–tubing–transducer system characteristics. Each combination of an intra-arterial catheter, a length of fluid-filled tubing, and a pressure transducer is equivalent to a harmonic oscillator with a characteristic resonant frequency (f_o) and damping coefficient ζ [2]. This study from 1980 [2] of 17 different pressure monitoring systems has not been repeated with today's disposable transducer-tubing systems. However, the newer systems in common use today are reported to have resonant frequencies on the order of 20 Hz. Although the human heart rate never approaches this frequency (20 Hz = 1200 cycles per minute), the arterial pressure waveform contains "harmonics," or Fourier components, at up to 10 times the heart rate, which is very close to f_o. (*see* Fig. 3-5). These higher frequency components will be amplified, thus distorting the shape of the pressure waveform. (*Adapted from* Barker and Tremper [3].)

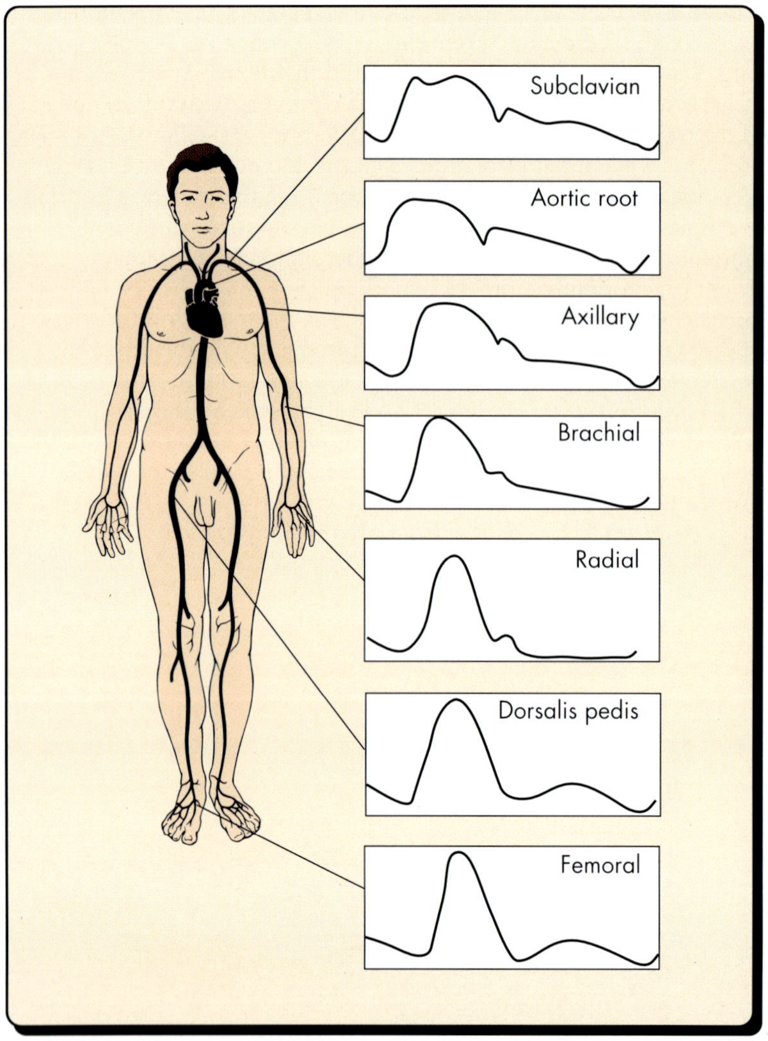

Figure 3-5. The arterial pressure versus time waveform. This figure shows the evolution of the pressure waveform from the aortic root to the distal periphery. The upstroke phase tends to steepen and become more narrow as the pulse wave propagates distally. This complex waveform shape accounts for the higher harmonics (high frequency Fourier components) as described in Figure 3-4. As the waveform gradually steepens in the periphery, the systolic pressure becomes higher while the diastolic and mean pressures become lower. (*Adapted from* Lake [4].)

INDIRECT MONITORS: PROBLEMS AND LIMITATIONS

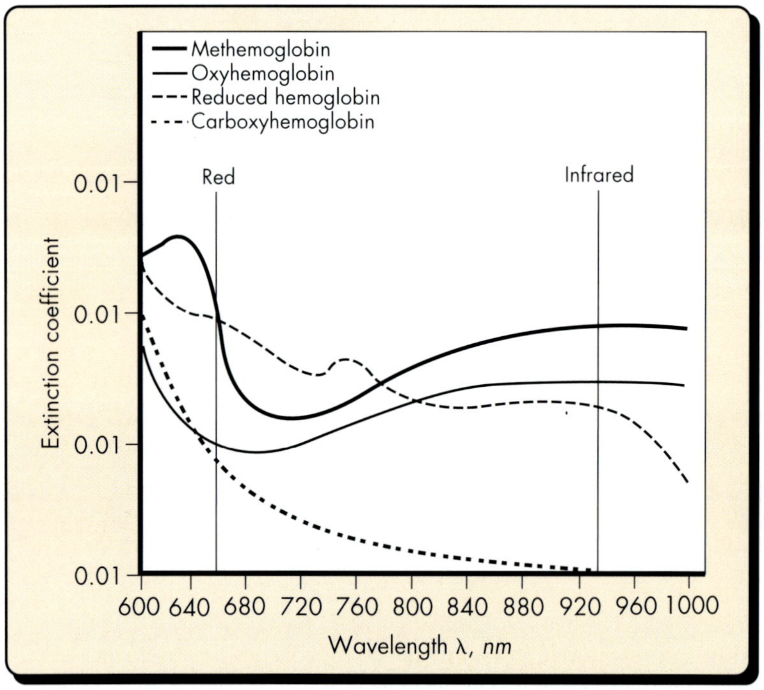

Figure 3-6. Fundamental principle of the pulse oximeter. The pulse oximeter is a good example of an "indirect" monitor. The pulse oximeter measures the light absorbance of the arterial blood at two wavelengths: 660 nm and 940 nm. This figure shows the light extinction coefficients (absorbances) of various hemoglobin species as functions of wavelength. If only two light absorbers are present in the blood (reduced hemoglobin and oxyhemoglobin), then measurements of absorbance at two wavelengths should permit the calculation of the fractions of the two species. This monitor is indirect because the "transducer" actually measures light intensity, which is then used to calculate hemoglobin saturation by a method that relies on experimental data. If more than two light absorbers are present (*eg*, intravenous methylene blue dye), then measurements at two wavelengths are insufficient data and the pulse oximeter cannot calculate hemoglobin saturation [5]. Theoretically, a pulse oximeter with four wavelengths could function accurately in the presence of all four hemoglobin species shown in the figure. (*Adapted from* Barker and Tremper [6].)

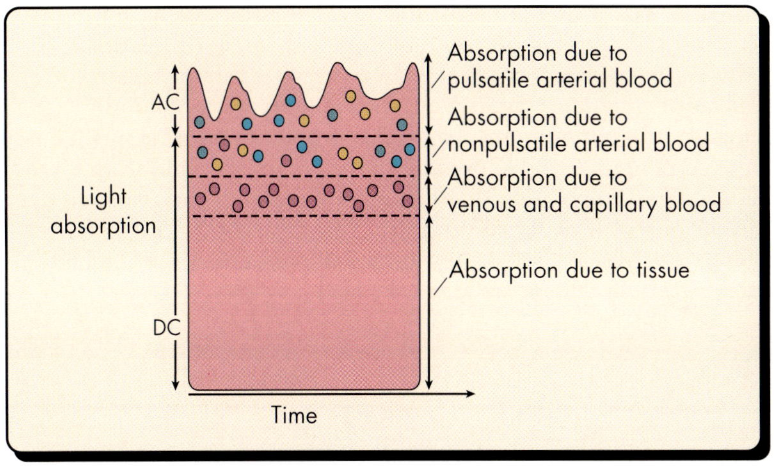

Figure 3-7. The tissue light-absorbance waveform. The pulse oximeter distinguishes the absorbance of the arterial blood from the absorbances of tissues and venous blood by making use of the pulsatility of the former. The oximeter assumes that the pulsatile or alternating current (AC) component of the light absorbance signal is caused entirely by oscillations in the arterial blood volume, as shown in this illustration of light absorbance versus time. The instrument calculates the ratio of the fluctuating AC component to the fixed direct current (DC) component to generate a "pulse-added absorbance" for each of its two wavelengths. It then calculates the ratio (R) of the two pulse-added absorbances, and from the value of R it finds a corresponding value of saturation in a "look up table" derived from experimental data [7]. Therefore, the pulse oximeter's estimate of arterial hemoglobin saturation is empirically based. (*Adapted from* Barker and Tremper [6].)

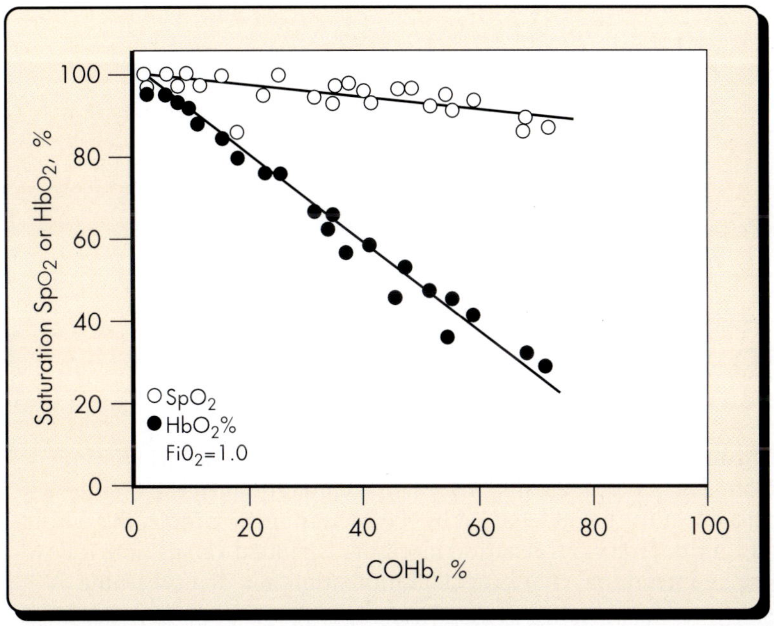

Figure 3-8. Pulse oximeter errors in carbon monoxide poisoning. Errors can occur in indirect monitors when any of the underlying assumptions are violated. This figure shows arterial hemoglobin saturation measured by pulse oximetry (SpO_2) and simultaneously by *in vitro* cooximetry (HbO_2%) plotted as functions of carboxyhemoglobin levels (COHb) in dogs exposed to carbon monoxide. The cooximeter (*closed circles*) shows the actual hemoglobin saturation decreasing linearly with rising COHb, whereas the pulse oximeter (*open circles*) shows little change in saturation. The animals died with COHb levels of approximately 80%, while the pulse oximeter still indicated a saturation of about 90%. In the presence of significant concentrations of dyshemoglobins, an underlying assumption of pulse oximetry (the presence of only two light-absorbing species) is violated. The oximeter's behavior is unpredictable under these circumstances. (*Adapted from* Barker and Tremper [8].)

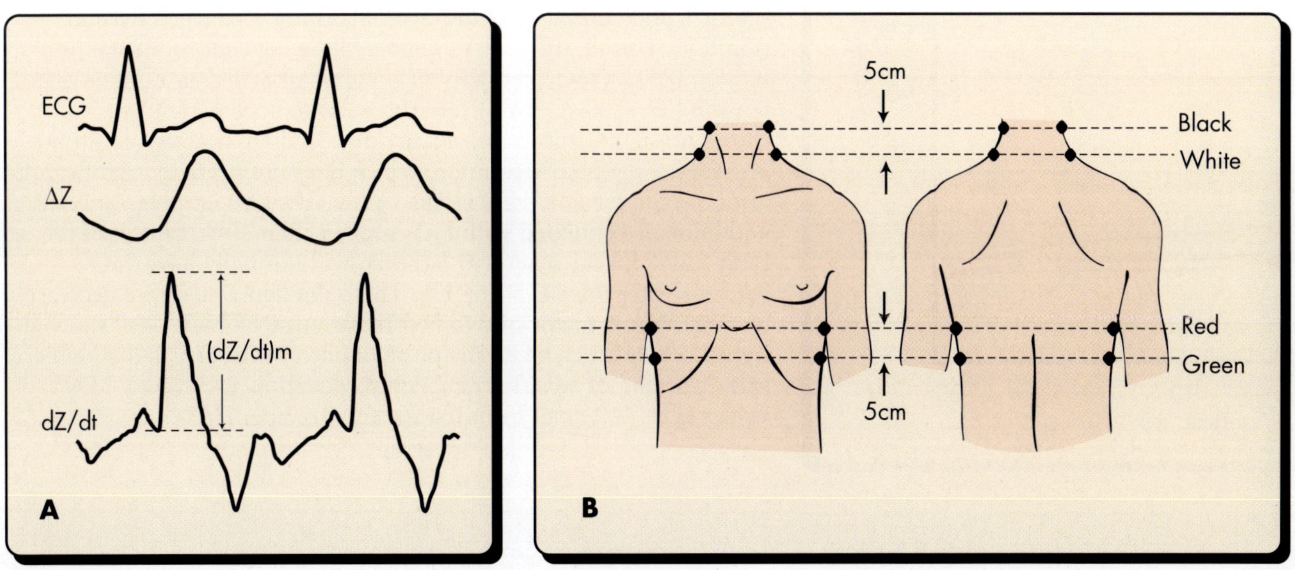

Figure 3-9. The bioimpedance cardiac output monitor. When the relationship between the actual measured variable and the "indirect" calculated variable is complex and unpredictable, the monitor is less likely to provide accurate and reliable data. The noninvasive measurement of cardiac output is an excellent example of this problem. One approach is the transthoracic bioimpedance technique, which measures changes in the electrical impedance of the chest and relates these changes to pulsations in aortic blood volume. If Z is the thoracic electrical impedance, then the Kubicek formula relates its time derivative, *dZ/dt*, to the stroke volume. **A**, The waveforms of Z and dZ/dt versus time compared with the electrocardiogram. **B**, The electrode placement for the BoMed NCCOM, a bioimpedance cardiac output monitor (BoMed, Irvine CA). Although this technology may have promise for the future, several clinical studies have indicated that it is not accurate or reliable enough to replace invasive thermodilution monitoring [9]. Several clinical conditions tend to deteriorate the performance of the device, including sepsis, high cardiac output, or increased lung water. ECG—electrocardiogram. (Part A *adapted from* Perrino *et al.* [10]. Part B *adapted from* Perrino *et al.* [10]; with permission.)

THERMODILUTION METHOD: SOURCES OF ERROR

Patient Variables
- Motion (shivering, extremity movement)
- Respiration (panting, Valsalva maneuver, sighing)
- Alterations in ventricular performance/dysrhythmias
- Valvular regurgitation
- Intracardiac shunts
- Inaccurate temperature measurement

Injectate Factors
- Wrong substance
- Wrong temperature or rewarming of injectate
- Wrong volume of injectate
- Rapid repetition of measurements
- Insufficient mixing with blood

Thermistor Factors
- Thermistor malposition
- Thermistor thrombus
- Intracatheter shunts
- Rapid volume effusion
- Concurrent electrocautery use
- Improper constants

Figure 3-10. Sources of error for thermodilution cardiac outout. This table shows that indirect monitors with complex relationships between the measured and calculated variables can have many sources of error. (*See* Figure 3-9.) Intermittent thermodilution remains our gold standard for cardiac output monitoring, yet it has an uncertainty near 20% because of the complex relationship between the temperature dilution curve (measured variable) and the cardiac output (calculated variable). This table lists 17 possible sources of error for bolus injection pulmonary artery thermodilution cardiac output. (*Adapted from* Lake [11].)

THE PHYSIOLOGY OF THE MONITORED VARIABLE

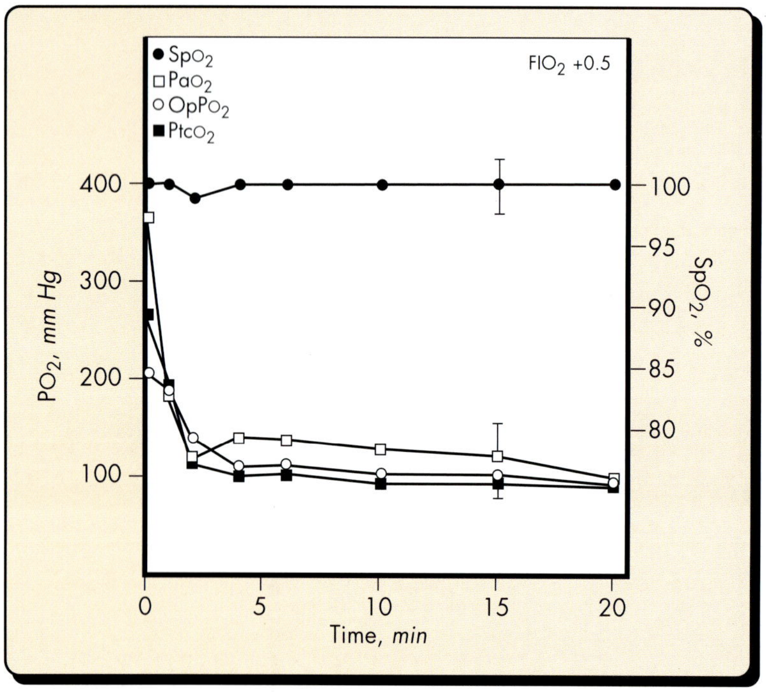

Figure 3-11. Four oxygen monitors during endobronchial intubation. The physiologic implications and limitations of the monitored variable must be understood by the user. In this example, the output of four different oxygenation monitors is plotted versus time following an intentional endobronchial intubation in a dog breathing 50% oxygen. The monitors shown are pulse oximeter (SpO_2), sequential arterial blood gas analysis (PaO_2), transcutaneous oxygen tension ($PtcO_2$), and continuous intra-arterial "optode" oxygen tension ($OpPO_2$). During the first 3 minutes following endobronchial intubation, PaO_2, $PtcO_2$, and $OpPO_2$ exhibit large decreases in oxygen tension (left y axis). SpO_2 from the pulse oximeter (right y axis) shows no significant change at any time. Pulse oximetry monitors arterial hemoglobin saturation, which does not decrease significantly until oxygen tension (PaO_2) falls below about 80 mm Hg. Animals and humans ventilated with F_IO_2 greater than 30%, typical of the range used during general anesthesia, will normally have PaO_2 values greater than 175 mm Hg. This value must therefore decrease by more than a factor of two before the pulse oximeter will show a significant SpO_2 change. The pulse oximeter thus does not provide early warning of adverse trends in oxygenation at elevated F_IO_2 values [12]. (*Adapted from* Barker and Tremper [6].)

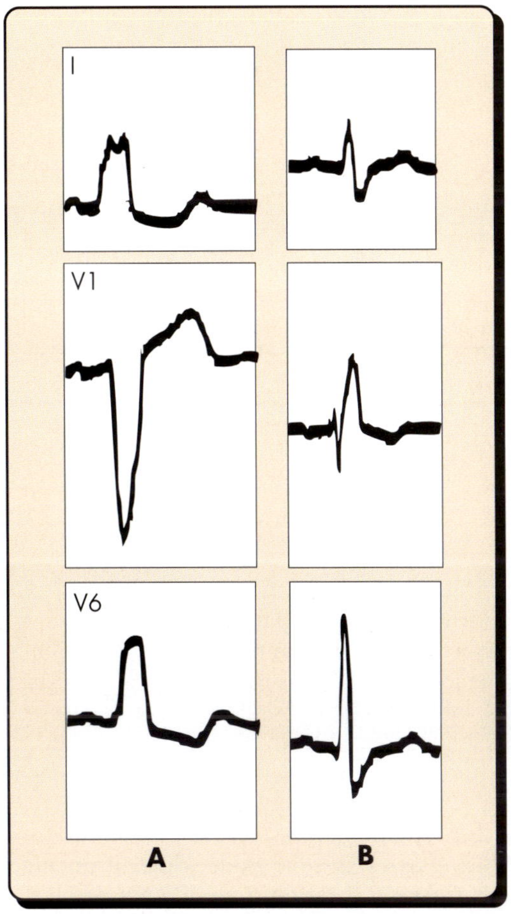

Figure 3-12. Electrocardiogram pattern recognition. Whereas some monitors provide numbers as their final output (*eg*, SpO_2), others merely display a waveform that must be interpreted by the astute clinician. The electrocardiogram (ECG) is the most common pattern recognition waveform used in the operating room. For example, this figure illustrates the characteristic patterns of left (**A**) and right (**B**) bundle branch blocks, which should be easily recognized by the anesthesiologist. Although computerized ECG analyzers can identify these patterns, this level of automated analysis is not usual in the operating room, where the ECG waveform is often distorted by artifact. (*Adapted from* Zaidan [13].)

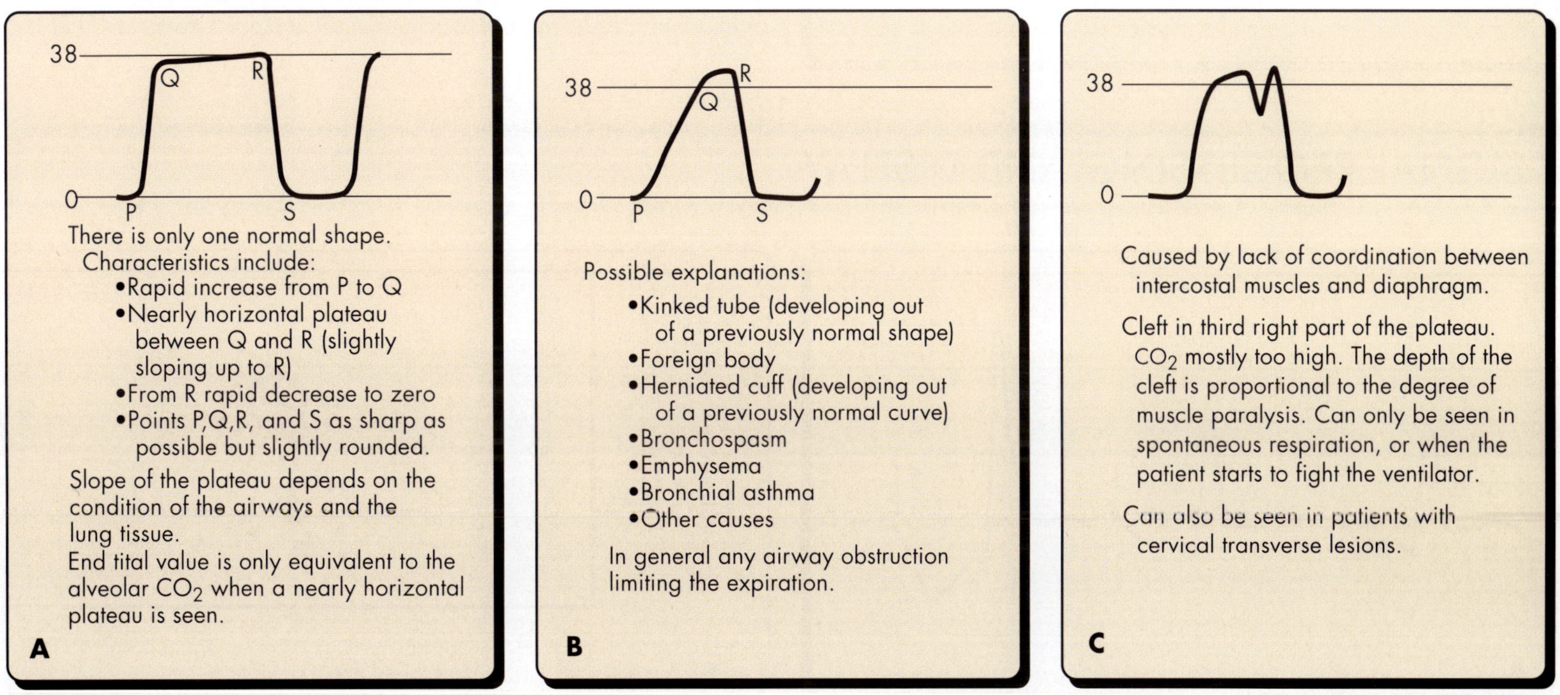

Figure 3-13. Capnogram pattern recognition. Although the capnograph monitor provides three important numeric values (end-tidal CO_2, inspired CO_2, respiratory rate), much of the diagnostic value of this monitor comes from skillful recognition of various capnogram patterns. The following patterns should be easily recognized by the anesthesiologist. A, Normal capnogram. B, Expiratory problems, which include obstruction of the endotracheal tube, bronchospasm, chronic obstructive pulmonary disease, and pulmonary aspiration. C, "curare cleft" capnogram, most often seen during mechanical ventilation when a patient attempts to inspire before the ventilator inspiratory cycle. This can indicate light anesthesia, hypercarbia, or incomplete muscle paralysis. (*Continued on next page*)

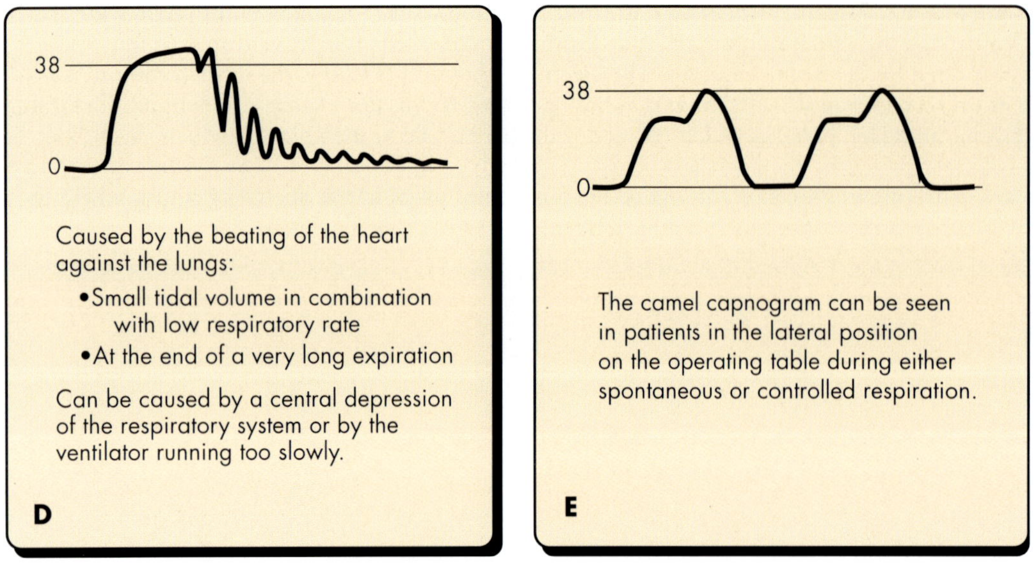

Figure 3-13. (*Continued*) D, Cardiogenic oscillations, which occur at the end of the expiratory plateau and are synchronous with the heartbeat. They are usually seen at low respiratory rates, and sometimes indicate decreased intravascular volume. E, "Camel capnogram," caused by the two lungs emptying asynchronously. This can occur in normal patients in the lateral decubitus position, or in patients with unilateral lung pathology (*eg*, endobronchial tumor). P, Q, R—expiratory phase; R, S, P—inspiratory phase. (*Adapted from* Smallhout [14].)

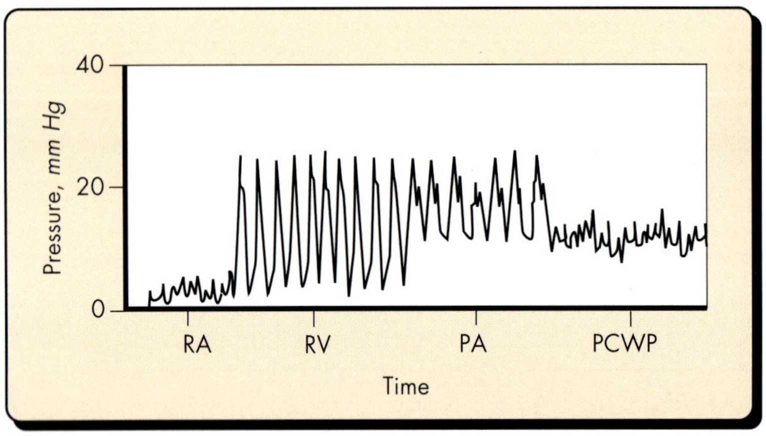

Figure 3-14. Pulmonary artery waveform patterns. This is a normal tracing of the pressure recorded from the tip of a Swan-Ganz catheter plotted versus time as the catheter is advanced. The changes in the shape and amplitude of the pressure oscillations are diagnostic of the catheter location as it is advanced from the internal jugular vein into the right atrium, the right ventricle, the pulmonary artery, and finally into the "wedge" position. The skilled anesthesiologist can safely and reliably perform pulmonary artery catheterization using only this pressure tracing as a real-time guide while advancing the balloon-tipped catheter. Catheter location is usually not confirmed by radiography until the postoperative period. PA—pulmonary artery; PCWP—pulmonary capillary wedge pressure; RA—right atrium; RV—right ventricle. (*Adapted from* Schwenzer [15].)

SIGNAL PROCESSING AND DISPLAY

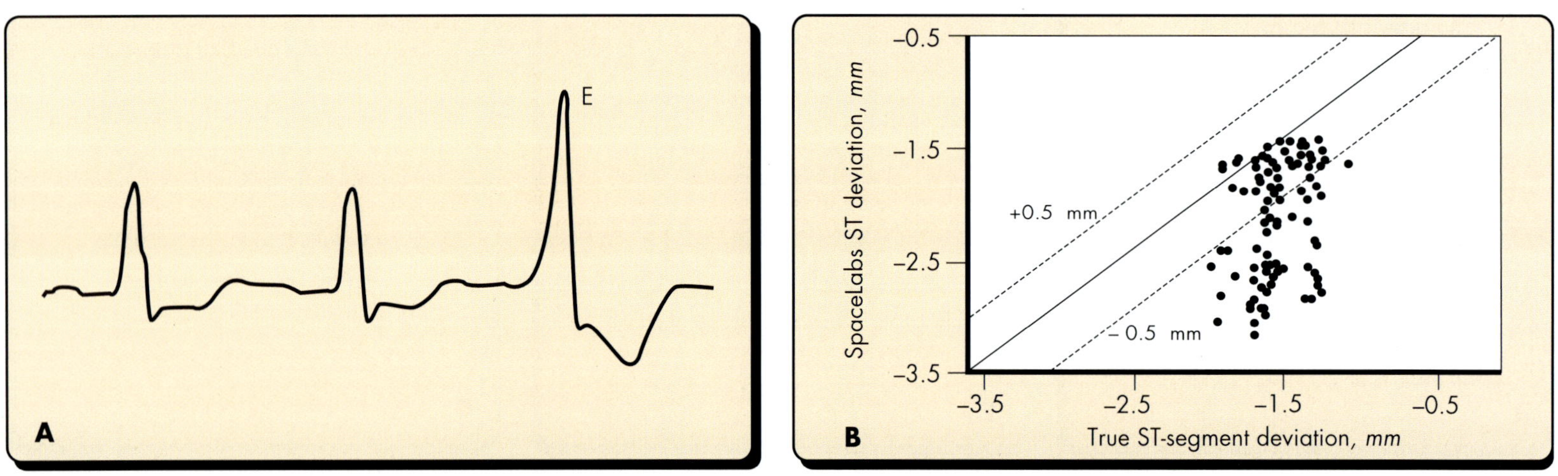

Figure 3-15. Automated analysis: ST-segment monitoring. Newer operating room physiologic monitors often include automated ST-segment analysis, which provides both current and trended ST-segment elevation and depression data for three electrocardiogram (ECG) leads. Although this is a valuable addition to our monitoring repertoire, it is not foolproof, as illustrated in this figure. The ST-segment deviation interpreted by an ST-segment monitor is plotted (**B**) versus the true ST-segment deviation for an ECG (**A**) containing frequent ectopic complexes (*E* in *panel A*). The analyzer incorrectly classified the frequent ectopics as dominant complexes, and therefore recorded significant false ST depressions, as shown [16]. Automated ST-segment analysis is thus a helpful supplement, but it does not replace the ECG waveform. (*Adapted from* Smith *et al.* [17].)

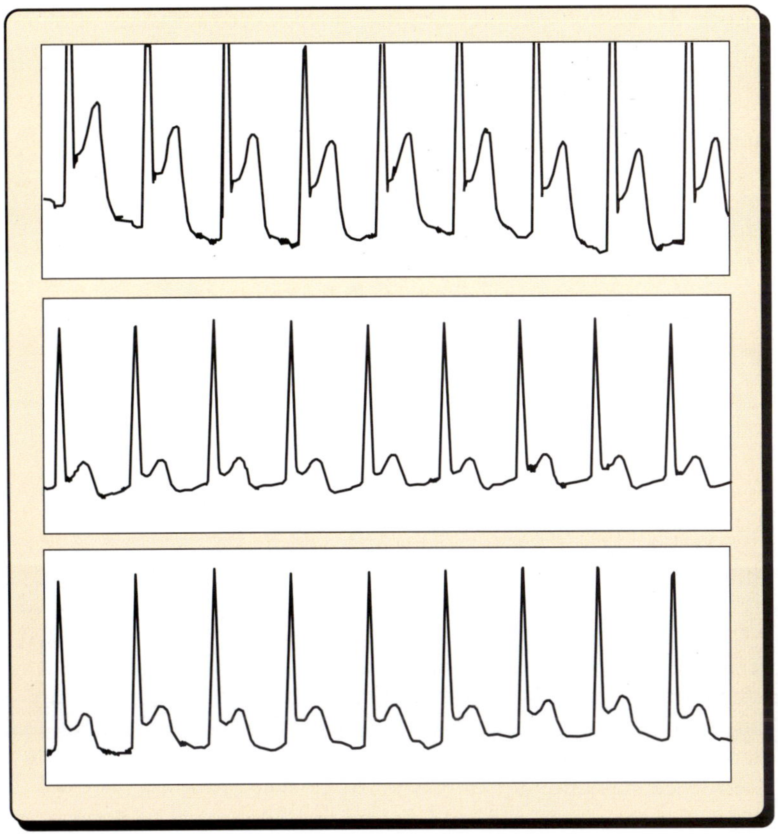

Figure 3-16. Electrocardiogram waveform calibration. This figure illustrates the importance of optimum waveform processing. The displayed electrocardiogram (ECG) must be properly calibrated and filtered for valid interpretation. The upper tracing is an uncalibrated ECG (note that the R wave goes off scale), which suggests that the patient has a 9-mm ST-segment elevation. The second tracing is the same ECG with proper amplitude calibration (1 mV/cm), processed through a 0.5- to 50-Hz bandpass filter. This filtering is inappropriate for ischemia diagnosis as it obliterates most of the ST elevation. The third tracing is correctly calibrated and filtered in the 0.05- to 100-Hz band; it reveals an actual 4-mm ST-segment elevation. (*Adapted from* Zaidan [13].)

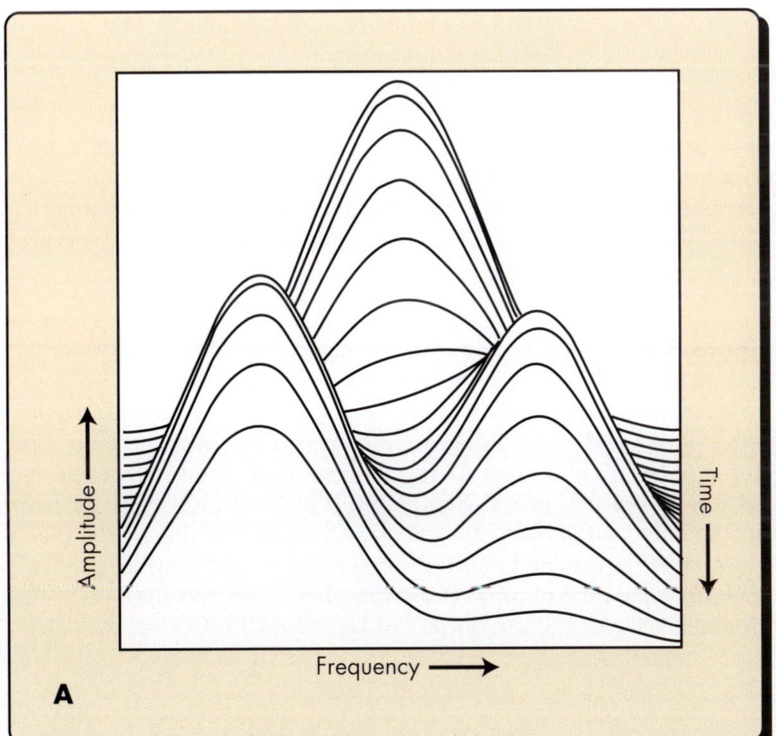

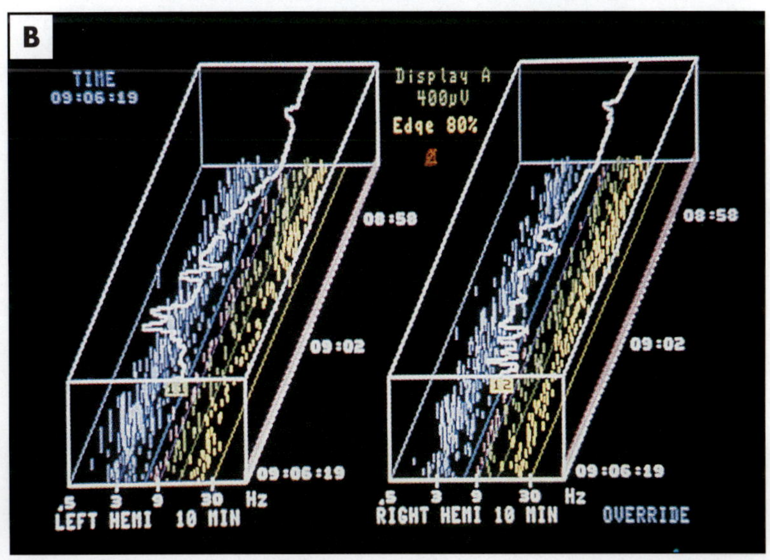

Figure 3-17. Monitors with three-dimensional displays: the processed electroencephalogram (EEG). An excellent example of challenging data displays is the "processed electroencephalogram," which is a display of EEG power spectral density versus frequency and time. This three-dimensional plot must be displayed on a two-dimensional screen in a manner easily interpreted by the average clinician. **A**, A traditional "compressed spectral array" display, in which successive amplitude versus frequency curves are plotted over one another, with more recent data being placed in front. **B**, The more innovative "telephone pole" display of the Lifescan (Diatek, Inc., San Diego), in which the pole height represents amplitude, horizontal axis represents frequency, and the oblique z-axis represents time with older data moving to the rear. This display allows quick left-versus-right hemisphere comparisons for asymmetry, and also shows the "spectral edge frequency," or frequency below which 80% of the EEG energy lies. Compare this display with that of *panel A* for ease and speed of interpretation, information content, and clinical relevance. Although this display has won widespread approval throughout the anesthesia community, the manufacturer of this instrument is unfortunately no longer in business. (Part A *adapted from* Levy [18]. Part B *adapted from* Frost [19]; with permission.)

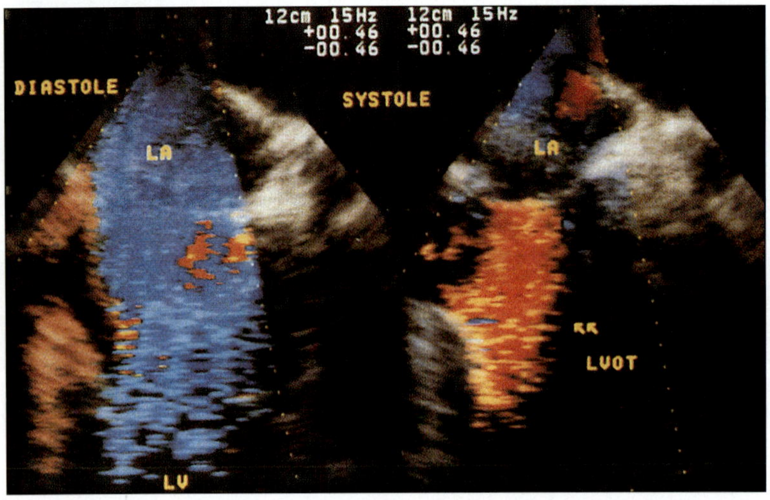

Figure 3-18. Color displays: transesophageal echocardiogram. One of the most useful applications of color in a monitor display is found in transesophageal echocardiography with color Doppler. These ultrasound images are from the level of the mitral valve and the left ventricular outflow tract. The left image was obtained during diastole, and the blue color represents flow away from the transducer (top of the triangle) during left ventricular filling. The right image was obtained during systole, with the red color representing flow toward the transducer during left ventricular ejection. Another application of color is seen in Figure 3-17B; the color does not itself convey important additional information, but makes the display easier to read. LA—left atrium; LVOT—left ventricular outflow tract. (*Adapted from* Thys and Reich [20]; with permission.)

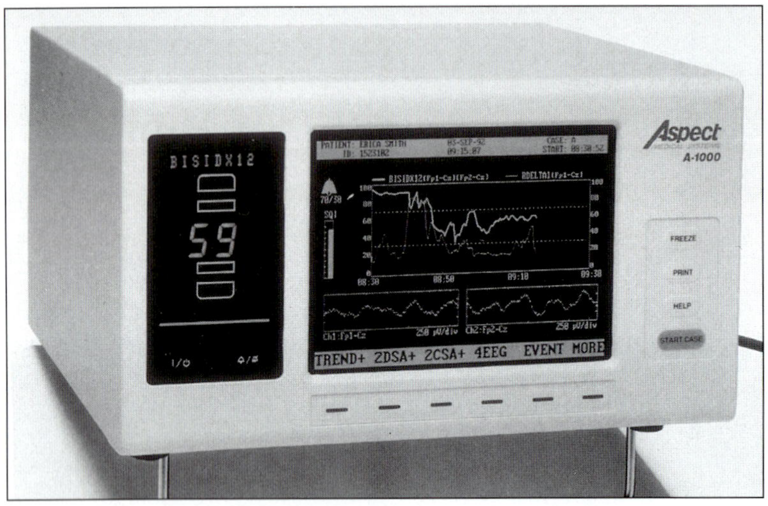

Figure 3-19. New varieties of signal processing: bispectral density. New calculated variables or displays are being invented or developed every year. Many of these eventually prove useless and the associated devices disappear: for example, consider esophageal manometry "depth of anesthesia" monitoring. Only time and clinical experience can separate the winners from the losers in the monitoring marketplace. Bispectral analysis is a recent technique for processing the raw electroencephalogram into a "bispectrum." The bispectral density is a measure of the phase coupling between two frequencies of the power spectrum. That is, if two prominent components in the spectrum are unrelated (*ie*, independent fundamentals), the bispectral density will be zero. However, if the two frequencies are harmonics of the same fundamental, then the bispectral density at the corresponding frequency values will be high. Some recent studies suggest that the bispectrum and the "bispectral index," a numeric value derived from the bispectrum, may be predictors of anesthetic depth. More studies and widespread clinical experience are required to determine the practical value of the bispectrum as a continuous monitor [21]. This figure shows the Aspect A-1000 Bispectral Analyzer. (Courtesy of Aspect Medical Systems, Inc., Framingham, MA.)

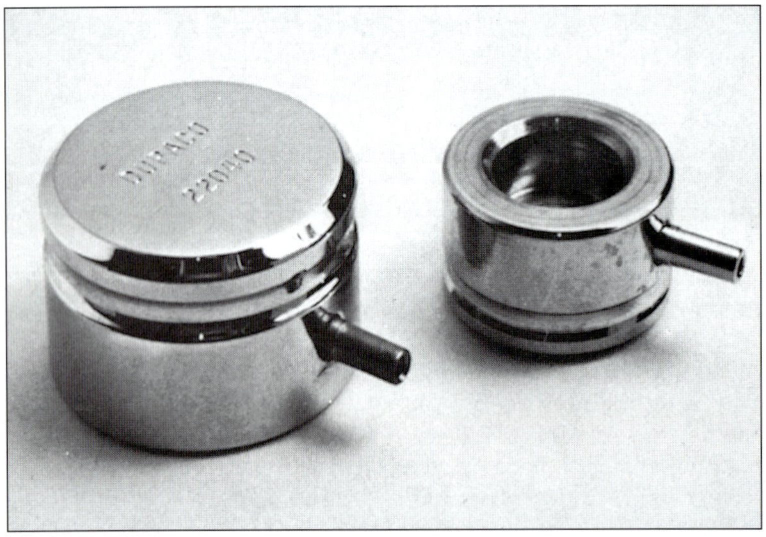

Figure 3-20. A simple monitor that never fails. The most useful and reliable monitors are often the most simple. This device requires no electricity, no three-dimensional displays, and no computerized processing; yet the precordial stethoscope provides continuous monitoring of breath and heart sounds, giving moment-to-moment information on ventilation and circulation. When combined with palpation of pulses and observation of chest movements, this can be the most important single monitor during anesthesia induction, particularly from the time of intravenous anesthetic injection until the airway is secured [10]. (Courtesy of Dupaco-MPI, Oceanside, CA.)

REFERENCES

1. Tremper KK, Barker SJ: Fundamental principles of monitoring instrumentation. In *Anesthesia*, edn 4. Edited by Miller RD. New York: Churchill Livingstone; 1994:1095–1126.
2. Gardner RM: Direct blood pressure measurement: dynamic response requirements. *Anesthesiology* 1981, 54:227.
3. Barker SJ, Tremper KK: Physics applied to anesthesia. In *Clinical Anesthesia*, edn 2. Edited by Barash PG, Cullen BF, Stoelting RK. Philadelphia: JB Lippincott Company; 1992:141–181.
4. Lake CL: Monitoring of arterial pressure. In *Clinical Monitoring for Anesthesia & Critical Care*, edn 2. Edited by Lake CL. Philadelphia: WB Saunders Company; 1994:101–118.
5. Barker SJ, Tremper KK: Effects of methemoglobinemia on pulse oximetry and mixed venous oximetry. *Anesthesiology* 1989, 70:112–117.
6. Barker SJ, Tremper KK: Pulse oximetry. In *Anesthesia Equipment Principles and Applications*. Edited by Ehrenwerth J, Eisenkraft JB. St. Louis: Mosby-Year Book; 1993:249–263.
7. Tremper KK, Barker SJ: Monitoring of oxygen. In *Clinical Monitoring for Anesthesia & Critical Care*, edn 2. Edited by Lake CL. Philadelphia: W.B. Saunders Company; 1994:196–212.
8. Barker SJ, Tremper KK: The effect of carbon monoxide inhalation on pulse oximetry and transcutaneous PO_2. *Anesthesiology* 1987, 66:677–679.
9. Wong DH, Tremper KK, Stemmer EA, *et al.*: Noninvasive cardiac output: simultaneous comparison of two different methods with thermodilution. *Anesthesiology* 1990, 72:784–792.
10. Perrino AC Jr, Feldman JM, Barash PG: Noninvasive cardiovascular monitoring. In *Monitoring in Anesthesia*, edn 3. Edited by Saidman LJ, Smith NT. Boston: Butterworth-Heinemann; 1993:101–143.
11. Lake CL: Monitoring of ventricular function. In *Clinical Monitoring for Anesthesia & Critical Care*, edn 2. Edited by Lake CL. Philadelphia: WB Saunders Company; 1994:172–194.
12. Barker SJ, Tremper KK, Hyatt J, Heitzmann H: Comparison of three oxygen monitors in detecting endobronchial intubation. *J Clin Monit* 1988, 4:240–243.
13. Zaidan JR: Electrocardiography. In *Clinical Anesthesia*, edn 2. Edited by Barash PG, Cullen BF, Stoelting RK. Philadelphia: JB Lippincott Company; 1992:771–805.
14. Smalhout B: A quick guide to capnography. Hewlett-Packard; 1983:9–13.
15. Schwenzer KJ: Venous and pulmonary pressures. In *Clinical Monitoring for Anesthesia & Critical Care*, edn 2. Edited by Lake CL. Philadelphia: WB Saunders Company; 1994:119–148.
16. Burns PN, Downs WG: Clinical evaluation of a bedside ST segment monitor. *Proc Comput Cardiol* 1988, 97–100.
17. Smith MS, Clements F, Debruijn N: Electrocardiography: monitoring for ischemia. In *Clinical Monitoring for Anesthesia & Critical Care*, edn 2. Edited by Lake CL. Philadelphia: WB Saunders Company; 1994:44–58.
18. Levy WJ: Electroencephalography. In *Clinical Monitoring for Anesthesia & Critical Care*, edn 2. Edited by Lake CL. Philadelphia: WB Saunders Company; 1994:269–287.
19. Frost EAM: Electroencephalography and evoked potential monitoring. In *Monitoring in Anesthesia*, edn 3. Edited by Saidman LJ, Smith NT. Boston: Butterworth-Heinemann; 1993:203–223.
20. Thys DM, Reich DL: Invasive cardiovascular monitoring. In *Monitoring in Anesthesia*, edn 3. Edited by Saidman LJ, Smith NT. Boston: Butterworth-Heinemann; 1993:51–100.
21. Sigl JC, Chamoun NG: An introduction to bispectral analysis for the electroencephalogram. *J Clin Monit* 1994, 10:392–404.

4

Spinal, Epidural, and Caudal Anesthesia

Manbir Batra, Michael F. Mulroy, and Joseph Neal

Techniques for regional anesthesia are becoming increasingly popular in the operating room as their advantages for postoperative analgesia and accelerated recovery become evident. Epidural analgesia, in particular, has found an increasing role in providing postoperative pain management for surgical patients, with increasing evidence that it not only enhances pain relief compared with traditional methods but can also speed recovery and, eventually, hospital discharge. Spinal anesthesia, likewise, is recognized as being highly efficient and reliable and even is useful in the outpatient setting to avoid nausea, vomiting, and somnolence. Both of these techniques are technically easy to perform compared with the peripheral nerve blocks and, thus, are the most common regional techniques employed in the operating room. Caudal anesthesia has also seen increasing use, particularly in the pediatric population in which it has advantages for postoperative analgesia.

The successful use of these techniques requires familiarity with standard local anesthetic pharmacology, which is covered in several excellent texts. This chapter focuses primarily on the anatomy and techniques of the various blocks, rather than on the pharmacology.

ANATOMIC AND ANESTHETIC CONSIDERATIONS

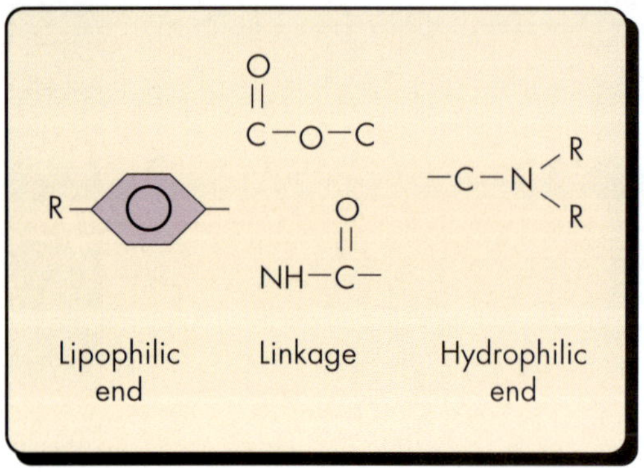

Figure 4-1. Structure of local anesthetics. All local anesthetics have three common features: a lipophilic end, a hydrophilic end, and an ester or amide linking the two. The primarily lipophilic end of the molecule most frequently, is some form of benzine ring. At the opposite end of the molecule is the more hydrophilic portion. This portion generally includes a tertiary amino group that can also exist as the charged quaternary salt, which is the molecular property that most enhances its water solubility. These two molecular ends are joined by either an ester or an amide linkage, thus providing the two major categories of local anesthetics. The length of the side chains in the hydrophilic portion are generally the primary determinants of the protein binding and of the lipid solubility of the compounds. Thus, the molecules with longer side chains are associated with greater potency and duration of action. [1].

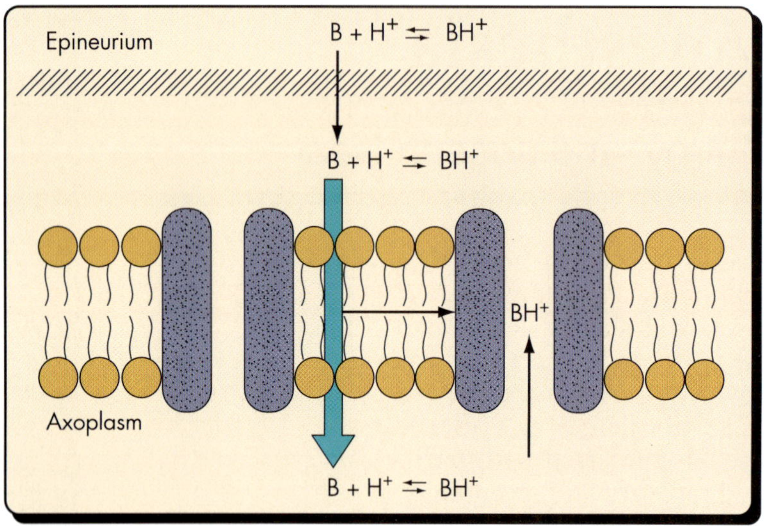

Figure 4-2. Neural cell wall with sodium channel. The primary target of the local anesthetic molecule is the sodium channel of the nerve membrane. The local anesthetic molecule does not enter the sodium channel directly from the outside. It must first penetrate through the lipid nerve membrane in its un-ionized form. Once inside the axoplasm of the nerve cell, the local anesthetic then diffuses rapidly into the sodium channel and appears to block conduction of sodium molecules through this channel by a deformation of the protein compounds within the channel wall. (*Adapted from* Mulroy [1].)

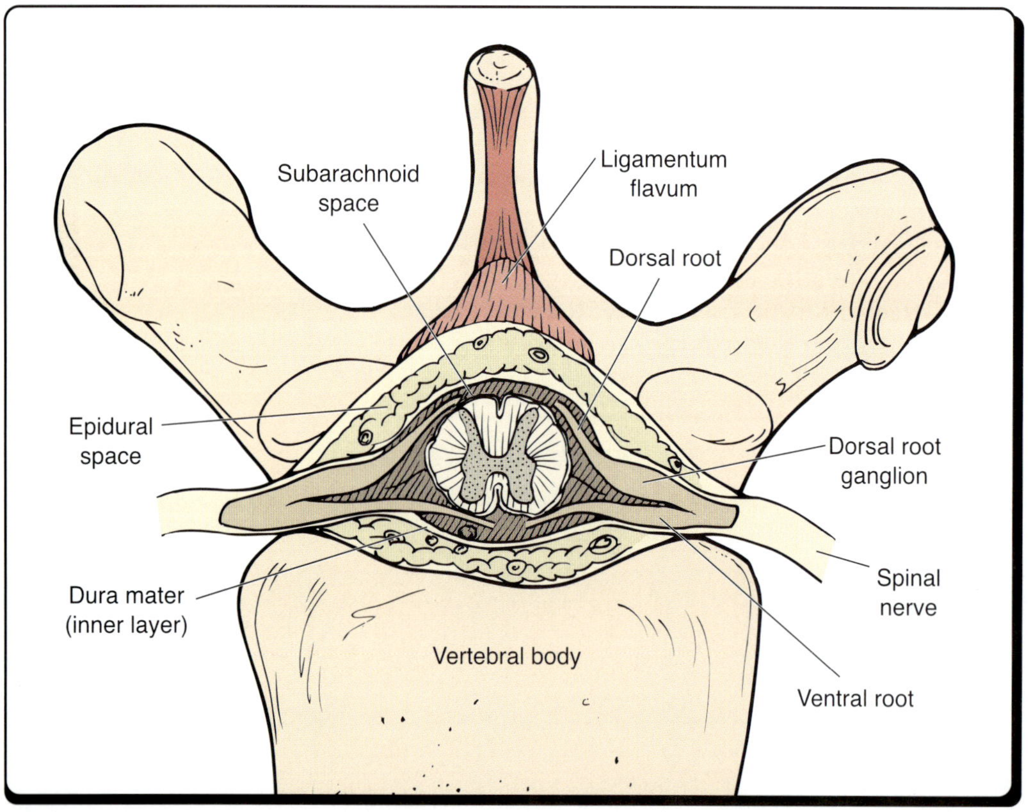

Figure 4-3. Cross section of spinal column. The target of the local anesthetic molecules in spinal epidural blockade are the neural pathways traversing the spinal column. The afferent fibers from the periphery enter the dorsal root ganglia at the lateral edges of the spinal canal and then connect with the dorsal root entry zone of the spinal cord itself before beginning their long journey upward to the cortex. The efferent fibers exit the cord along the ventral horns, and their ventral nerve roots join the afferent fibers to form the spinal nerves, which exit from the lateral foramina of the spinal column. The spinal column itself is composed of the dense solid vertebral bodies on the anterior surface, and the pedicles, laminae, and spinous processes, which provide protection for the delicate cord structures on the posterior side. Within the spinal canal itself, the cord is protected by the cushion of cerebral spinal fluid that is enclosed within the dural sac. Local anesthetics injected within this sac penetrate the nerve fibers rapidly and produce the dense rapid spinal profile of spinal anesthesia. Anesthetic solutions injected outside the dura produce the slower onset and segmental analgesia associated with the epidural blockade. (*Adapted from* Covino and Scott [2].)

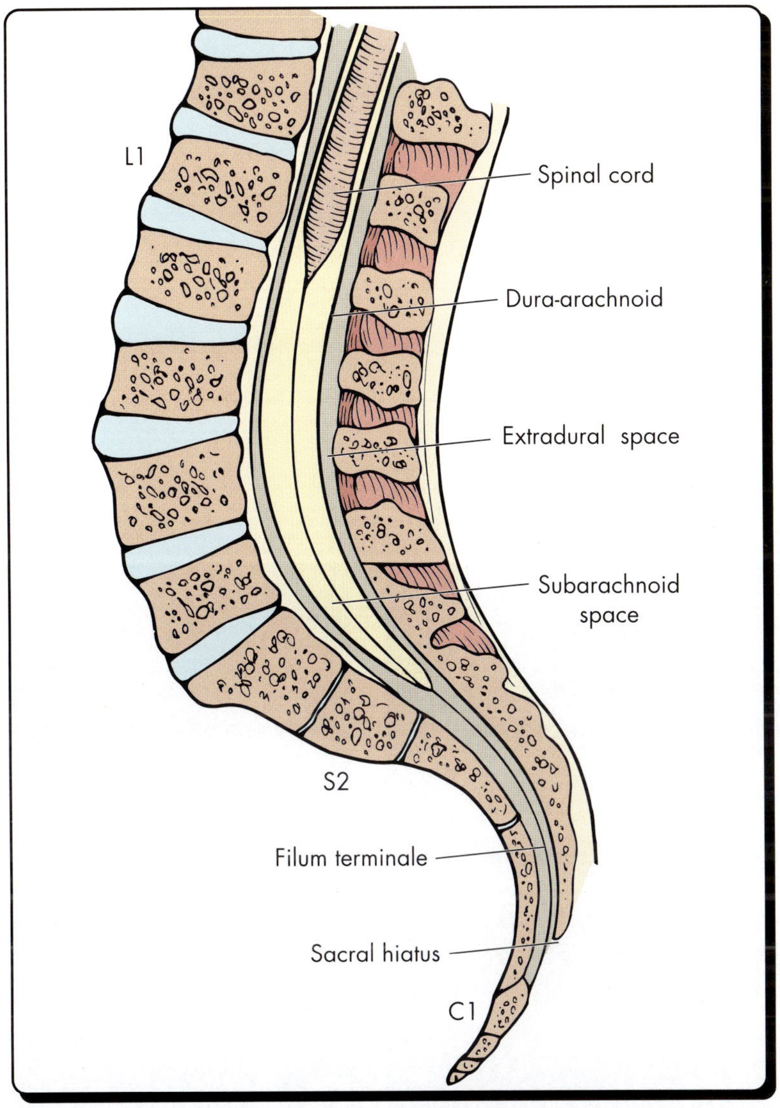

Figure 4-4. Lateral view of the spinal column. In the normal adult, the spinal cord itself ends at approximately the L1 level of the vertebral body. The dural sac surrounding the cord extends below to the sacral segment. Thus, the easiest application of spinal anesthesia is in the lower lumbar area. In this area, insertion of the needle into the dural sac avoids any direct contact with the spinal cord itself. The epidural space is at its largest in this lower lumbar area, and it is also a convenient place for the performance of epidural blockade. (*From* Lee and coworkers [3].)

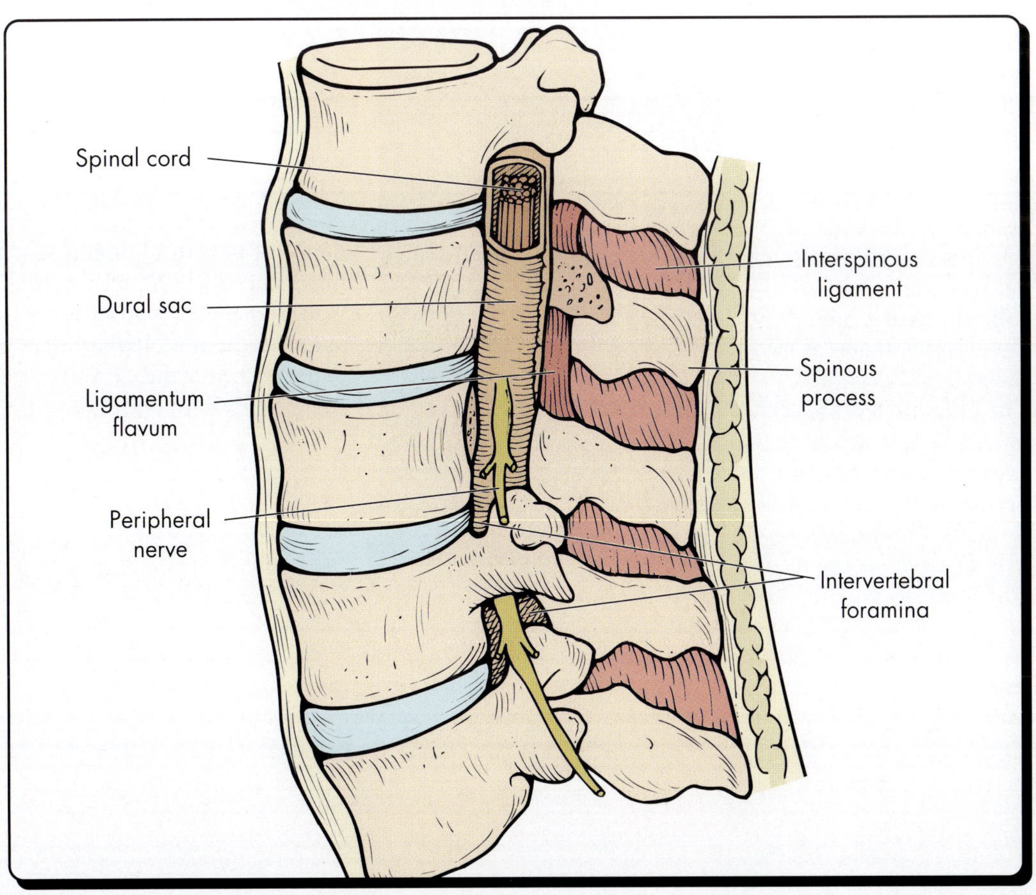

Figure 4-5. Lateral view of the lumbar vertebral column. The peripheral nerves depart the spinal cord and travel for a short distance within the dural sac before exiting from the vertebral column through one of the lateral vertebral foramina. The larger entrance to the center of the vertebral column itself, however, is the posterior approach through the ligamentum flavum. This dense ligament protects the dura and nerves from posterior entry by completely covering the posterior opening. The opening is further reinforced by the dense interspinous ligament that joins the adjacent spinous processes of each vertebral body, and also serves as a useful marker of the midline of the spinal column. (*From* Lee and coworkers [3].)

INDICATIONS FOR SPINAL ANESTHESIA
Lower segment blockade (saddle block)
Perirectal work, pilonidal cysts, vaginal procedures, childbirth
Lower level spinal (T10 level)
Foot surgery, knee surgery, transurethral prostatic resection
Upper thoracic level (T4–T6)
Hernia repair, open prostatectomy, lower abdominal surgery, hysterectomy, cesarean delivery

Figure 4-6. Indications for spinal anesthesia.

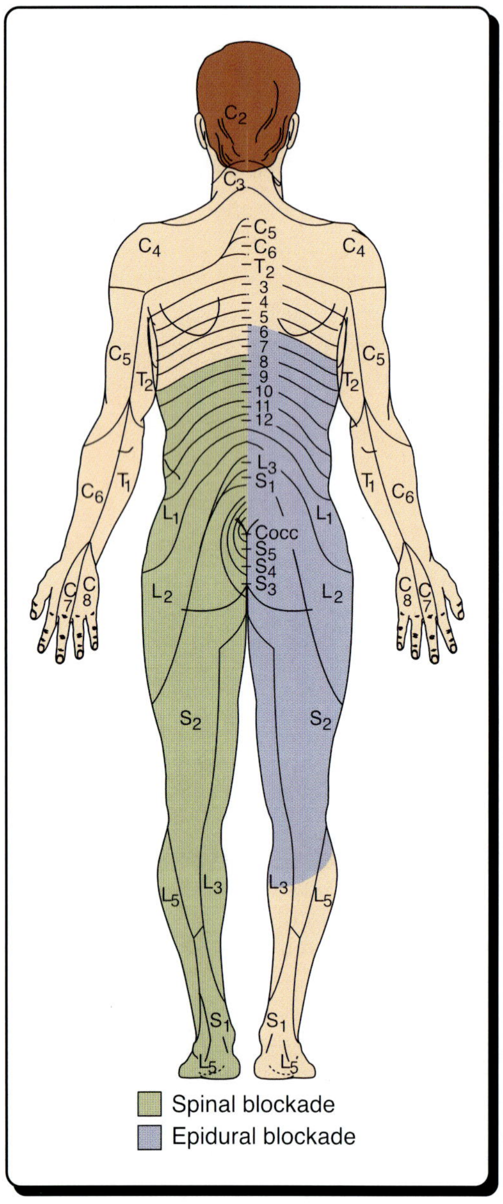

Figure 4-7. Spinal (subarachnoid) blockade produces dense anesthesia of all the peripheral nerves distal to the point of injection as well as a variable level of blockade above the point of injection, depending on the total dose and volume of the anesthetic solution involved. These effects are reflections of the anatomy of subarachnoid injection: all the peripheral nerves going to the caudad portions of the body must pass the point of injection on their way to their ultimate exit from the spinal canal. Epidural injection, on the contrary, can produce a *segmental* blockade of the dorsal nerve roots, because the injected solution bathes only the peripheral nerves in the area of injection. The ultimate level of blockade of epidural anesthesia is dependent on the total volume of the solution injected. (*Modified from* Covino and Scott [4].)

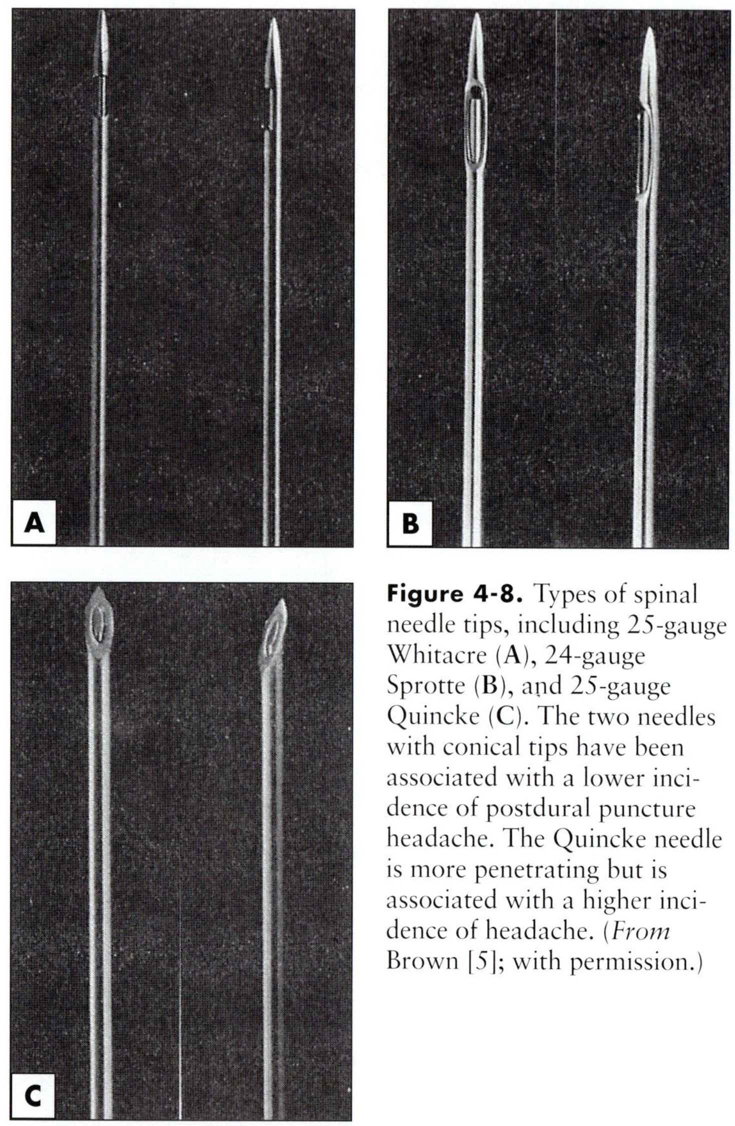

Figure 4-8. Types of spinal needle tips, including 25-gauge Whitacre (**A**), 24-gauge Sprotte (**B**), and 25-gauge Quincke (**C**). The two needles with conical tips have been associated with a lower incidence of postdural puncture headache. The Quincke needle is more penetrating but is associated with a higher incidence of headache. (*From* Brown [5]; with permission.)

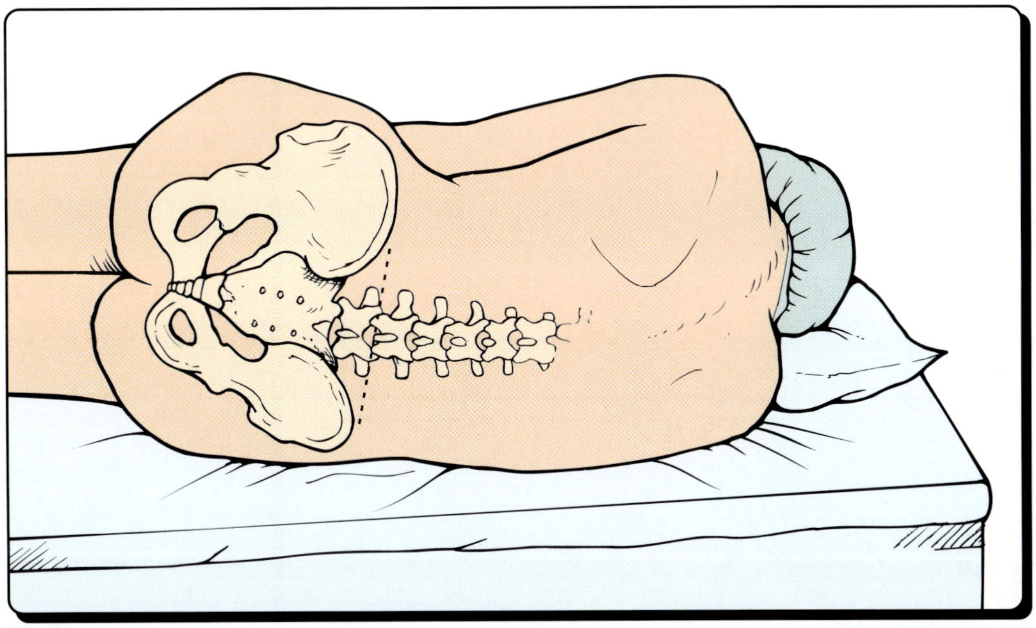

Figure 4-9. Lateral position for performance of spinal anesthesia. The patient is placed near the edge of the bed with the knees drawn up toward the chest and the head flexed down toward the knees. This position provides the maximum anterior flexion of the vertebral column. A pillow should be placed under the patient's head (but not under the shoulders) to maintain straight alignment of the spinal column. The patient should be encouraged to keep both the hips and shoulders perpendicular to the bed. A line drawn between the highest points of the iliac crest passes through the L4-5 interspace or the L4 spinous process. (*From* Mulroy [1].)

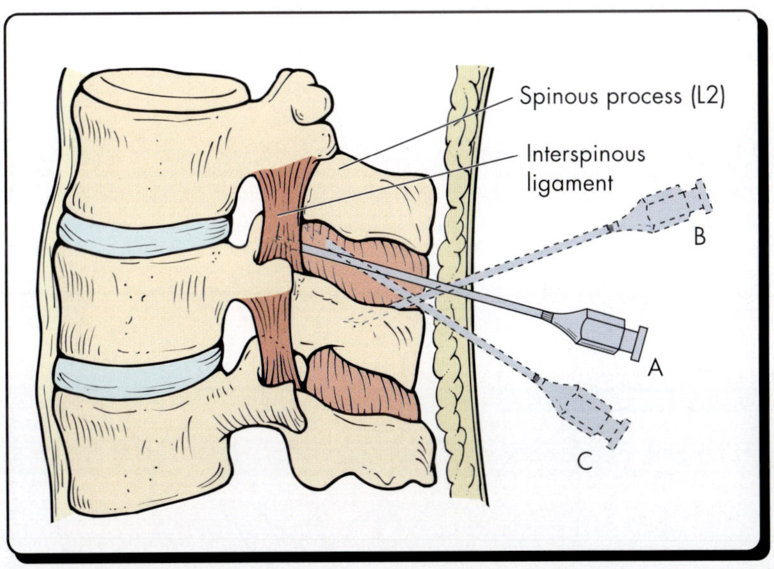

Figure 4-10. Lateral view of the spinal needle direction. In the classical midline approach, the needle is introduced between the two spinous processes with a slight cephalad angulation. When angled correctly (*A*), the needle passes through the interspinous ligament and into the ligamentum flavum. When the needle is directed too far inferiorly (*B*), it contacts the bony ridge of the inferior spinous process. Cephalad redirection allows the needle to pass further. When angling in the cephalad direction produces contact with the bone at a shallower level (*C*), the bone contacted is the inferior border of the superior spinous process, and more caudad redirection is needed. By adjusting the angle with each pass based on these observations, the interspace usually can be found. If bone is contacted at the same depth on repeated passes, the most likely explanation is that the needle is not in the midline position but has deviated laterally to contact the lamina. The identity of the true midline should then be reassessed (*From* Mulroy [1].)

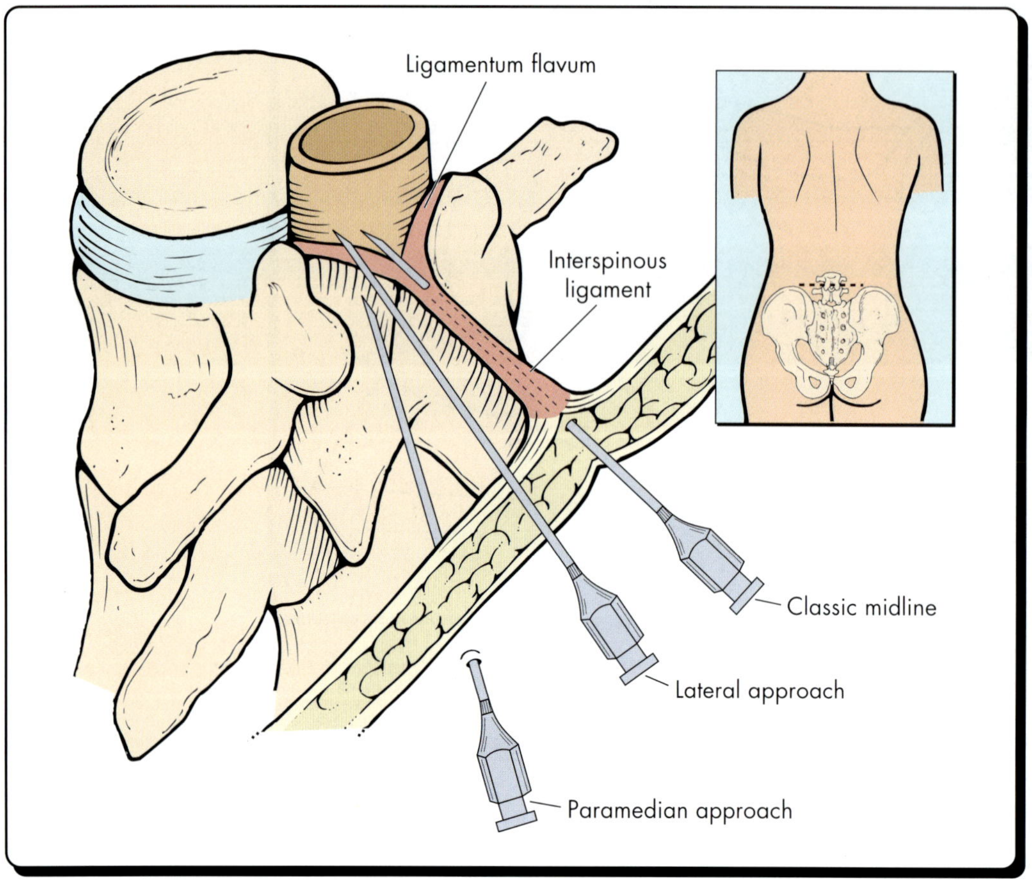

Figure 4-11. Paramedian and lateral approach of spinal needle insertion. In the classical midline spinal approach, the needle traverses the interspinous ligament and the ligamentum flavum before entering the dura. In patients with extremely calcified interspinous ligaments, the needle can be introduced 1 cm lateral to the midline and angled slightly toward the midline as it is advanced, thus avoiding the interspinous ligament and yet still piercing the ligamentum flavum and dura near the midline. In patients with more advanced osteoarthritis, it is sometimes useful to use a more paramedian approach in which the needle is actually introduced inferior and lateral to the interspace. Skin entry is performed 1 cm lateral to the spinous process, inferior to the space desired to be entered. The needle is advanced perpendicular to the skin until it contacts the lamina of the vertebral body and then walked upward and inward at 45° angles until it approaches the midline in the interspace. These approaches are suitable for both spinal and epidural blockade. (*Adapted from* Mulroy [1].)

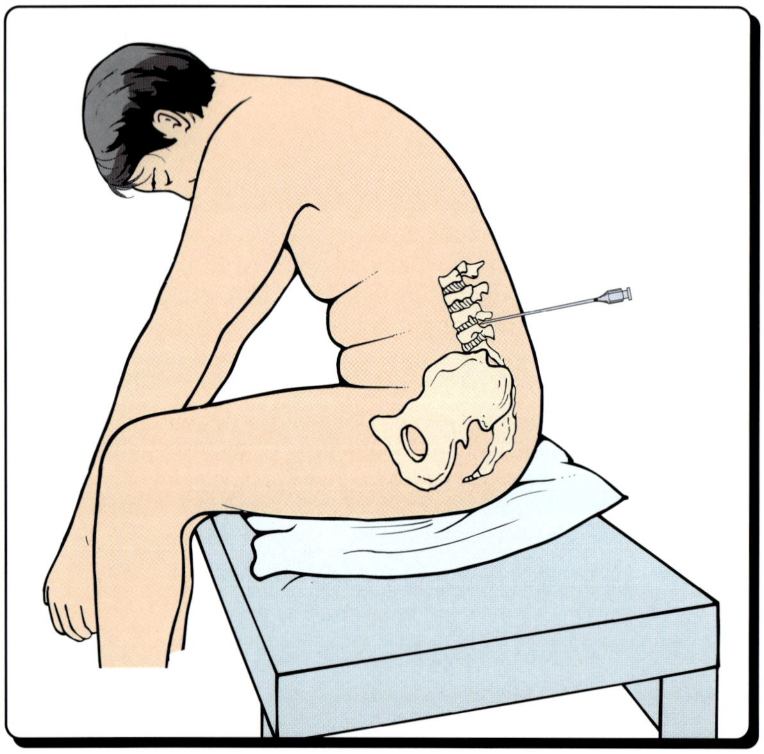

Figure 4-12. Sitting approach for spinal anesthesia. The patient is instructed to sit on the edge of the stretcher or operating table with the feet supported on a stool or bench that allows for more flexion of the lumbar spine. The shoulders are hunched forward, again contributing to increased flexion of the spine. Frequently, an assistant is needed to help the patient maintain this position and to monitor and provide support for the patient who has been given some sedation. This approach is particularly useful in the patient who is overweight in whom the midline is difficult to appreciate in a standard lateral decubitus position. (*Adapted from* Mulroy [1].)

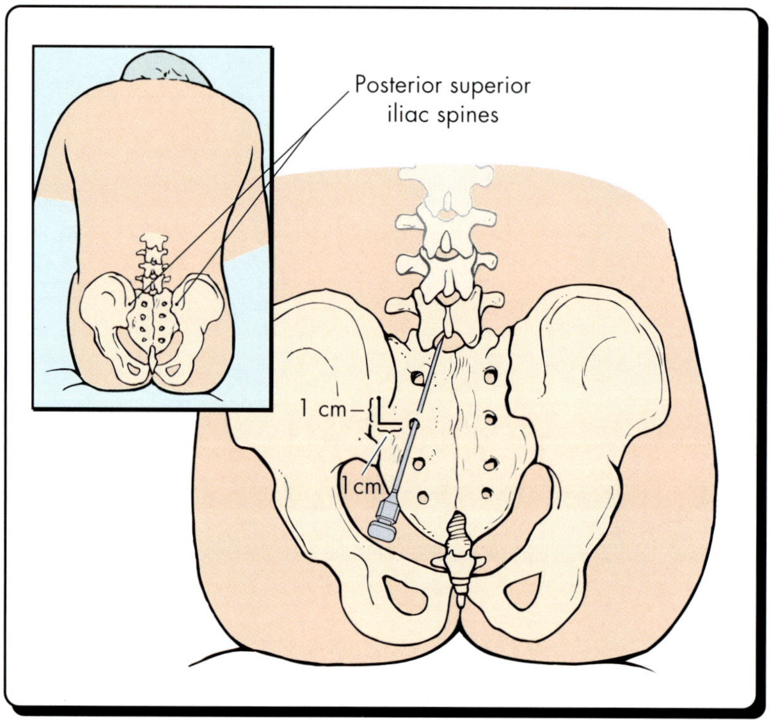

Figure 4-13. Taylor approach for spinal anesthesia. The L5-S1 interspace is the largest in the spinal column and easily can be approached from a paramedian direction with the patient in a sitting position. A skin mark is made 1 cm medial to and 1 cm inferior to the posterosuperior iliac spine. After adequate local infiltration, a 5-in needle is introduced in a 45° medial and 45° cephalad angle until bone is contacted. This bone is usually the lamina of the S1 vertebrae. The needle can then be walked superiorly and medially into the interspace. (*From* Brown [5].)

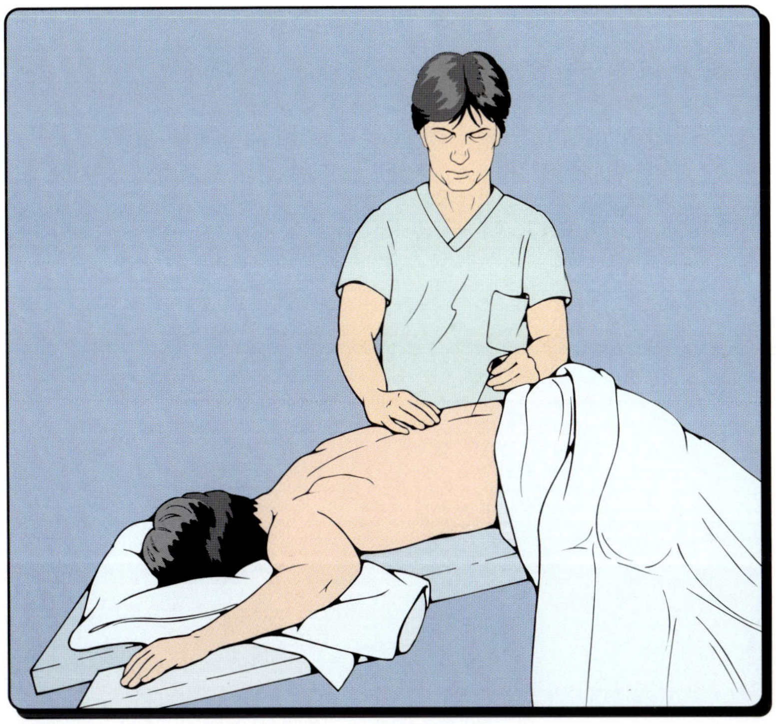

Figure 4-14. Spinal anesthesia in the jackknife position. The patient is placed in the prone position on the operating table. The table is then flexed to a maximum degree and turned in a slight head-down direction. The flexion point of the table should be directly under the patient's hips. The use of a pillow under the hips helps accentuate the flexion. The needle then can be introduced using the standard midline or paramedian approaches. Spinal fluid pressure is often negative in this area, and gentle aspiration may be needed to confirm identification of the subarachnoid space. Injection of a hypobaric location anesthetic solution produces excellent anesthesia for rectal procedures. (*From* Mulroy [1].)

RATE OF FAILED SPINAL ANESTHETICS RELATIVE TO THE LEVEL OF LUMBAR PUNCTURE

	Munhall et al. Failed		Tarkkila Failed	
Puncture site	Total	%	Total	%
T12-L2	0/0	NA	1/41	2.4
L2-3	0/56	0.0	7/541	1.3
L3-4	5/85	5.9	43/1197	3.6
L4-5	3/44	6.8	7/94	7.4
L5-51	0/15	0.0	0/3	0.0

Figure 4-15. Success rate of spinal anesthesia by vertebrae interspace. It appears that the L2-3 interspace has the highest probability of success for spinal anesthesia. NA—not applicable. (*Adapted from* Munhill and coworkers [6]; Tarkkila [7].)

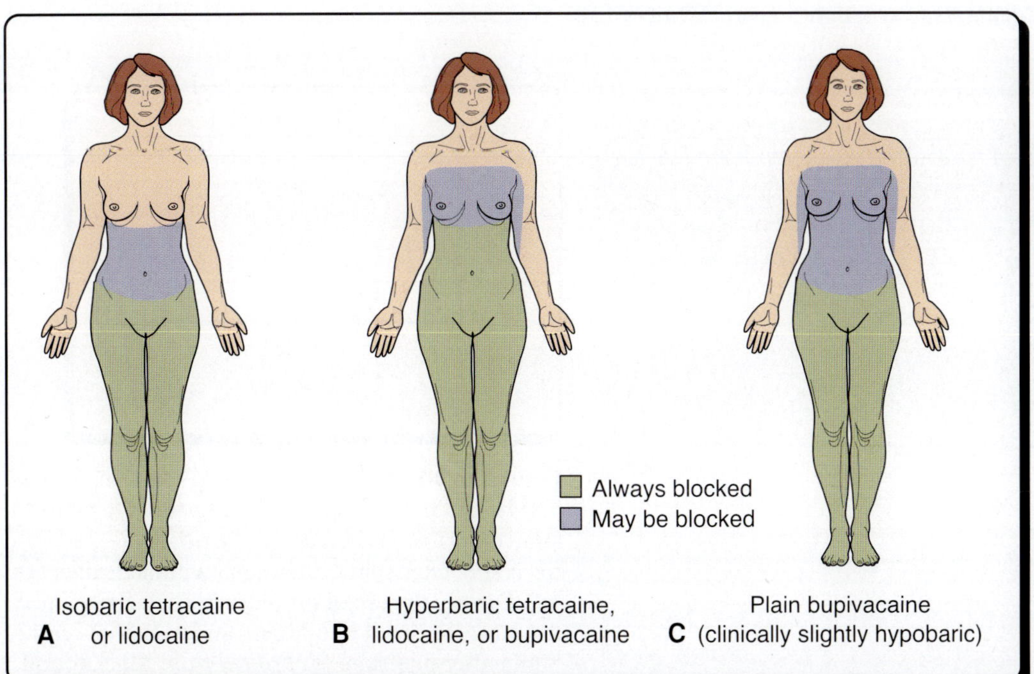

Figure 4-16. Spread of spinal anesthesia. The usual extent of spread of spinal anesthesia with different anesthetic solutions injected slowly at the L3-4 interspace in a classical midline position is demonstrated in A, B, and C. Isobaric solutions tend to produce lower blocks, but with much higher variability of spread. (*Adapted from* Wildsmith and Rocco [8].)

FACTORS AFFECTING SUBARACHNOID LOCAL ANESTHETIC INJECTIONS

Determinants of spread
- Major factors
  - Baricity of solution
  - Position of patient (except isobaric solution)
  - Dose and volume of drug injected (except isobaric)
- Minor factors
  - Level of injection
  - Speed of injection/barbotage
  - Size of needle
  - Physical status of patient
  - Intra-abdominal pressure

Determinants of duration
- Drug employed
- Dose injected
- Presence of vasoconstrictors
- Total spread of blockade

Figure 4-17. The influence of multiple factors on the duration and spread of a single dose of lidocaine, 50 mg. Epinephrine prolongs the blockade but also significantly prolongs the total recovery time. The addition of fentanyl also prolongs the sensory motor blockade and actually provides longer surgical anesthesia in the lower abdomen. Isobaric solutions tend to spread less far than do hyperbaric solutions, and in general, all hyperbaric solutions rise to the T3-4 level. (*Adapted from* Wildsmith and Rocco [8].)

DURATION OF SPINAL ANESTHESIA WITH LIDOCAINE, 50 mg

		Duration, *min* ± SD					
Solution	Block height	2-Segment Regression	T12 Surgical Anesthesia	Motor Block	L1 Regression	S2 Regression
1.5% Plain (isobaric)	T6 (T3-L2)	56±5	20±13	71±8	104±5	130±18
1.5% Dextrose	T3 (T7-L1)	39±5	29±10	30±8	73±10	99±11
5% with dextrose only	T3 (C8-T5)	50±16	49±30	88±20	109±6	150±8
5% with epinephrine	T4	56±11	45±30	108±30	96±42	156±43
5% with fentanyl	T3	70	75±32	89±31	100±31	157±11

Figure 4-18. Duration of spinal anesthesia with lidocaine, 50 mg, with various additives. SD—standard deviation. (*Adapted form data of* Chiu and coworkers [9] and Liu and coworkers [10]; *reprinted from* Mulroy [1].)

CARDIOVASCULAR RESPONSE TO SUBARACHNOID BLOCKADE AT 20 MINUTES

	T10 Level, %	T1 Level, %
Mean arterial pressure	−8	−22
Heart rate	Unchanged	−14
Peripheral resistance	−10	−7
Cardiac output	Unchanged	−19

Figure 4-19. Cardiovascular response to subarachnoid blockade at 20 minutes. (*Adapted from* Sivarajan and coworkers [11].)

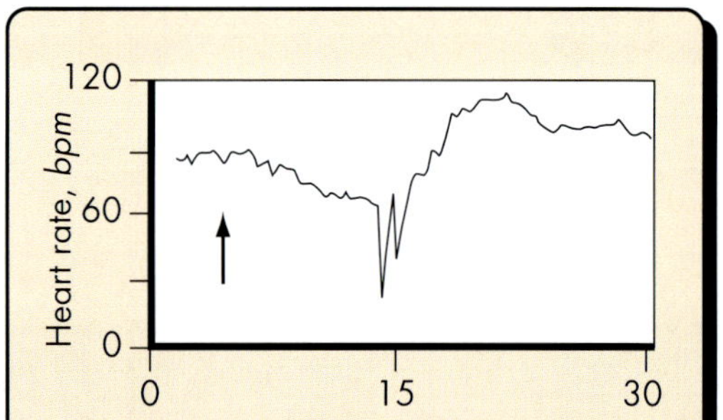

Figure 4-20. Bradycardia during spinal anesthesia. The heart rate of this 85-year-old patient demonstrated an abrupt decrease at the time indicated by the *arrow* after spinal anesthesia with lidocaine, 50 mg. Despite the use of prophylactic ephedrine, the heart rate declined to 68 bpm, and asystole occurred 8 min after injection. (*Reprinted from* Mackey and coworkers [12].)

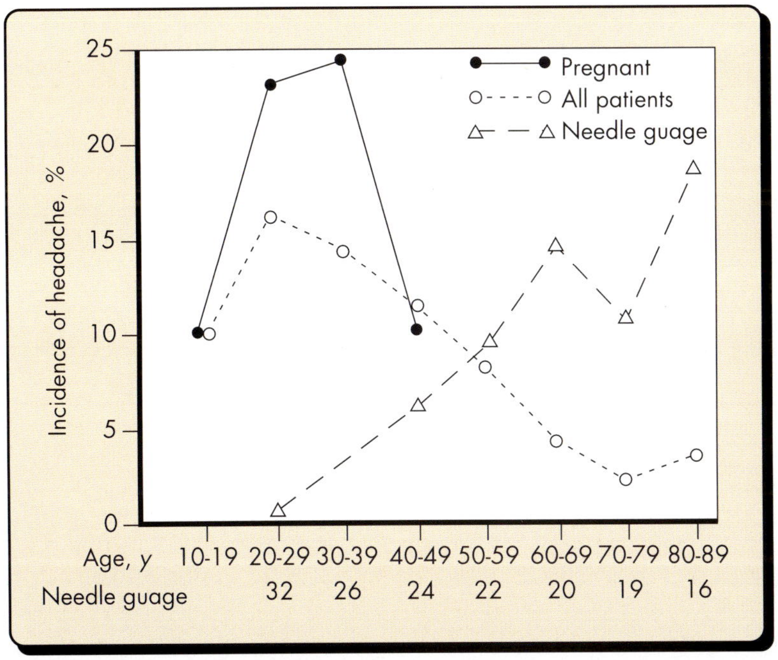

Figure 4-21. Factors affecting spinal headache. Larger needles are associated with a higher incidence of spinal headache than are smaller ones; however, the probability of spinal headache decreases with increasing age. The incidence is highest in pregnant patients. (*Reprinted from* Mulroy [13].)

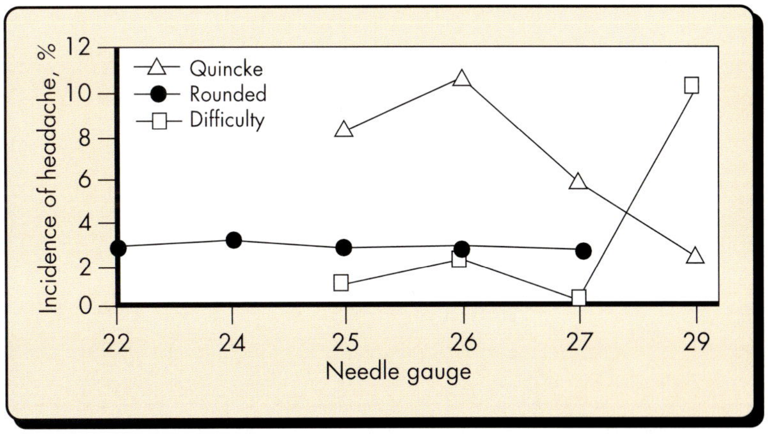

Figure 4-22. Needle design is a major factor in the incidence of spinal headache. Whereas the traditional standard-sized Quincke points are associated with an 8% to 10% incidence, the rounded bevel needles currently available are more commonly associated with a 2% to 3% incidence of headache, at most, in younger patients, and an even lower incidence in those over the age of 40. Smaller-gauge Quincke needles produce a lower incidence of headaches than do larger-gauge ones, but at the price of greatly increased technical difficulties and failures. (*Adapted from* Mulroy and Wills [14].)

EPIDURAL ANESTHESIA

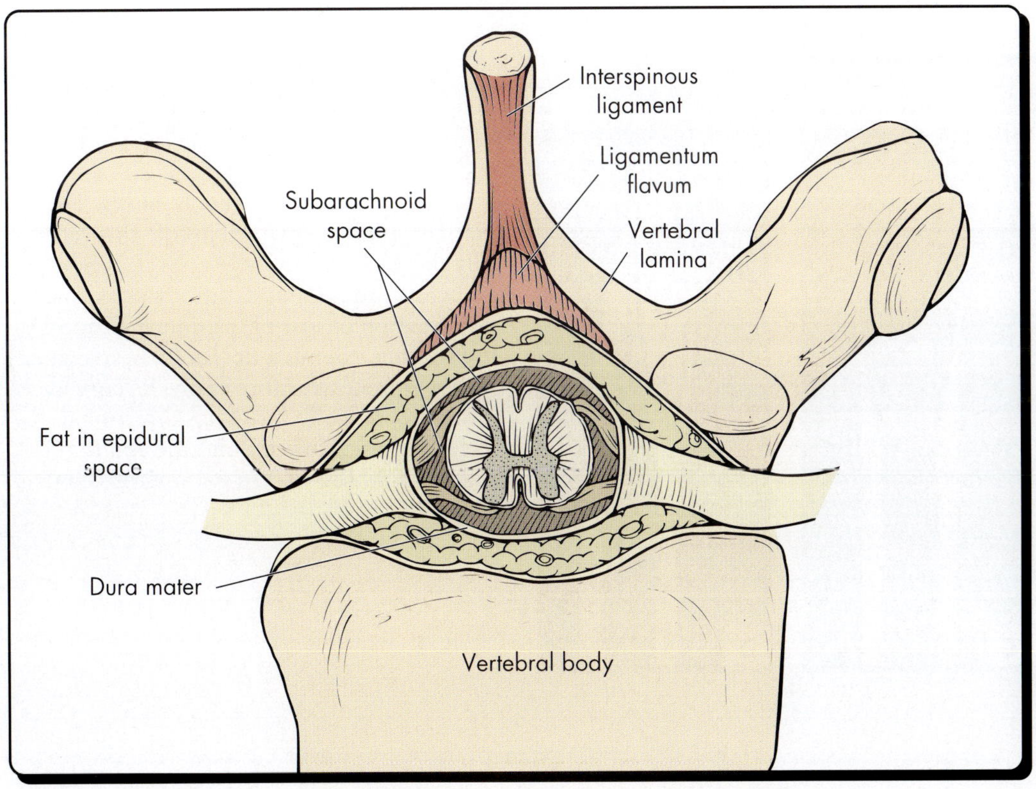

Figure 4-23. Epidural space. The epidural space circumferentially surrounds the dural sac. It is delimited anteriorly by the vertebral bodies and posteriorly by the spinal laminae, which are joined in the midline by the ligamentum flavum. The epidural space itself is filled with fat, areolar tissue, and veins. The epidural space is widest in its posterior midline between the ligamentum flavum and the dura. Proceeding from the cervical to the lumbar regions, the depth of the epidural space varies from 3 to 4 mm in the thoracic region to its widest size of 5 to 6 mm at the L2 interspace. (*From* Brown [15].)

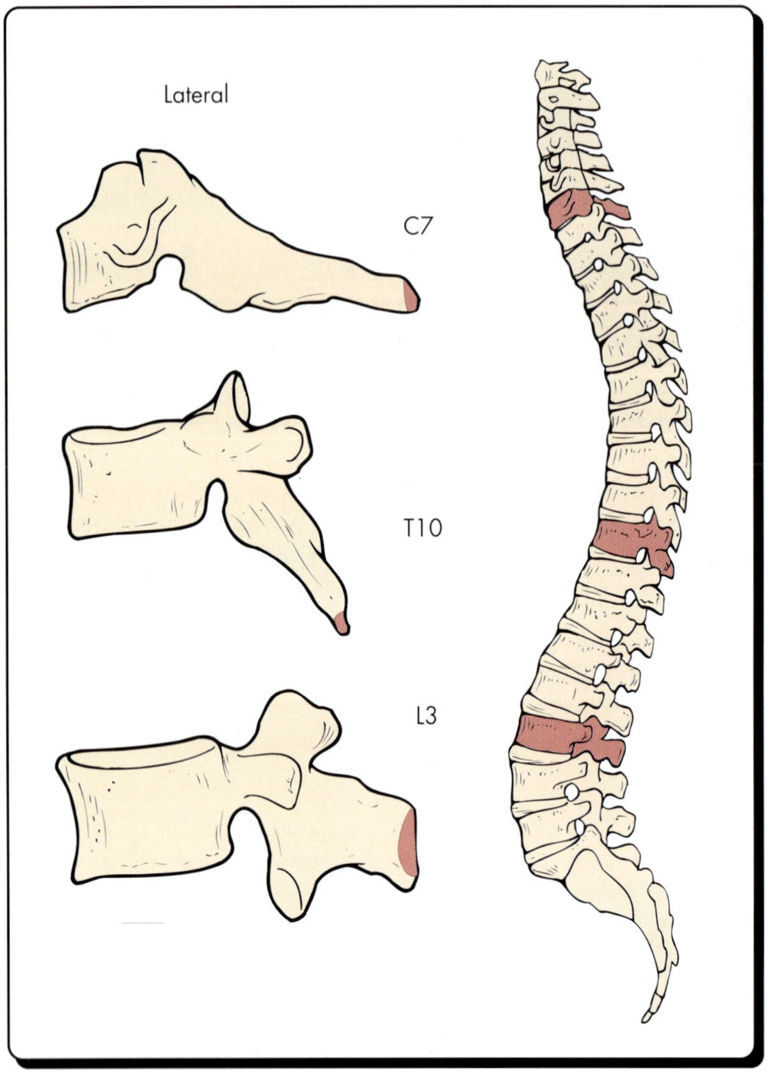

Figure 4-24. Spinal processes at various spinal levels. The angles of the spinal processes vary widely along the vertebral column. This anatomic feature has implications for determining whether to use a midline or paramedian approach to the epidural space. The relatively perpendicular orientation of cervical and lumbar spinous processes to vertebral bodies favors a midline approach, whereas the very acute angle of middle and upper thoracic spinous processes favors a paramedian approach. The intermediate angulation of lower thoracic spinous processes allows either approach. (*From* Brown [15].)

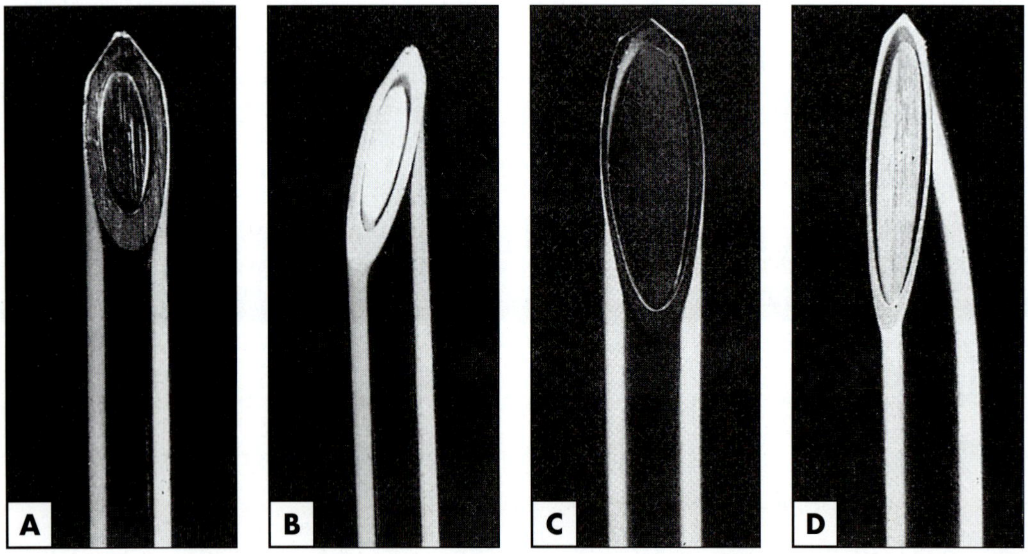

Figure 4-25. Various needle types for epidural anesthesia. Epidural needles are available in several designs. **A** and **B**, The relatively blunt Crawford needle theoretically increases resistance to passage through the ligamentum flavum, thus emphasizing the sensation of loss of resistance. **C** and **D**, The sharper, rounded tip Tuohy needle glides off bony processes more easily. Its curved outlet theoretically facilitates directional placement of a catheter into the epidural space. (*From* Brown [5]; with permission.)

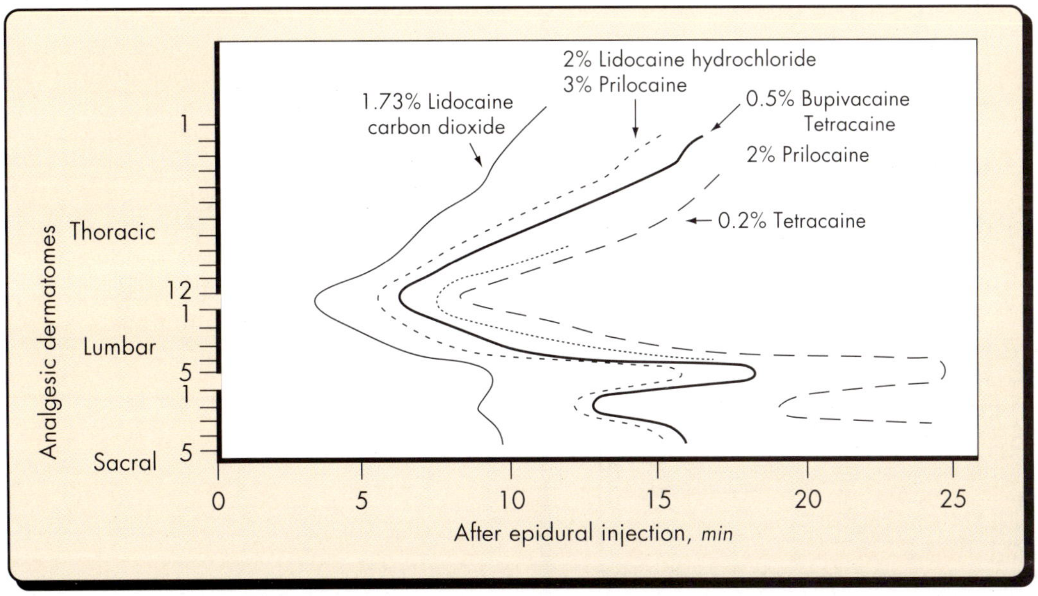

Figure 4-26. Epidural anesthesia classically spreads in a segmental fashion in both caudad and cephalad directions from the injection site. Sacral anesthesia is frequently slower in onset or even incomplete because of the thickness of the sacral nerve roots. Attachment of the dura to the foramen magnum limits anesthetic spread beyond the cervical regions. The dermatomal spread of analgesia as a function of time and type of local anesthetic is illustrated. (*From* Bromage [16].)

IDEAL CATHETER PLACEMENT FOR CONTINUOUS EPIDURAL ANESTHESIA AND ANALGESIA

Operation	Epidural Placement Site
Thoracotomy	High to mid thoracic epidural
Abdominal aortic aneursym repair	Mid to low thoracic epidural
Upper abdominal surgery	Mid to low thoracic epidural
Colectomy or exploratory laparotomy	Low thoracic epidural
Lower abdominal surgery	Low thoracic or high lumbar epidural
Ileoanal pull-through	Low thoracic or high lumbar epidural
Femoral-popliteal bypass	Lumbar epidural
Total hip or knee replacement	Lumbar epidural

Figure 4-27. Ideal catheter placement for continuous epidural anesthesia and analgesia. The choice of spinal level for epidural catheter placement is predicated on "centering" the injection site at the level of maximal surgical stimulus. The suggested epidural catheter placement site for various surgical procedures is given.

INDICATIONS FOR EPIDURAL ANESTHESIA AND ANALGESIA

Pre-existing disease indications:
- Patients with concurrent disease placing them at risk for postoperative complications—cardiac disease, pulmonary disease, hypercoagulation, morbid obesity

Surgical incision site indications:
- Upper abdominal and thoracic incisions

Peripheral vascular disease:
- Patients undergoing vascular surgery who have hypercoagulability and also are at risk for vaso-occlusive complications

Orthopedic procedures
- Patients undergoing hip repair, replacement, or both, who are undergoing knee replacement, who are at risk for postoperative thromboembolic complications

Figure 4-28. Indications for epidural anesthesia and analgesia, suggesting which patients may benefit most from perioperative epidural placement. (*From* Liu and coworkers [17].)

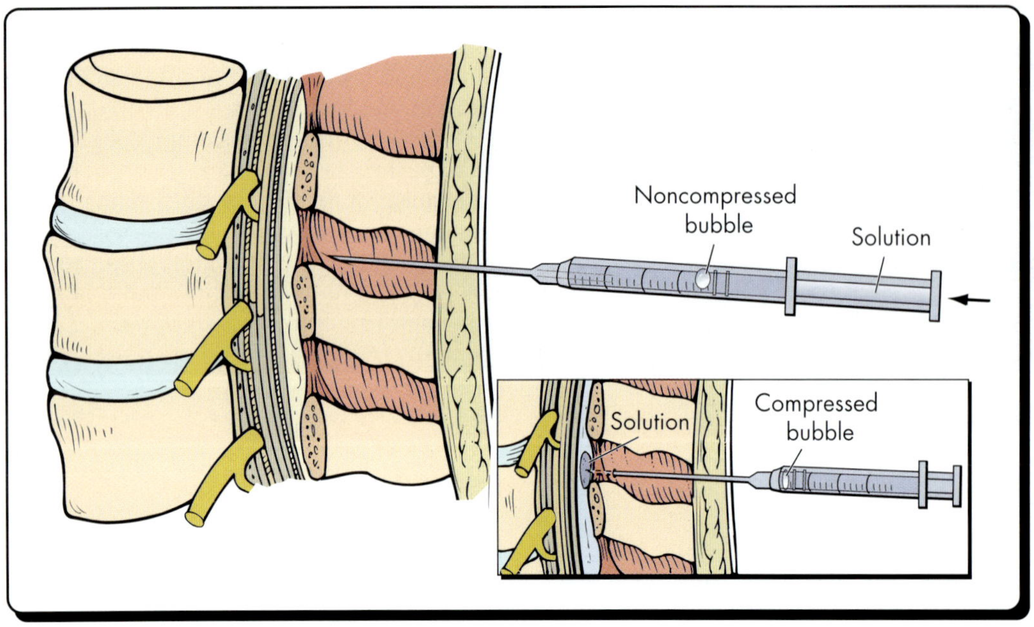

Figure 4-29. Loss-of-resistance technique. After the epidural needle is seated within the ligamentum flavum, the anesthesiologist notes strong resistance to compression of the syringe barrel. This resistance is best visualized by observing the compression of a small air bubble within the saline-filled syringe. As the epidural needle is advanced through the ligamentum flavum, a sudden loss of resistance occurs as the needle tip exits the tick ligament and enters the epidural space. (*From* Brown [15].)

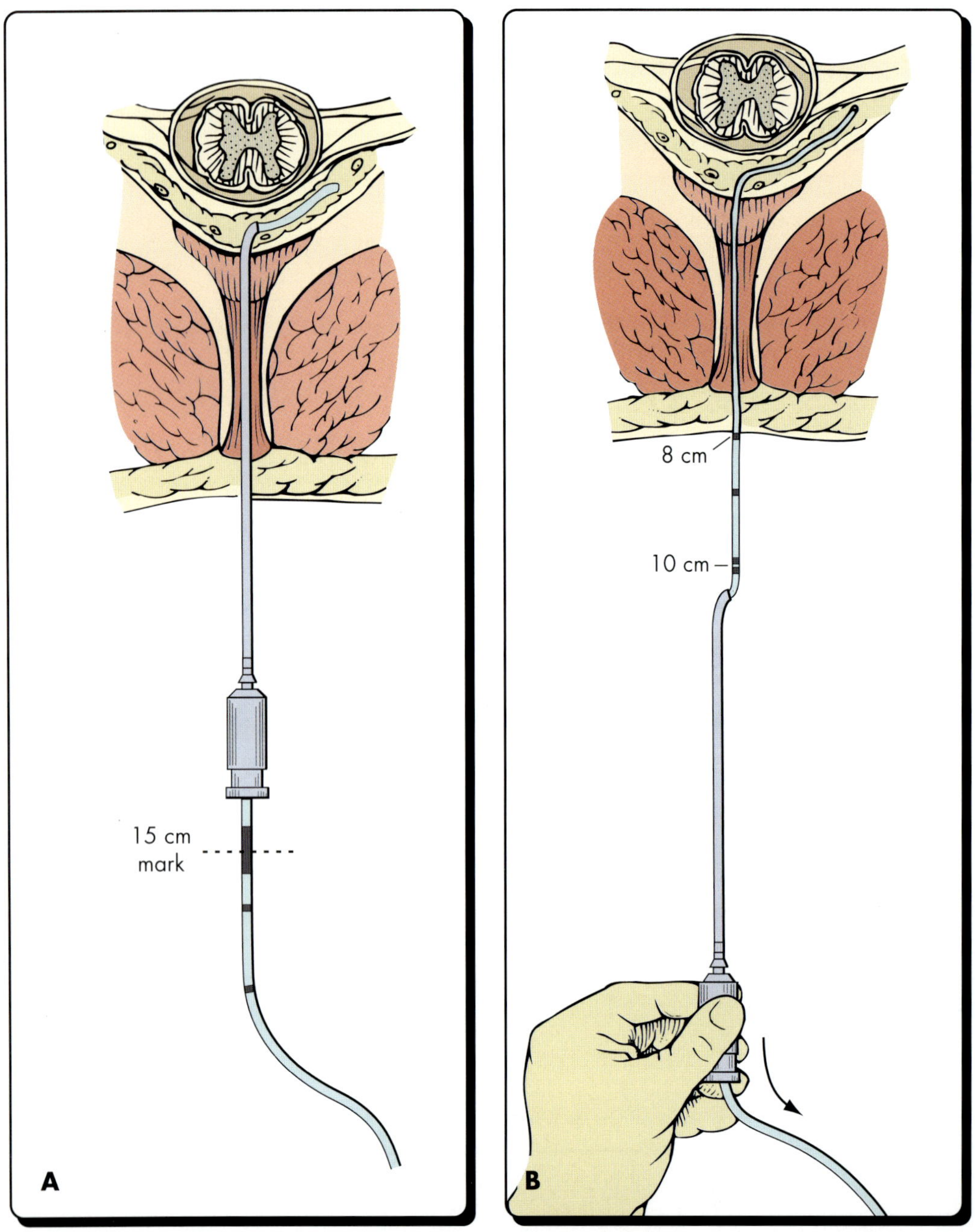

Figure 4-30. A marked epidural catheter being threaded through an etched epidural needle (**A** and **B**). This arrangement enables one to determine the distance a catheter is threaded into the epidural space. The distance at which loss of resistance is achieved is noted on the epidural needle, thus determining the distance between the skin and the epidural space. The epidural catheter is then threaded through the needle until a length of 4 to 5 cm is advanced into the epidural space. After removal of the epidural needle, the catheter is withdrawn until 2 to 4 cm of catheter length remains within the epidural space. This measurement is determined by adding 2 to 4 cm to the number of centimeters representing the skin-to-epidural space distance. For example, if loss of resistance is attained at 5 cm and the epidural catheter is withdrawn to the 8-cm mark, then 3 cm of catheter remains within the epidural space. (*From* Brown [15].)

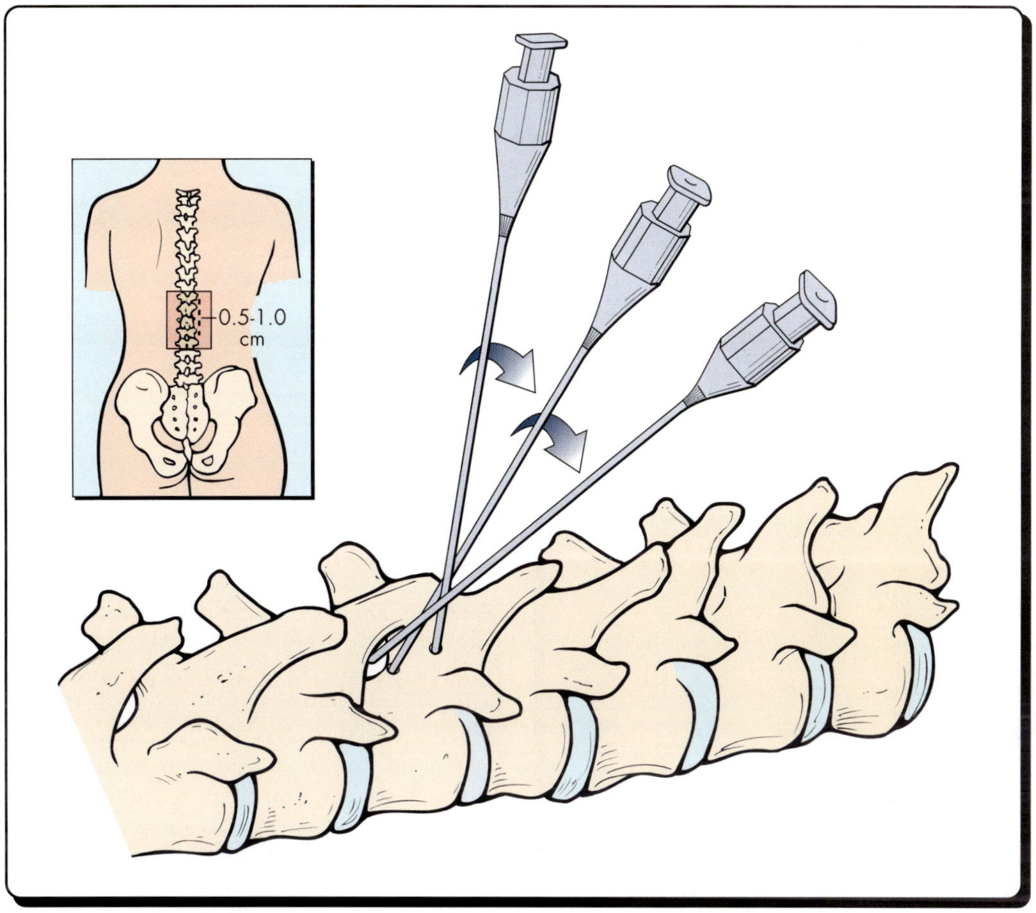

Figure 4-31. Paramedian approach for thoracic epidural anesthesia. This approach may avoid the difficulties inherent in midline needle placement between long and acutely angulated thoracic spinous processes. Furthermore, it may offer an extra degree of control as the needle approaches the narrow thoracic epidural space, at which point the spinal cord is only millimeters beyond the dura. To perform a paramedian approach, the skin is marked 0.5 to 1 cm lateral to a thoracic spinous process. After local anesthetic infiltration, the epidural needle is advanced until the underlying lamina is contacted. The needle is then "walked" in a cephalad and slightly medial direction until the needle tip is felt to slip off the lamina and encounter the firm lateral reflection of the ligamentum flavum. The epidural space is subsequently identified by slowly advancing the needle using the loss-of-resistance technique. (*From* Mulroy [1].)

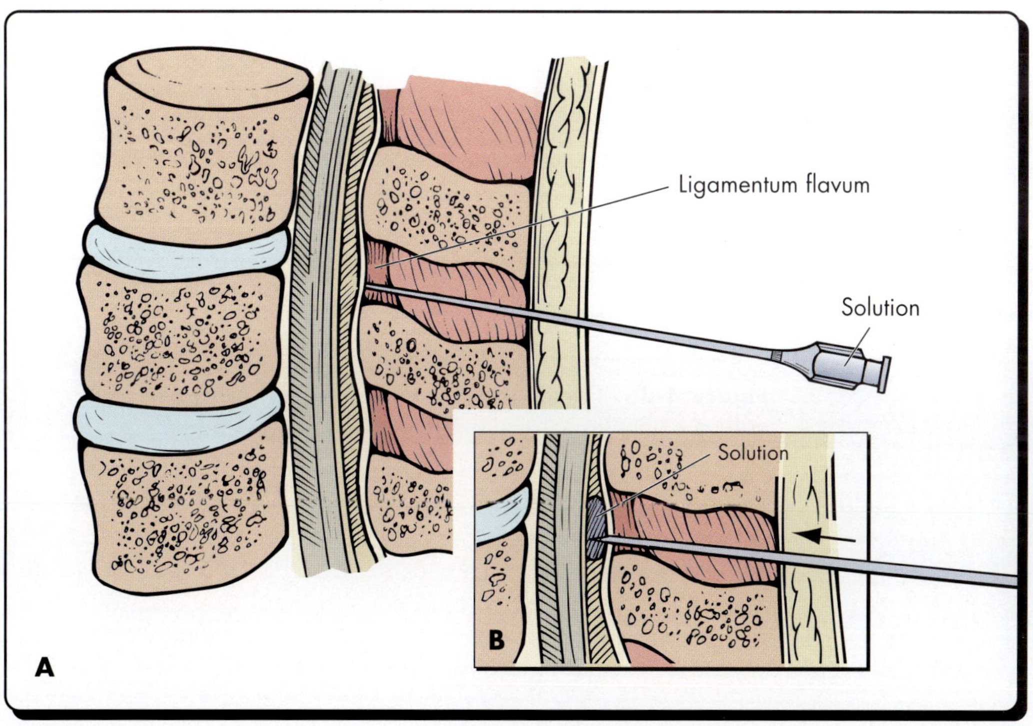

Figure 4-32. Hanging drop technique for cervical epidural space identification (**A** and **B**). Because negative pressure exists in the cervical epidural space, the anesthesiologist may use the hanging drop technique for cervical epidural space identification. The epidural needle is placed into the ligamentum flavum; however, instead of attaching a syringe, a drop of water is placed in the epidural needle hub. The drop of water is "sucked into" the needle hub by negative pressure as the needle tip enters the epidural space. (*From* Brown [15].)

EPIDURAL BLOOD PATCH TECHNIQUE

Identify the epidural space at the sight of the original dural puncture, or one or two spaces caudad.

Aseptically withdraw 20 mL of the patient's blood.

Slowly inject the blood into the epidural space until the patient complains of pressure or pain in the legs, buttocks, back, or head. Do not inject over 20 mL.

Have the patient remain supine for approximately 20 minutes.

Have the patient avoid Valsalva maneuvers for the next 24 hours.

Figure 4-33. The epidural blood patch technique is a common one. (*Adapted From* Mulroy [13].)

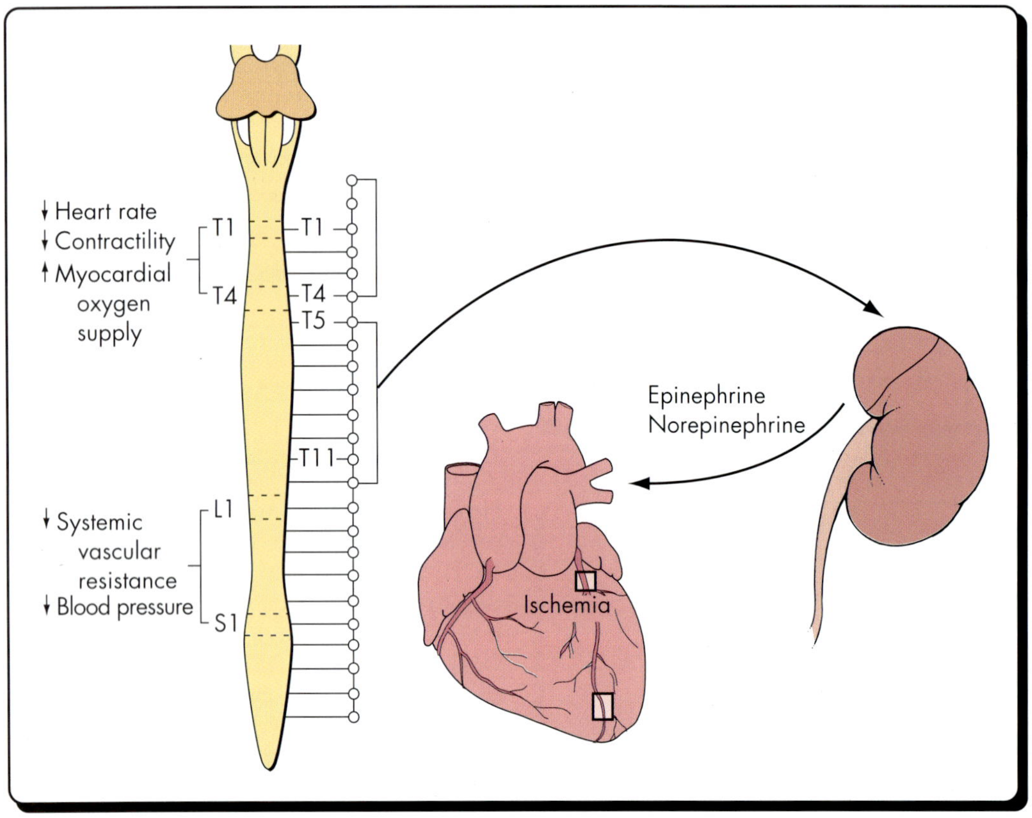

Figure 4-34. Cardiovascular changes with epidural anesthesia. Cardiovascular changes associated with epidural anesthesia are largely the result of which spinal cord segments are anesthetized. When thoracic sympathetic segments (T1-5) are blocked, the result is decreased sympathetic output to the heart. This is manifested by decreased heart rate, decreased contractility, and increased myocardial oxygen supply in those patients with ischemic myocardium. Blockade of lumbar spinal segments (L1-4) results in diminished systemic vascular resistance and, consequently, lower blood pressure. (*From* Liu and coworkers [17].)

EFFECTS OF EPIDURAL EPINEPHRINE

Prolongs local anesthetic duration

Decreases local anesthetic uptake, potentially limiting toxicity

Intensifies the effect of local anesthetic blockade

May reduce tachyphylaxis

Essential component of the intravenous epidural test dose

Figure 4-35. Effects of epidural epinephrine. Advantages of adding epinephrine to epidural local anesthetic solutions. (*From* Mulroy [1].)

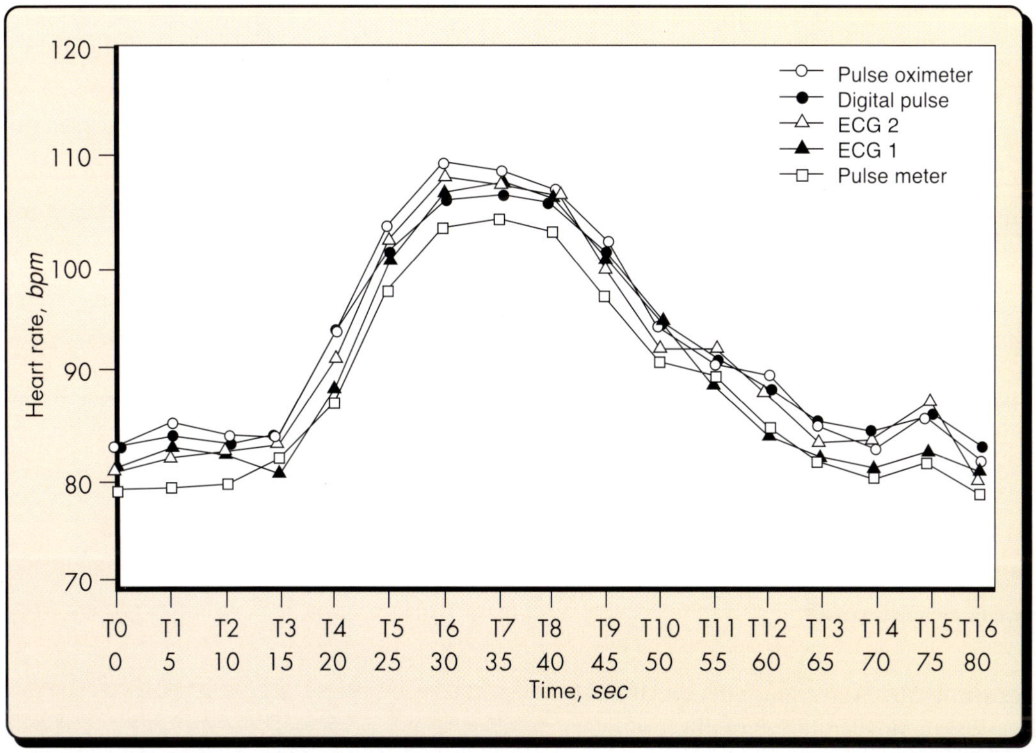

Figure 4-36. Epinephrine test dose response. There is always the risk of unintentionally injecting local anesthetic into an epidural vein with an epidural needle or catheter, thereby causing systemic local anesthetic toxicity. The intravenous epidural test dose uses the hemodynamic effects of epinephrine to identify when such unintentional intravenous placement has occurred. Injection of 15 μg of epinephrine into an epidural vein consistently elevates the heart rate by 30% within 30 seconds, in the normal patient. The epidural test dose is not effective in patients who are taking beta blockers, women who are experiencing labor contractions at the time of test dose injection, or in some circumstances when patients are receiving high MAC levels of inhalational general anesthetics. The ease of detecting a positive epinephrine intravenous test dose with the use of pulse oximetry or digital pulse counters is illustrated. ECG—electrocardiogram. (*From* Mulroy [1]; with permission.)

CAUDAL ANESTHESIA

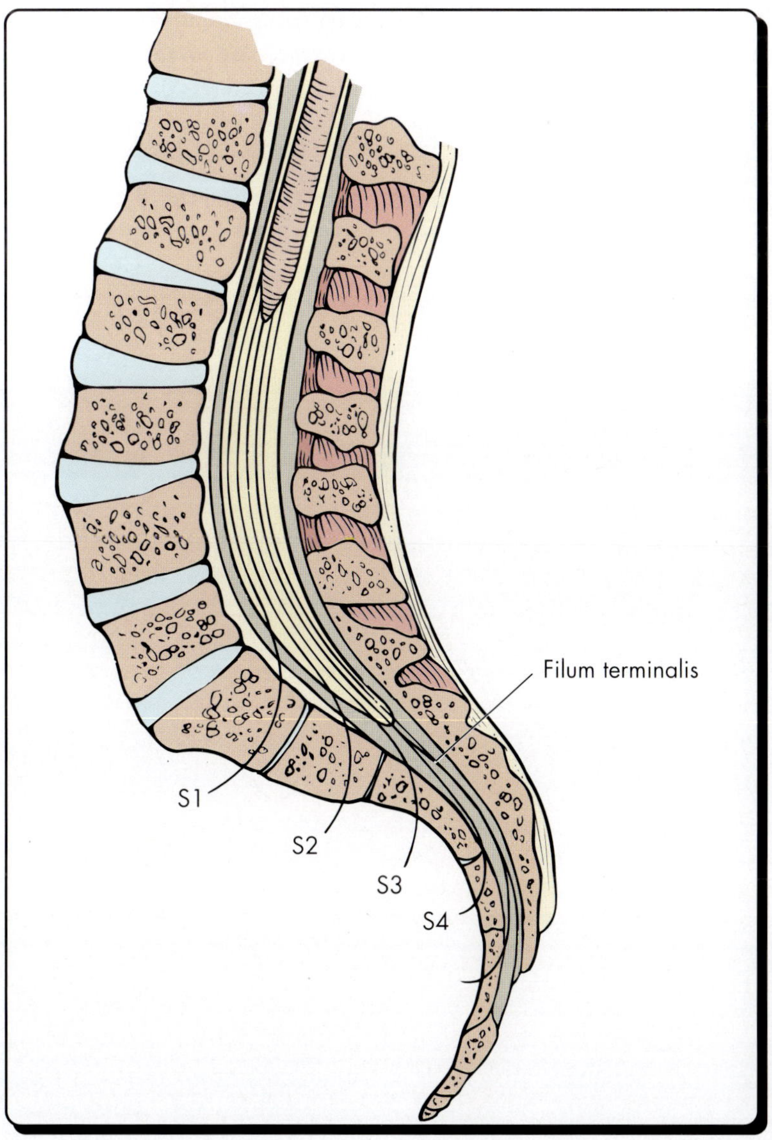

Figure 4-37. Lateral view of the sacral anatomy. The caudal canal is the lowermost extension of the spinal canal. The dorsal roof is the fused posterior laminae of the sacral vertebral bodies. The only direct opening into the canal normally occurs at the level of the fifth sacral vertebra, at which point the failure of development of the spinous process and the laminae leaves a hiatus in the bony roof of the canal. This opening is bounded laterally by the prominent cornu (the incompletely developed articular processes) and covered by the thick sacrococcygeal ligament. Along the lateral border of the canal itself are openings both anterior and posterior in the sacral bone at the S1 through S4 levels. The sacral nerve roots emerge both posteriorly and anteriorly through these modified intervertebral foramina. The canal is concave anteriorly but basically flat at the point of entry from the sacral hiatus. The angle of the canal to the skin surface varies with sex and race. In whites, the canal is at an angle of approximately 35° to the skin surface; in blacks, the angle may be 45°; In women, the angle is slightly less steep than in their male counterparts. The degree of bone fusion is variable, and the canal is absent in 5% to 7% of the population. (*Adapted from* Mulroy [1].)

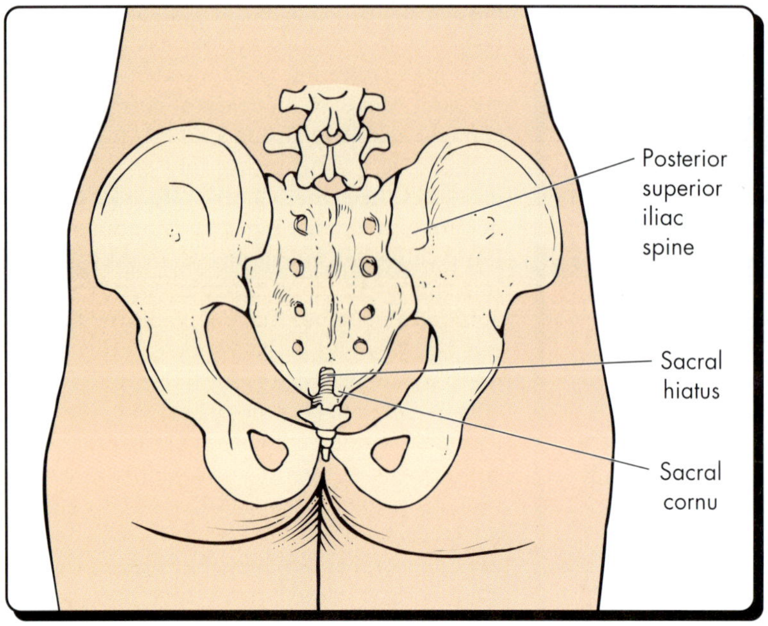

Figure 4-38. Posterior view of the sacral anatomy. The sacral hiatus is covered by a thick ligament that lies between and slightly inferior to the two prominent sacral cornua. (*Adapted from* Mulroy [1].)

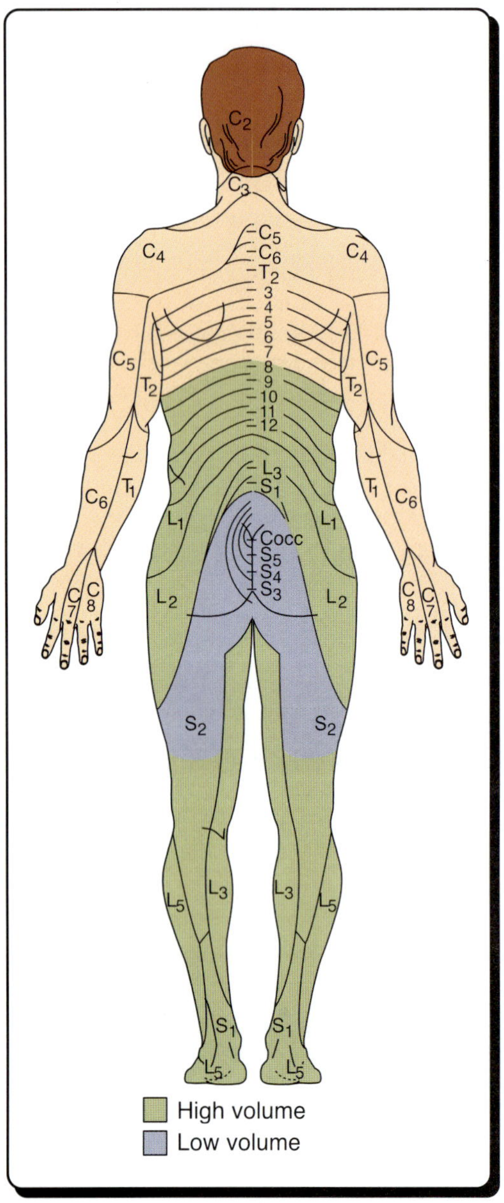

Figure 4-39. Distribution of caudal anesthesia. Small volumes of injection, such as 10 to 15 mL in an average adult, provide primarily perianal and lower leg anesthesia. Larger volumes, such as 25 mL, may be associated with leg and lower abdominal anesthesia. In pregnant patients, even these volumes may extend to the upper abdomen and allow for performance of cesarean delivery. In general, however, caudal anesthesia is limited to the perineal and lower abdominal areas.

OPERATIONS SUITABLE FOR CAUDAL ANESTHESIA

- Low-dose perianal operations, such as fistulas, hemorrhoids, and anal warts
- Vaginal procedures
- Perineal procedures
- High-dose lower extremity surgery
- Cesarean delivery (advisable only if caudal catheter is already present)

Figure 4-40. Operations suitable for caudal anesthesia.

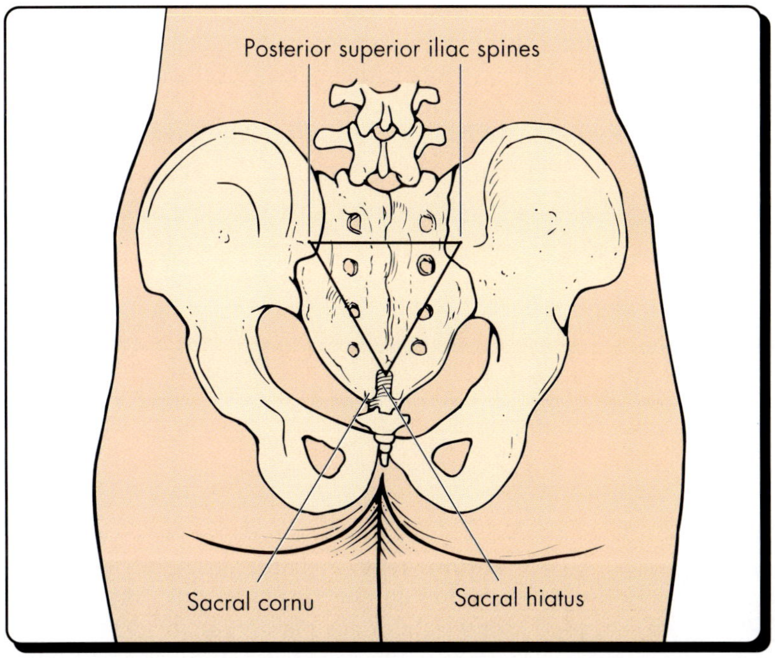

Figure 4-41. Surface anatomy for caudal blockade. In most patients, the prominent sacral cornua can be felt on either side of the sacral hiatus. This hiatus forms a valley or trough between these prominent bones. A triangle drawn between the hiatus and the two posterior superior iliac spines should produce an equilateral structure. (*Adapted from* Brown [5].)

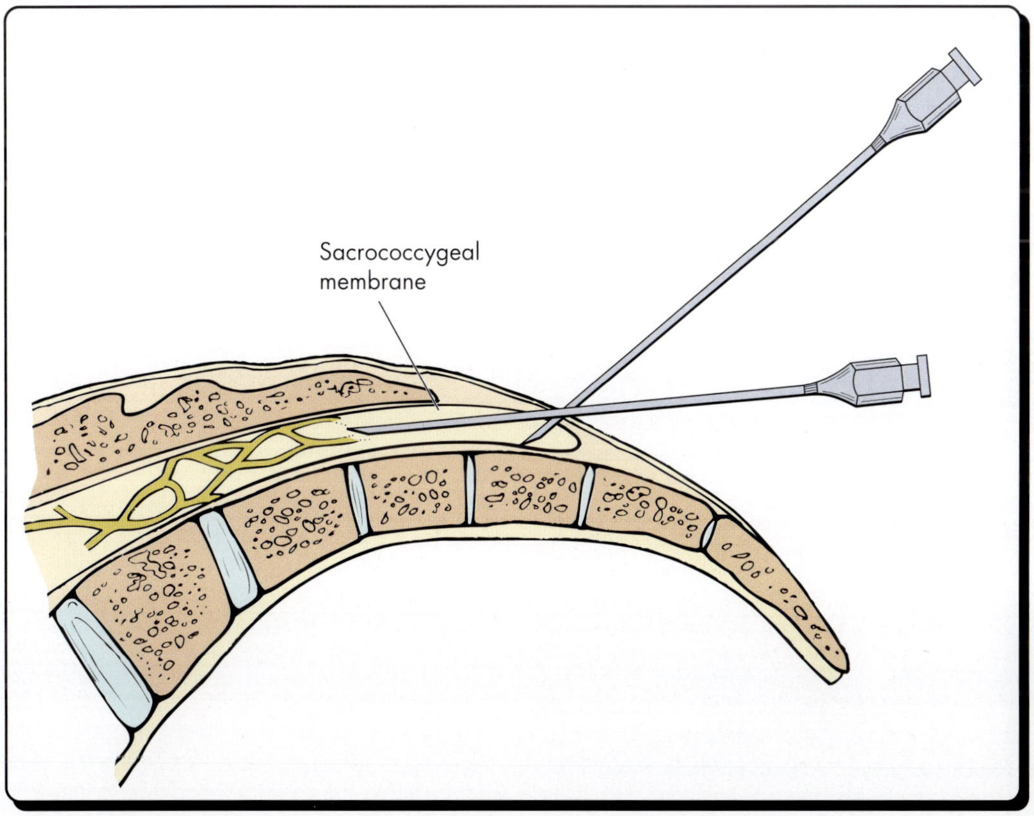

Figure 4-42. A needle directed through the sacrococcygeal membrane at a 45° angle will usually enter the ligament with a "pop" and contact the anterior bone of the sacral canal. The needle needs to be rotated so that the bevel does not scrape the periosteum of this layer. The angle of advancement also needs to be changed to allow direct passage 2 to 3 cm up the canal without contacting bone again. This space is generously endowed with blood vessels, and the terminal point of the dural sac extends a variable distance into the sacral canal, but usually lies at the S2 level. (*Adapted from* Mulroy [1].)

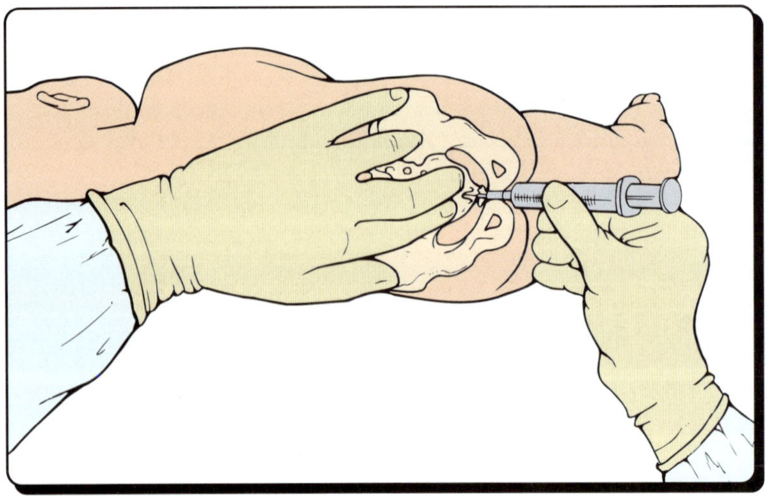

Figure 4-43. Pediatric caudal anesthesia in the lateral position. This technique is performed after the induction of general anesthesia and placement of an intravenous catheter. It is easily done in either the lateral or the prone position in children. The sacrococcygeal membrane is easily identified by the characteristic "pop," and the injection is made after advancing the needle 1 to 2 mm. (*Adapted from* Mulroy [1].)

DOSAGE IN CHILDREN FOR CAUDAL BLOCK

	Dose, mL, for block to	
Age, *y*	T12	T7
2	4	6
3	5	7.5
4	5.5	8
5	6	9
6	7	10.5
7	8	12
8	9	13.5
9	10	15
10	11	16.5

	Dose, mL, for block to	
Body weight, *kg*	T12	T7
10	3	4.5
12.5	4	6
15	5	7.5
17.5	6	9
20	7	10.5
22.5	8	12
25	9	13.5
27.5	10	15
30	11	16.5

Figure 4-44. Pediatric dosing. Doses for children can be calculated either on the basis of weight or age but are usually expressed in volumes injected. The two drugs most commonly used are 1% lidocaine and 0.25% bupivacaine. (*Adapted from* Covino and Scott [4].)

SUMMARY

SUMMARY TABLE		
	Advantages	**Disadvantages**
Spinal Anesthesia	Technically easiest	Postdural puncture headache
	Rapid onset	Fixed duration
	Dense anesthesia	Dense anesthesia
Epidural Blockade	Variable duration	Technically more difficult
	Variable intensity	Less reliable
	Segmental blockade	Risk of toxicity
Caudal Blockade	Limited spread	Technically most difficult
	Possible if lumbar anatomy is distorted	Anatomy variable

Figure 4-45. Summary of the advantages and disadvantages of spinal anesthesia and epidural and caudal blockade.

REFERENCES

1. Mulroy MF: *Regional Anesthesia: An Illustrated Procedural Guide*. edn. 2. Philadelphia: Lippincott-Raven; 1996:2, 4, 73–85, 112–126, 254.
2. Covino BG, Scott DB: Handbook of Epidural Anaesthesia and Analgesia. London: Grune & Stratton; 1985:16, 107.
3. Lee JA, Atkinson RS, Watt MJ: *Lumbar Puncture and Spinal Analgesia: Intradural and Extradural*. Edinburgh, London: Churchill Livingstone; 1985:56, 67.
4. Scott DB: *Techniques of Regional Anaesthesia*. Norwalk, CT: Appleton & Lange; 1989:161.
5. Brown DL: Spinal, epidural and caudal anesthesia. In *Anesthesia*. edn. 4. New York: Churchill Livingstone; 1994:1508, 1513, 1516, 1517.
6. Munhill R, Sukhani R, Winnie A: Incidence and etiology of failed spinal anesthetics in a university hospital: a prospective study. *Anesth Analg* 1988, 67:843–848.
7. Tarkkila P: Incidence and causes of failed spinal anesthetics in a university hospital: a prospective study. *Reg Anesth* 1991, 16:48–51.
8. Wildsmith JAW, Rocco AG: Current concepts in spinal anesthesia. *Reg Anesth* 1985, 10:119–124.
9. Chiu AA, Liu S, Carpenter RL, *et al.*: The effects of epinephrine on lidocaine spinal anesthesia: a crossover study. *Anesth Analg* 1995, 80:735–739.
10. Liu SL, Pollock JE, Mulroy MF *et al.*: Comparison of 5%, 1.5% with dextrose, and 1.5% dextrose free lidocaine solutions for spinal anesthesia in human volunteers. *Anesth Analg* 1995, 81:697–702.
11. Sivarajan M, Amory DW, Lindbloom LE, Schwettmann RS. Systemic and regional blood-flow changes during spinal anesthesia in the rhesus monkey. *Anesthesiology* 1975, 43:78–88.
12. Mackey DC, Carpenter RC, Thompson GE, *et al.*: Bradycardia and asystole during spinal anesthesia: a report of three cases without morbidity. *Anesthesiology* 1989, 70:866–868.
13. Mulroy MF: Spinal headaches: management and avoidance, In *Problems in Anesthesia: Regional Anesthesia at the Virginia Mason Medical Center: A Critical Perspective*. Edited by Brown DL. Philadelphia, PA: Lippincott; 1987:602–611.
14. Mulroy MF, Wills RP: Spinal anesthesia for outpatients: appropriate agents and techniques. *J Clin Anesth* 1995, 7:622–627.
15. Brown DL: *Atlas of Regional Anesthesia* Philadelphia, PA: WB Saunders; 1992:260, 286, 288, 289, 292.
16. Bromage PR: *Epidural Analgesia*. Philadelphia, PA: WB Saunders; 1978:119–159.
17. Liu SS, Carpenter RL, Neal JM: Epidural anesthesia and analgesia: examining their role in post-operative outcome. *Anesthesiology* 1995, 82:1474–1506.

5

Peripheral Nerve Blocks

Vildan Mullin

Nerve blocks are an important part of the practice of anesthesiology. However, they have been neglected for years because of a lack of appreciation of applied anatomy, pharmacology, and physiology and because of poor training.

When properly applied, nerve blocks can be very rewarding procedures for pain management and anesthesia practice. First hand experience and observation cannot be replaced; however, one can learn a great deal from photographs and graphical representation of techniques.

To be successful in performing regional anesthesia, the following are necessary: knowledge of applied anatomy, knowledge of physiology, and the ability to visualize the relationships between anatomy and physiology.

Good rapport and communication between the anesthetist and the patient are very important both before and during the nerve block. These assets will ensure good cooperation and assist in the correct placement of the needle, while alerting the anesthetist to potential complications.

Regional anesthesia alone or in combination with sedation or light general anesthesia can provide excellent analgesia and physiologically advantageous conditions.

The expansion of acute and chronic pain management has given new life and a bright future to regional anesthesia in recent years.

LOCAL ANESTHETICS

MOST COMMON LOCAL ANESTHETICS USED FOR NERVE BLOCKS

Anesthetic Agent *	Usual Concentration, %	Average Onset Time, *min* ± SE	Average Analagesic Duration†	Addition of Epinephrine % Change		Recommended Maximal Doses	
				Duration	C max	Plain, *mg/kg*	With Epinephrine, *mg/kg*
Major Nerve Blocks:							
Lidocaine	1.0	14 ± 4	200	+50		7	9
Mepivacaine	1.0	15±6	250			7	9
Bupivacaine	0.25–0.5	10–25	575			2	3
Local Infiltration and Minor Nerve Blocks:							
Lidocaine	0.5		75 (35–340)	+200	-50		
Mepivacaine	0.5		108 (15–240)	+120			
Bupivacaine	0.25		200±33	+115			
Ropivacaine‡	0.2–0.5	15–25	400			2	

*Local anesthetic toxicity: bupivacaine > mepivacaine > lidocaine.
†Duration depends on location and local absorption.
‡These are estimated numbers based on limited clinical experience to date.

Figure 5-1. Most common local anesthetics used for nerve blocks. The use of mixtures of local anesthetics for nerve blocks has become relatively popular in recent years. However, there does not appear to be any significant advantages to the use of these mixtures [1]. Performing nerve blocks using the lowest possible concentration of local anesthetics may offer some advantages, including (1) the ability to increase the volume of local anesthetic (an important factor in achieving successful plexus block) and (2) a reduction in systemic local anesthetic toxicity. Conc—concentration; SE—standard error.

COMMONLY USED NEEDLES IN NERVE BLOCKS

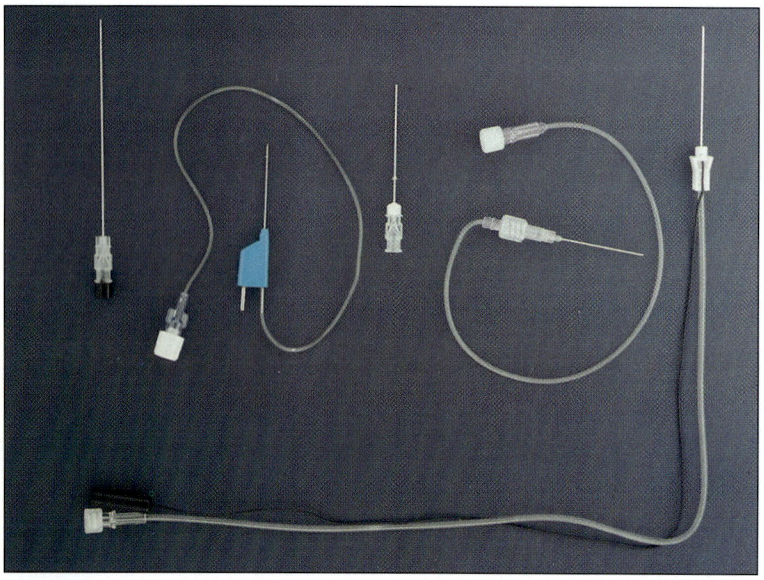

Figure 5-2. Commonly used needles in nerve blocks. The depth of the tissue to be penetrated determines the length of the needle required. If the needle is to pass through the fascia, a blunt needle may give a more distinct feeling of resistance and penetration. If a nerve stimulator is to be used, an insulated needle is more appropriate because it requires the application of less voltage and locates the nerve with more precision [1].

NERVE STIMULATORS

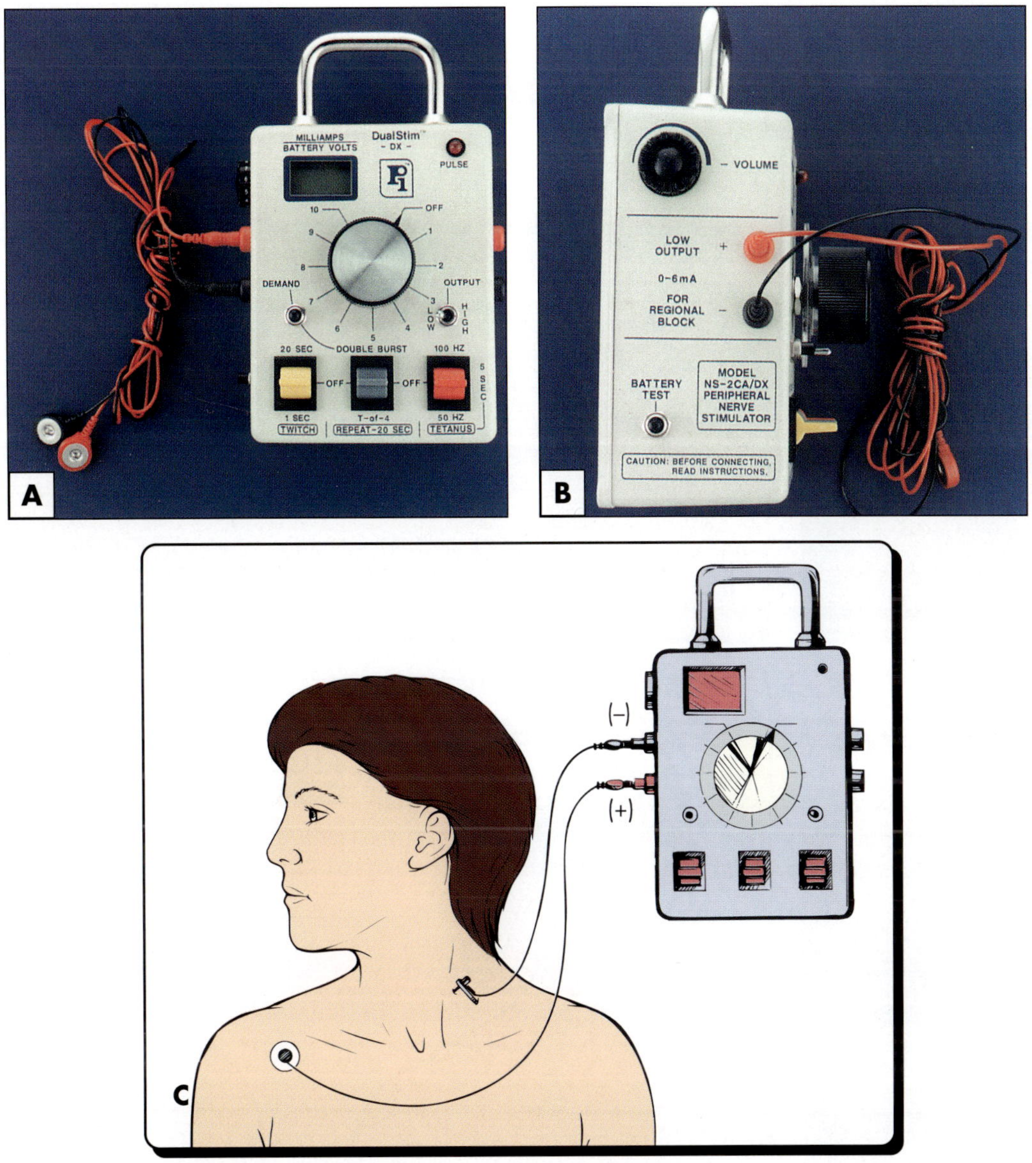

Figure 5-3. Nerve stimulators (**A**, front view, **B**, side view, and **C**). Nerve stimulators should be used only as adjuncts to a sound regional techniques based on comprehensive knowledge of anatomy. Nerve stimulators may play an important role (1) in a patient who is uncooperative, disoriented, or unable to communicate and report a paresthesia; (2) in a child or an adult already under general anesthesia, and (3) in confirming paresthesia and location of the needle with the lowest possible level of stimulation.

A peripheral nerve stimulator should have a current of 0.1 to 10 mA and a frequency of l pulse per second (1 Hz). **C**, The negative lead should be attached to the nerve block needle [2]. During stimulation the current should be set at 2 to 4 mA. As the needle advances toward the nerve, the current should be reduced to 0.5 to 0.1 mA. After injection of 1 to 2 mL of local anesthetic solution, if the needle is in the right position, muscle contraction will disappear. (**A** and **B** courtesy of Life-Tech, Inc., Houston, TX.)

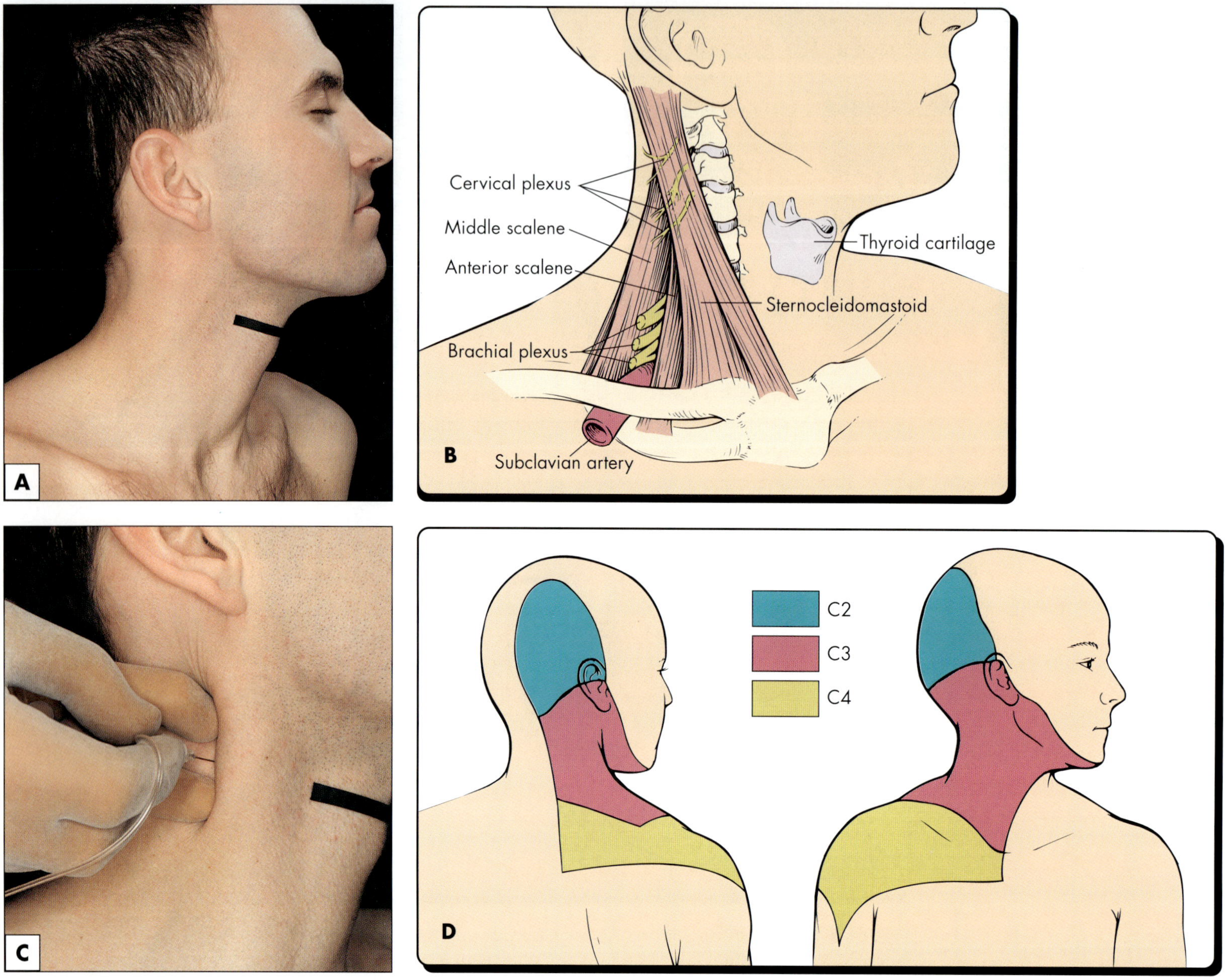

Figure 5-4. Cervical plexus blocks. When properly performed, a deep cervical plexus block is sufficient to produce anesthesia for most surgical procedures in the neck and eliminates the need for a superficial cervical plexus block [3]. **A** and **B**, The landmarks to be used as guides for needle insertion include the (1) sternocleidomastoid (SCM) muscle; (2) upper border of the thyroid cartilage, which corresponds to the level of the fourth vertebra (C4); and (3) interscalene groove. The cervical plexus is situated between the anterior scalene and middle scalene muscles.

C, The technique for cervical plexus block is as follows. With the patient in the supine position and the upper body inclined at an angle of 30° to 45°, the patient is asked to raise his head to make the SCM muscle more prominent. The anesthetist places his fingers at the C4 level behind the SCM muscle, and the patient is asked to lower his head to relieve the tension in the SCM muscle while the interscalene groove is palpated. When it is difficult to palpate the groove (the interscalene groove is narrower at this level than at the C6 level), one should attempt to locate it at the C6 level and follow the groove to the C4 level. With the anesthetist's fingers in position, a 1.25-in (3-cm) 22-gauge needle is inserted and advanced slowly between the two fingers—as they are palpating—into the interscalene groove, perpendicular to all planes and slightly caudad. When paresthesia is produced or when the transverse process of the fourth cervical vertebra is contacted (it should be no more than 3 cm deep), the local anesthetic is injected. Careful aspiration during injection is mandatory because of the proximity to the vertebral artery. *The recommended local anesthetics include 1% lidocaine, 15 to 20 mL, or 0.25% to 0.5% bupivacaine, 15 to 20 mL.* **D**, Distribution of cutaneous anesthesia.

The anesthetist should keep in mind the following points while administering the nerve block. (1) The block should be performed only on one side to avoid bilateral phrenic nerve paralysis. (2) During injection, the anesthetist should keep his fingers firmly in place to prevent inadvertent movement of the needle.

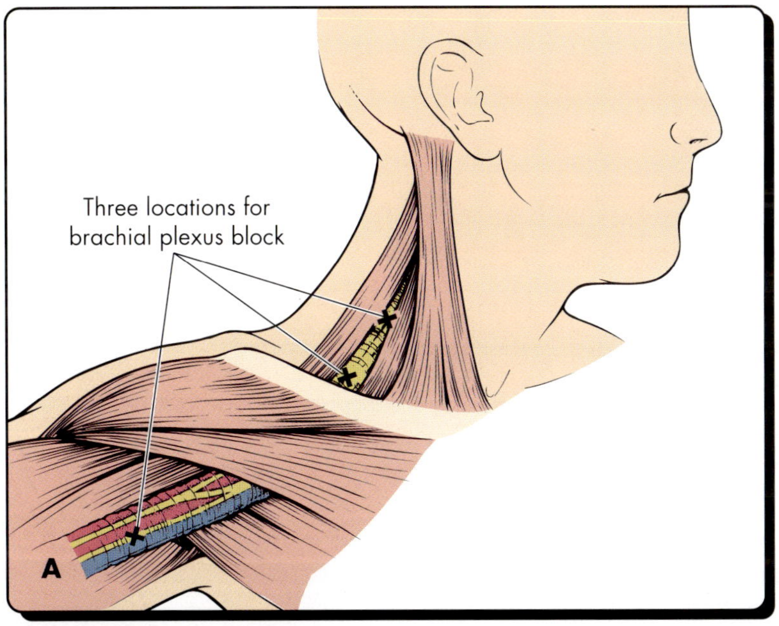

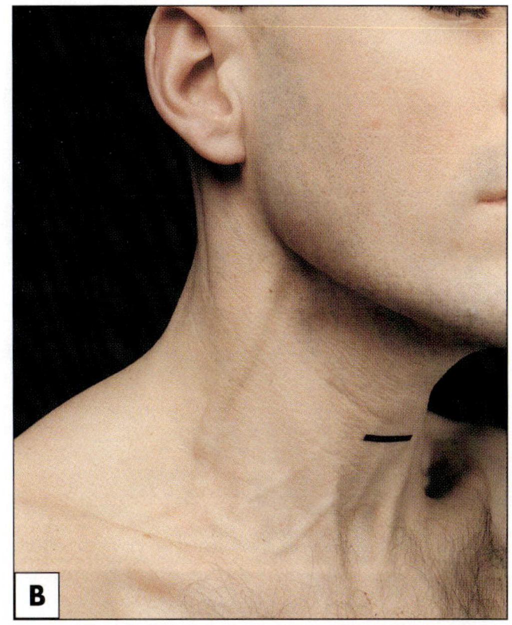

Figure 5-5. A and B, Brachial plexus blocks. There are three locations for brachial plexus block. The site and extent of the surgical procedure determines which of the three techniques is indicated [4]. (1) Interscalene plexus block is used in surgery of the clavicle, shoulder, and upper arm; (2) supraclavicular plexus block is used in surgery of the upper arm, elbow, forearm, and radial aspect of the hand; (3) axillary plexus block is used in surgery of the forearm and hand (areas innervated by the ulnar and median nerves).

The anesthetist should keep in mind the following points while performing brachial plexus blocks. (1) In 90% of successful brachial plexus blocks signs of the block appear within 5 minutes of injection. The absence of visible signs of motor blockade at this time indicates a failed block [4]. (2) With all three techniques, motor blockade develops faster than does sensory blockade [4]. (3) With supraclavicular and interscalene techniques, the intercostal brachial nerve may be blocked by depositing 4 to 5 mL of anesthetic solution subcutaneously over the axillary artery [5]. (4) With the exception of the axillary approach, the production of paresthesia is essential for a successful block [6]. (5) Pain on injection may be a sign of an intraneural injection.

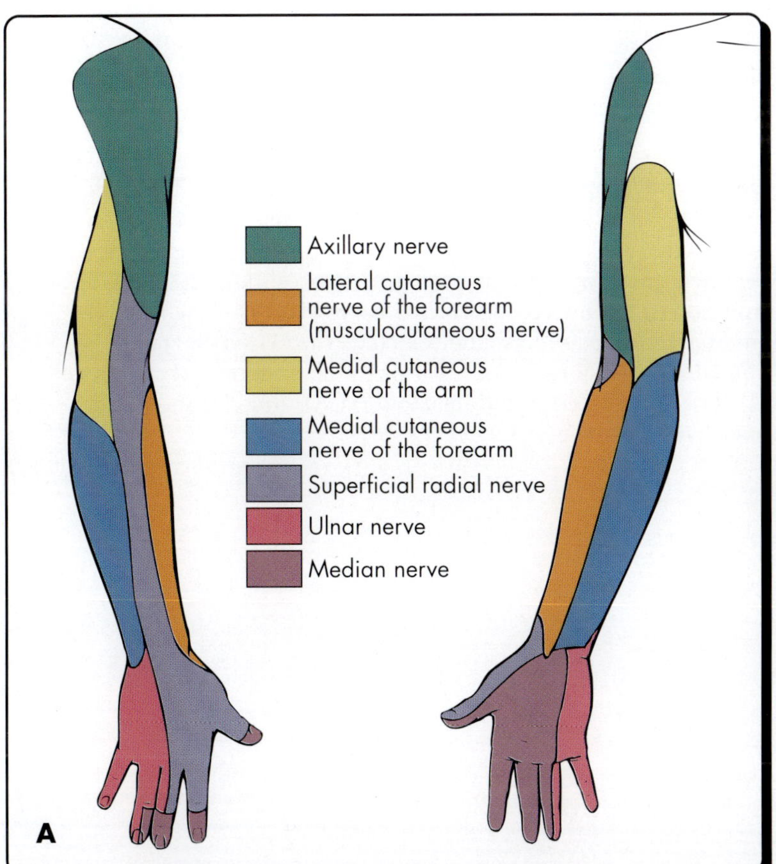

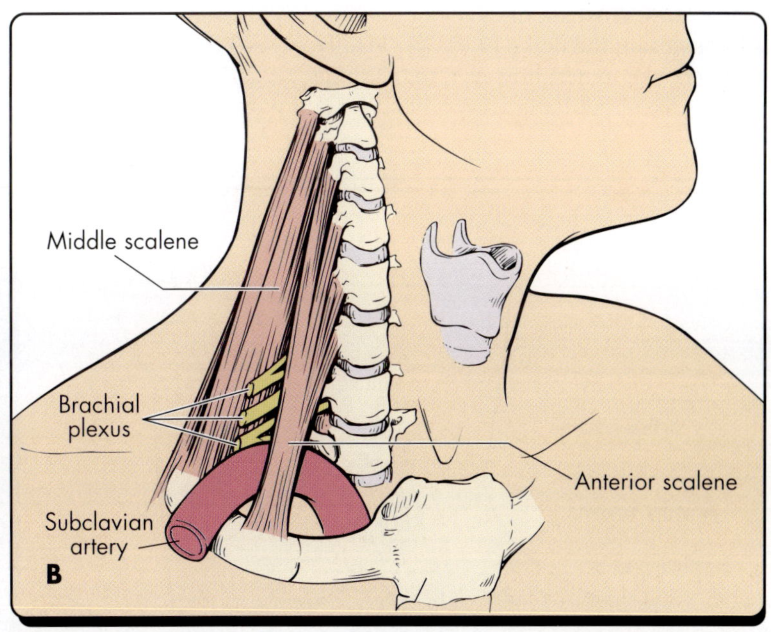

Figure 5-6. Interscalene brachial plexus block. This type of brachial plexus block is indicated for surgery of the shoulder and upper arm [7]. Increasing the volume of local anesthetic to 30 to 40 mL produces anesthesia of the entire arm, except for the ulnar nerve distribution in about half of all patients [5]. **A** and **B**, The major landmarks to be used as guides include the (1) cricoid cartilage corresponding to the level of the sixth cervical vertebra, (2) sternocleidomastoid (SCM) muscle, and (3) interscalene groove. The interscalene groove is fairly easy to palpate at the C6 level. The brachial plexus is found at an average depth of 2 to 2.5 cm [8].

(Continued on next page)

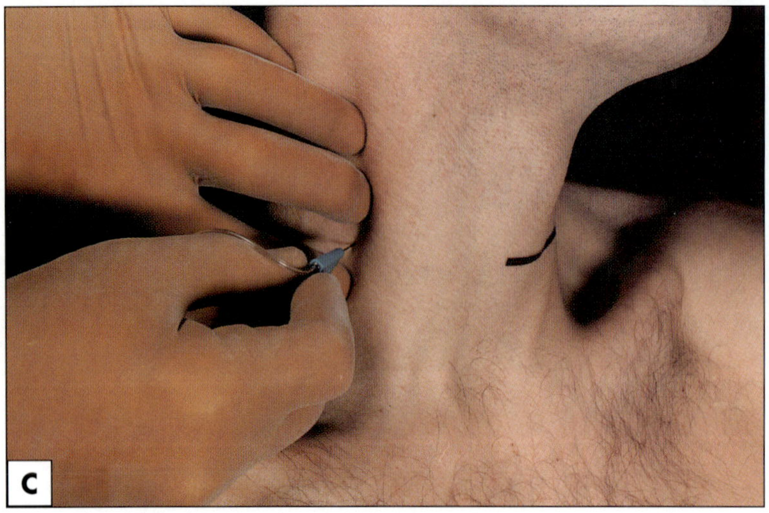

Figure 5-6. (*Continued*) C, The technique for intrascalene block is as follows. The patient is placed in the supine position with the upper body inclined 30° to 45° upward and the head turned slightly to the contralateral side. The patient is asked to elevate his head so that the anesthetist can identify the SMC muscle. At the level of the sixth cervical vertebra the anesthetist places two fingers behind the SCM muscle and rolls his fingers back and forth into the interscalene groove. Once the groove is identified and fixed by the fingers, a 5-cm 22-gauge needle is inserted perpendicularly to all planes, directed caudally, and advanced slowly. (Paresthesia should be explained to the patient in advance to determine the location accurately.) Once the patient experiences paresthesia, the operator stops and holds the needle firmly while an assistant injects the local anesthetic with frequent aspiration. *The recommended local anesthetics include 1% lidocaine, 20 to 25 mL, or 0.25% to 0.5% bupivacaine, 20 to 25 mL.* With successful block, cutaneous distribution of anesthesia will occur as shown in **D**.

The anesthetist should keep in mind the following points while administering the nerve block. (1) Ideally, paresthesia should be below the shoulder; however, for shoulder surgery, paresthesia around the shoulder is acceptable [9]. (2) If paresthesia cannot be elicited, the needle should be withdrawn and redirected gradually until it comes into contact with the plexus.

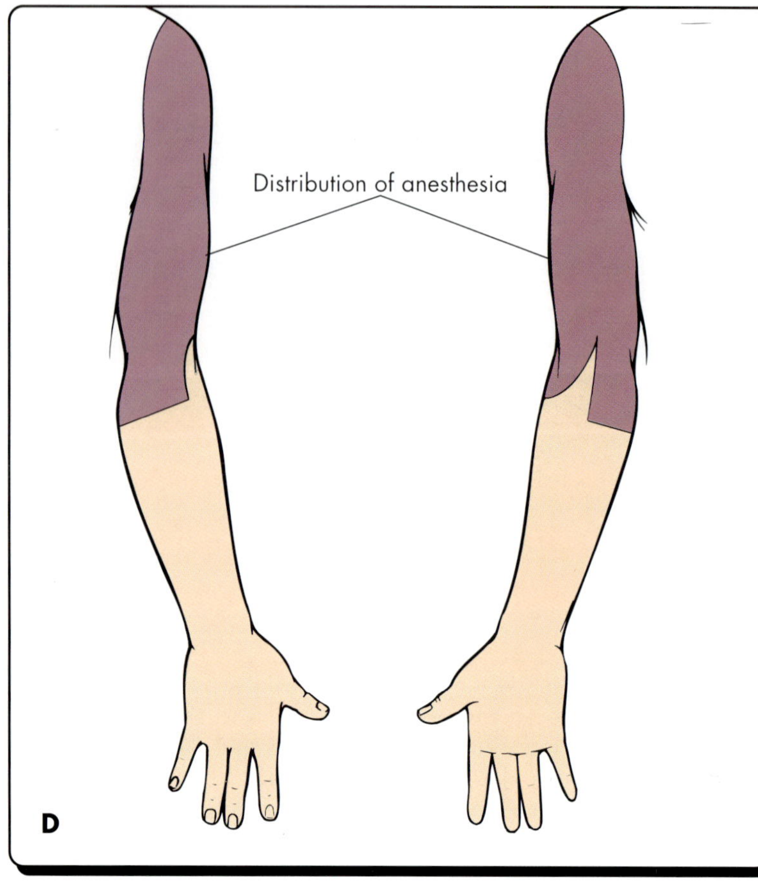

Complications of the intrascalene approach include (1) blocking of the phrenic nerve in almost all cases (this can be problematic in a patient with significant lung disease), (2) intravascular injection (aspiration is required after every 2 to 3 mL of injection of anesthetic agents), (3) recurrent laryngeal nerve block, (4) sympathetic chain block (cervical portion), (5) Horner's syndrome, and (6) subarachnoid or epidural injection.

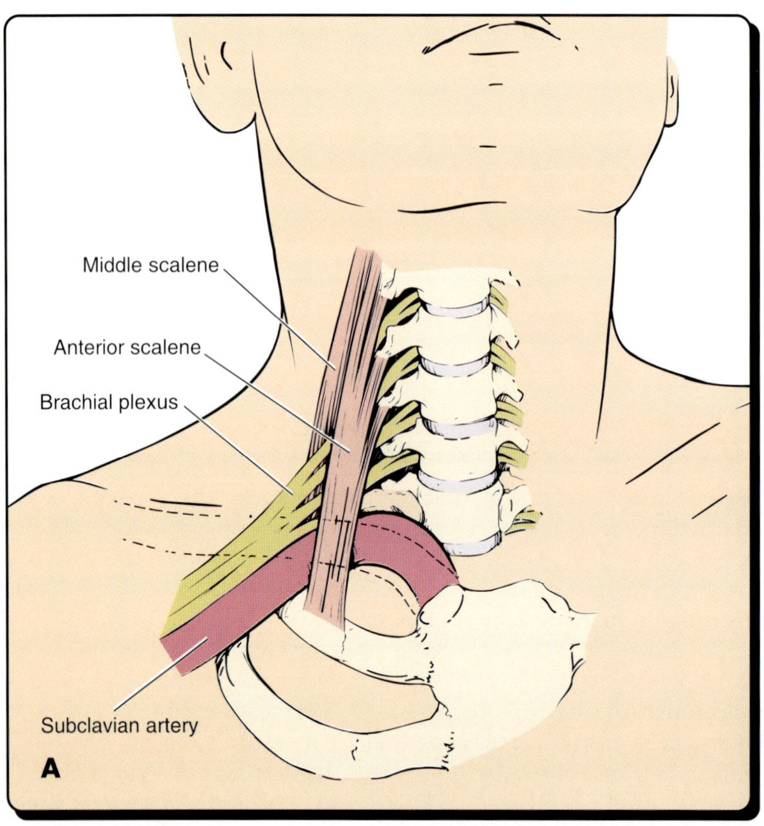

Figure 5-7. Supraclavicular brachial plexus block. This type of brachial plexus block is the most consistently effective approach to the brachial plexus. It anesthetizes the arm, with the exception of the skin over the shoulder and in some instances the skin in the dis tribution of the intercostobrachial nerve [10,11]. **A**, The major landmarks to be used as guides include the (1) subclavian pulse immediately posterior and superior to the midpoint of the clavicle, (2) clavicle, (3) sternocleidomastoid (SCM) muscle, and (4) interscalene groove.

(*Continued on next page*)

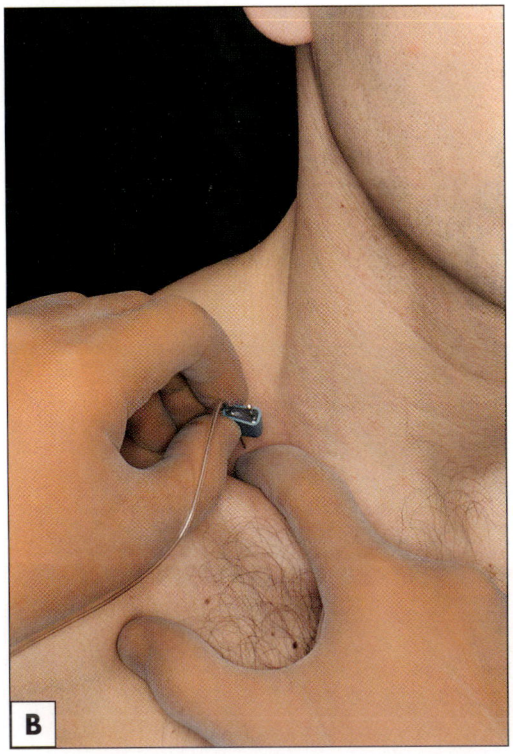

B

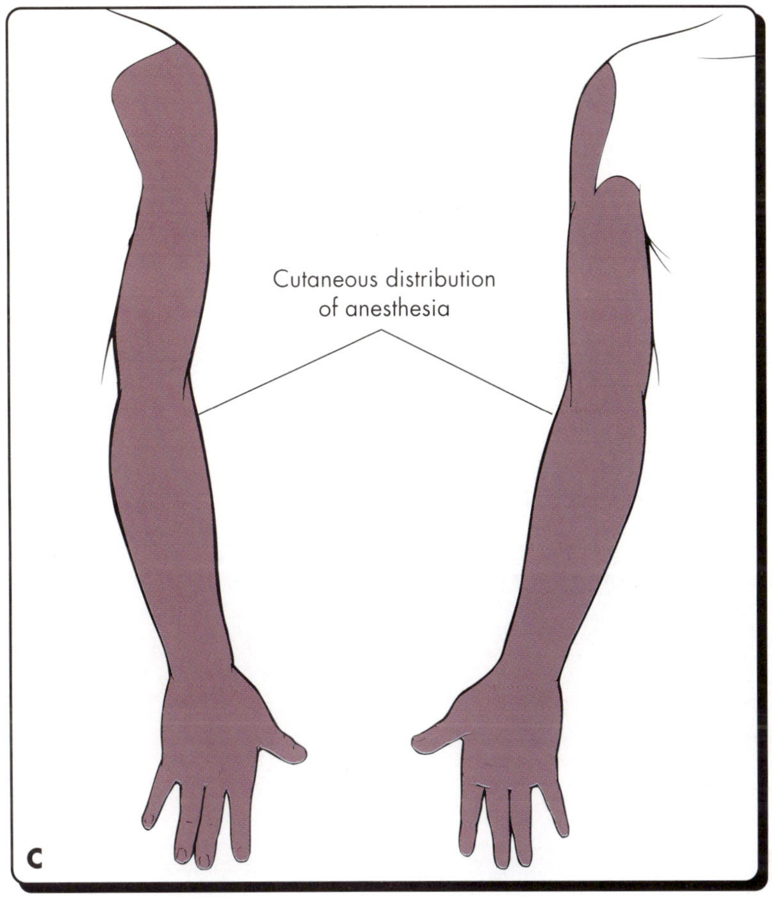

Figure 5-7. (*Continued*) B, The technique for supraclavicular block is as follows. The patient is placed in the semisitting position, with his head tilted to 45° angle and in the neutral position. The anesthetist faces the patient and palpates the subclavian pulse just posterior and superior to the clavicle. A 3-cm, 22-gauge needle is inserted perpendicular to all planes at 2 cm above the clavicle and slightly lateral to the subclavian artery. An attempt to elicit paresthesia should be made to guarantee a successful block. The local anesthetic is then injected with frequent aspiration. During all stages of the procedure, the palpating finger must stay firmly in place. *The recommended local anesthetics include 1% lidocaine, 20 to 25 mL, or 0.25% to 0.5% bupivacaine, 20 to 25 mL.* C, Cutaneous distribution of anesthesia with supraclavicular approach.

The anesthetist should keep in mind the following points while administering the nerve block. (1) The brachial plexus is superficial and is found at an average depth of 2.7 cm [8,12]. (2) Paresthesia indicative of stimulation of the middle trunk results in the highest success rate in blocking all three trunks of the brachial plexus (paresthesia in the distribution of the median nerve may represent stimulation of the middle trunk) [13]. (3) In some patients the subclavian pulse may be difficult to feel with the patient's head in the neutral position. The patient should be asked to turn and tilt his head toward the side to be blocked. This maneuver may release tension in the scalene muscles and make the pulse palpable. (4) In addition, if there is no palpable subclavian pulse, the interscalene groove should be identified and marked. The entry point of the needle should be 2 cm above the clavicle on this line. In essence, this is a modified interscalene approach to the brachial plexus.

Complications of the supraclavicular approach include (1) pneumothorax (recognition of the superficial position of the brachial plexus and use of a short needle should make this complication a rarity), (2) Horner's syndrome, (3) phrenic nerve block, (4) intravascular injection, and (5) hematoma formation.

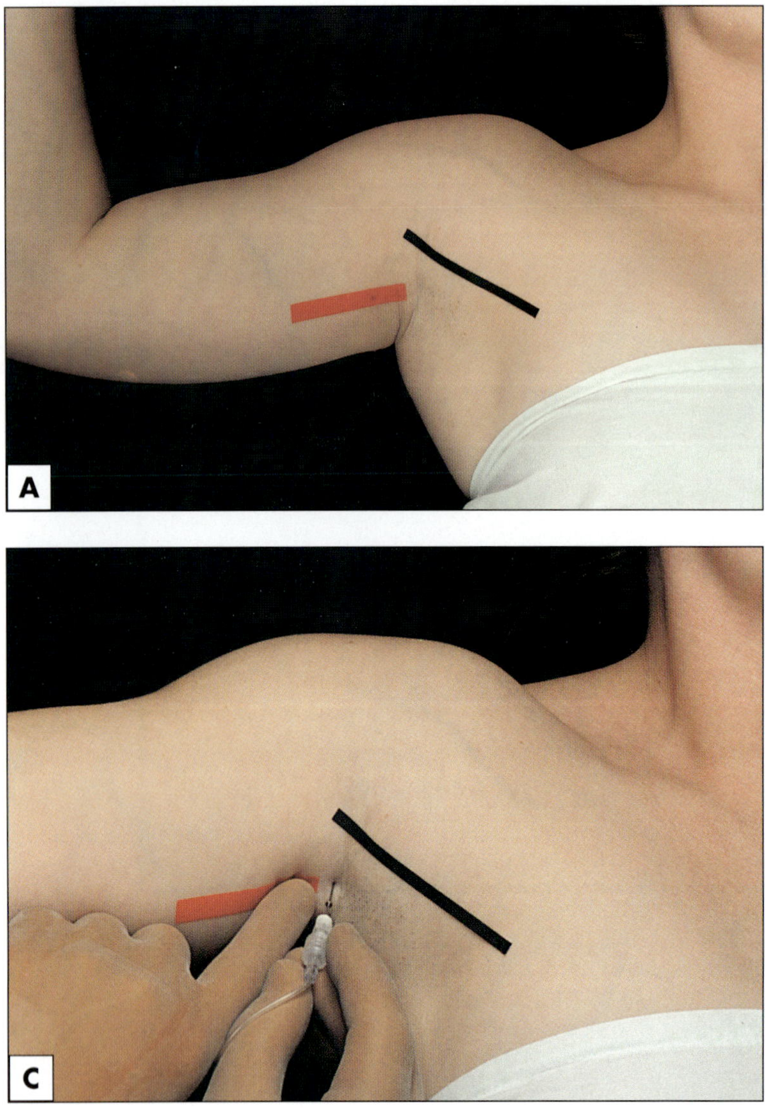

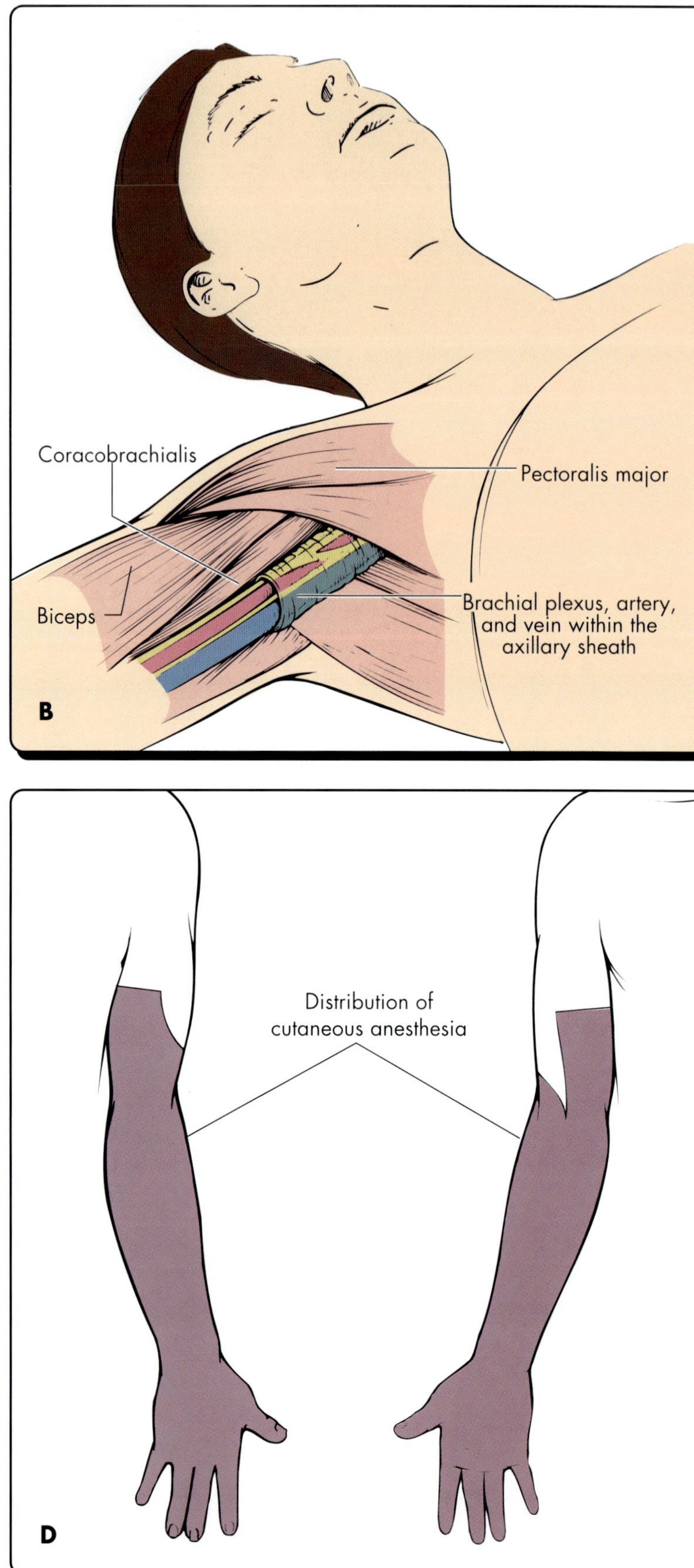

Figure 5-8. Axillary brachial plexus block. This type of brachial plexus block produces a reliable block of the medial aspect of the arm, forearm, and hand; however, it may fail to block the musculocutaneous and radial nerves in approximately 25% of patients, with resultant lack of anesthesia in the lateral aspect of the arm [14]. A and B, The major landmarks to be used as guides include the pectoralis major muscle and axillary artery. C, The technique for axillary approach is as follows. The patient is placed in the supine position, with the arm to be blocked abducted to 90° and the dorsum of the hand resting on a table. The axillary artery is palpated at the highest point in the axilla. The anesthetist's finger should locate the pulse and a 1.25-in (4-cm) 22- or 23-gauge needle is inserted in front of the palpating finger perpendicular to the skin in all directions and toward the artery. On insertion of the needle two distinct clicks are felt; the first click is heard as the needle passes through the skin and the second as the needle enters the fascia of the neural sheath. If the needle is in the fascia, pulsations of the needle should be evident. While holding the needle firmly, the local anesthetic solution is injected slowly with frequent aspiration to prevent intravascular injection. *The recommended local anesthetics include 1% lidocaine, 35 to 50 mL, or 0.25% to 0.5% bupivacaine, 35 to 50 mL.* D, Distribution of cutaneous anesthesia with the axillary approach.

The anesthetist should keep in mind the following points while administering the block. (1) Use a blunt needle to be able to identify penetration of the skin and fascia. (2) Try to reach the highest possible point in the axilla at which the pulse can be palpated. Most of the time, approach will block the musculocutaneous nerve. Local anesthetics diffuse easily through the loosely organized tissues [15,16]. (3) Apply pressure with a finger over the artery below the injection site to facilitate proximal spread [15]. (4) A subcutaneous ring below the axilla, 3 to 4 cm to each side of the artery will block the intercostobrachial and medial cutaneous nerve block, which will help decrease tourniquet pain. (5) Hold the needle firmly in place to prevent it from moving away from the fascia. (6) Try to avoid seeking paresthesia, if possible [17]. (7) The earliest sign of a successful axillary block is the patient's inability to extend the elbow [14].

Complications of the axillary approach include (1) hematoma formation and (2) nerve injury with temporary or permanent sensory deficit. Nerve injury is a rare but possible complication.

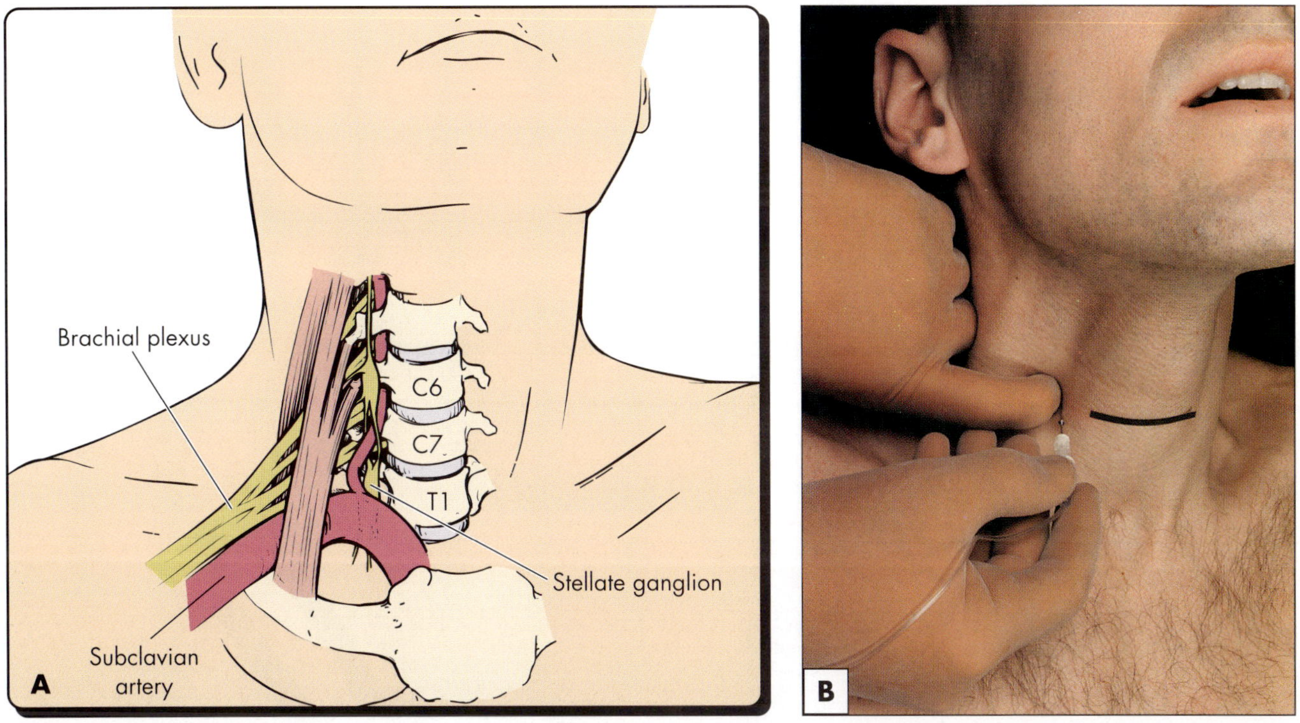

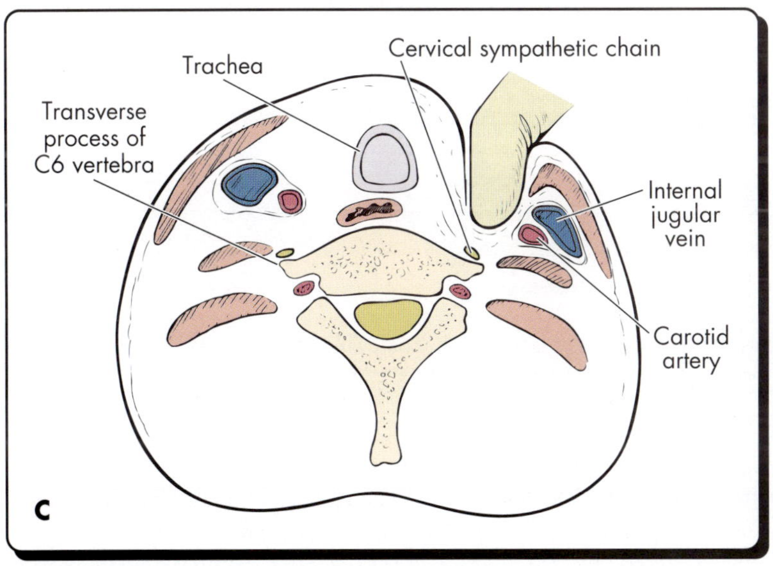

Figure 5-9. Stellate ganglion block. This block is used to diagnose and treat sympathetically mediated painful conditions of the upper extremity, upper chest wall, and face. **A**, The major landmarks to be used as guides for needle insertion include the (1) cricoid cartilage corresponding to the level of the sixth cervical vertebra (C6), (2) sternocleidomastoid (SCM) muscle, and (3) carotid artery.

B and **C**, The technique for stellate ganglion block is as follows. The patient lies in the supine position without a pillow under his head, with his neck maximally extended. The patient is asked to open his mouth slightly to decrease tension in the platysma muscle, thereby aiding palpation of the C6 transverse process. The anesthetist locates the cricoid cartilage with his index finger, retracts the SCM muscle and carotid artery, and palpates the C6 transverse process. The finger must remain firmly in that position. Using the other hand, the operator inserts a 1.5-in (4-cm) 22- or 23-gauge needle perpendicular to the horizontal plane immediately in front of the palpating finger until contact with the C6 transverse process is made (usually at a depth of about 1 to 2 cm) [18]. The local anesthetic is then injected carefully, while aspirating frequently to avoid intravascular injection. *The recommended local anesthetics include 1% lidocaine, 10 to 15 mL, or 0.25% bupivacaine, 10 to 15 mL.* The signs of a successful block are (1) Horner's syndrome, (2) increased blood flow to the upper extremity (the temperature should increase several degrees), (3) positive sweat test, and (4) absence of the skin conduction response [19].

The anesthetist should keep in mind the following points while administering the block. (1) The palpating finger must stay firmly in place to avoid moving the needle from the plane of injection. The needle should maintain continuous contact with the C6 transverse process. (2) Immediately after the injection is completed, the patient should sit up to facilitate downward flow of the anesthetic solution to reach the second and third thoracic dermatomes.

Complications of stellate ganglion block include (1) recurrent laryngeal nerve block, (2) hematoma, (3) brachial plexus block, (4) injection into the vertebral artery, and (5) subarachnoid injection.

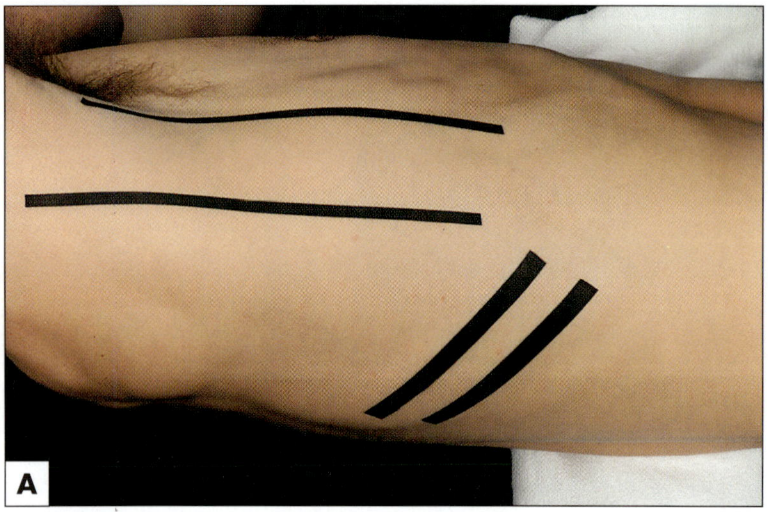

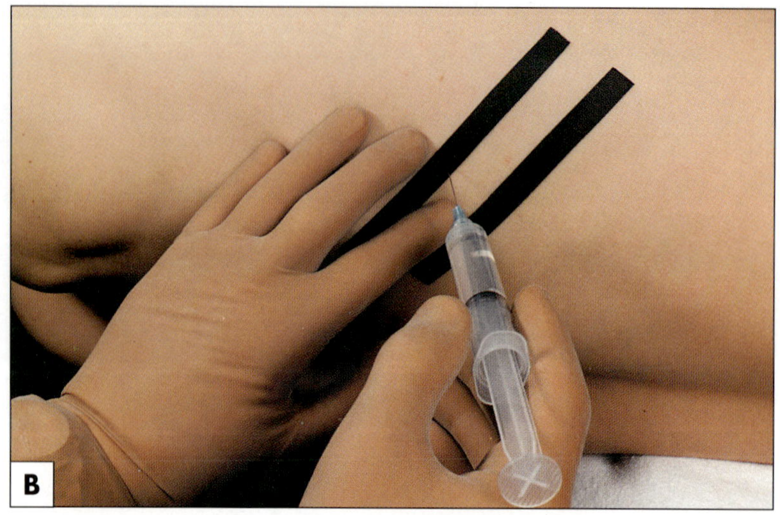

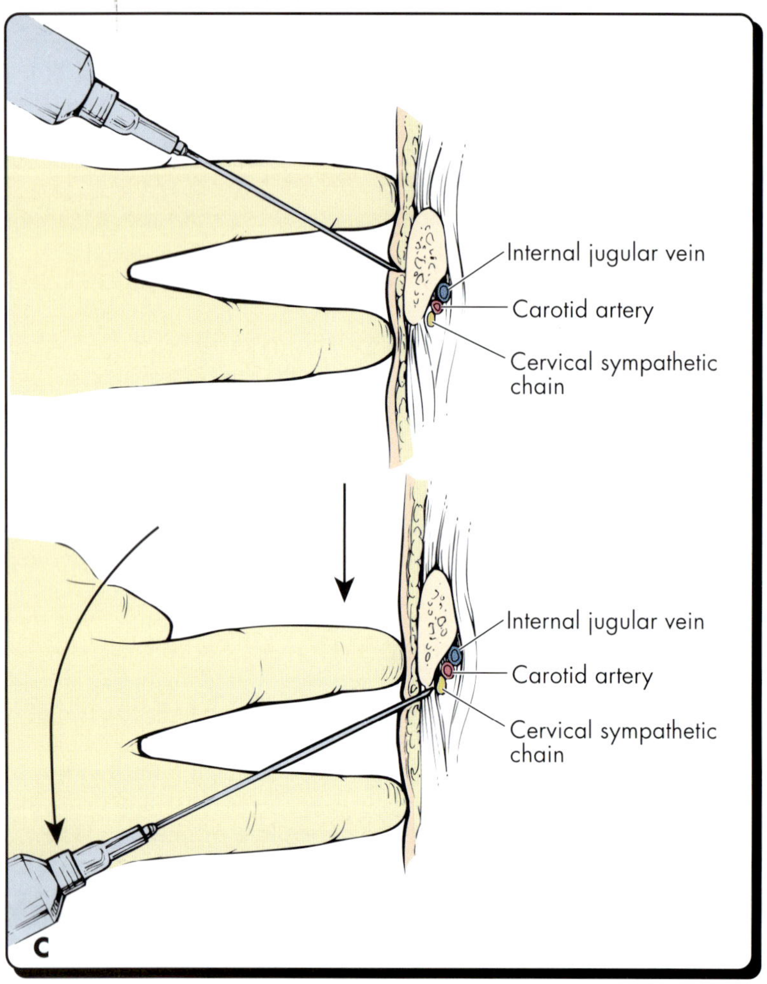

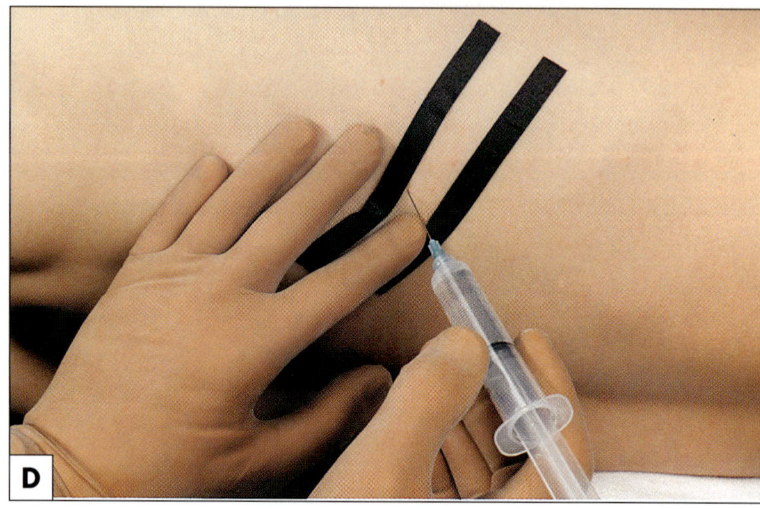

Figure 5-10. Intercostal nerve block. This nerve block is usually administered for the diagnosis and control of pain in the corresponding dermatomes. **A**, The local anesthetic solution usually spreads from the point of injection along the length of the rib [20], making possible intercostal nerve blocks at the anterior and posterior axillary lines. At these locations the ribs are more readily palpable than they are in the posterior paravertebral approach in which the ribs are deeper.

B, C, and D, The technique for intercostal nerve block is as follows. The patient is placed in either the prone or the lateral position with a pillow under the flank. The patient's arm is abducted and held over his head on the side to be blocked. The anesthetist palpates the rib between his index and middle fingers and inserts a 1-in 25-gauge needle until it reaches the rib. The anesthetist then uses the finger palpating the rib to pull the skin, muscle, and needle—as one unit—in a caudad direction until the needle drops into the intercostal space. Once the needle is in the intercostal space, it should be advanced no more than 0.5 to 1 cm forward under the rib. This move prevents inadvertent pleural puncture. The anesthetist's fingers must remain firmly in place until the completion of the injection. Pneumothorax is the most serious complication of the intercostal nerve block [21]. *The recommended local anesthetics include 0.5% to 1% lidocaine, 3 mL, or 0.25% bupivacaine, 3 mL with epinephrine.*

The anesthetist should keep in mind the following while administering intercostal nerve block. (1) Use the shortest possible needle depending on the patient's chest wall thickness [20]. (2) Try to hit the lower portion of the rib. This decreases the distance between the point of insertion and the location of the intercostal space.

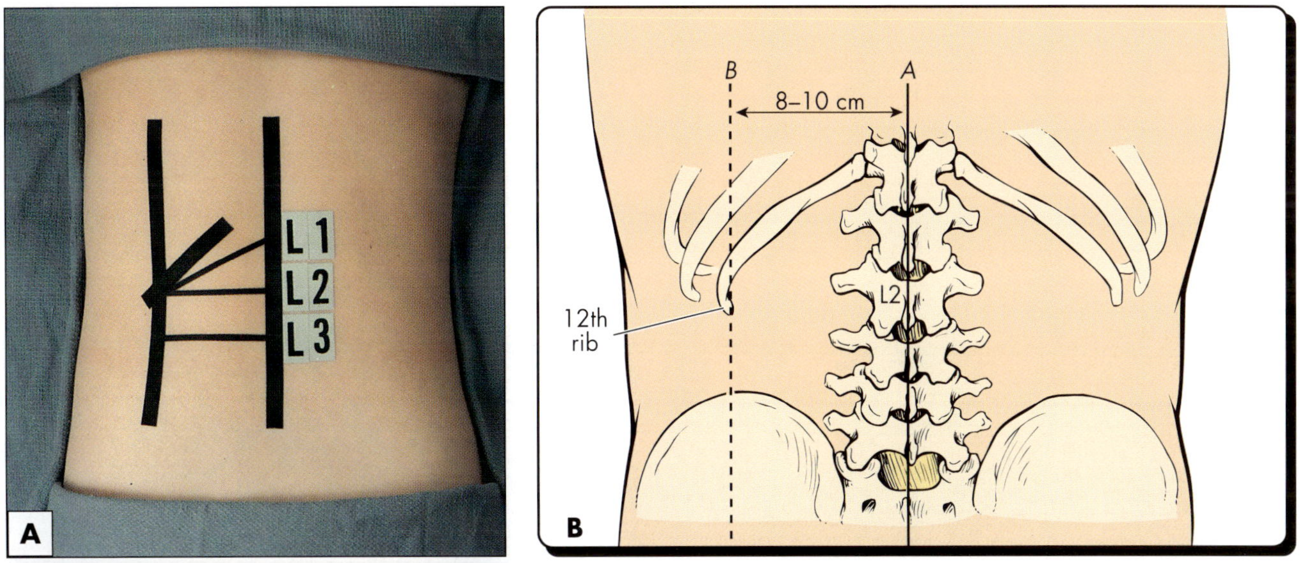

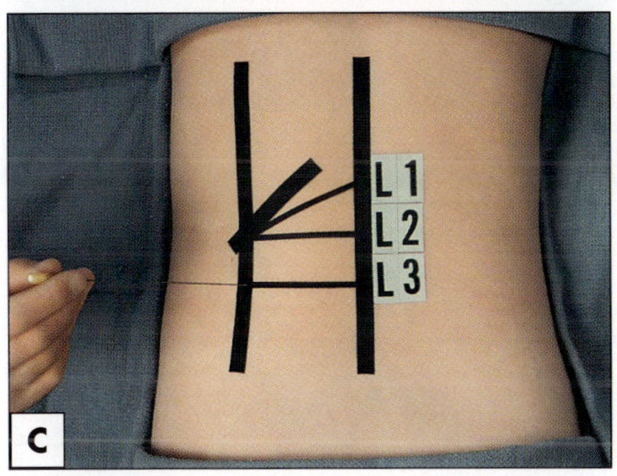

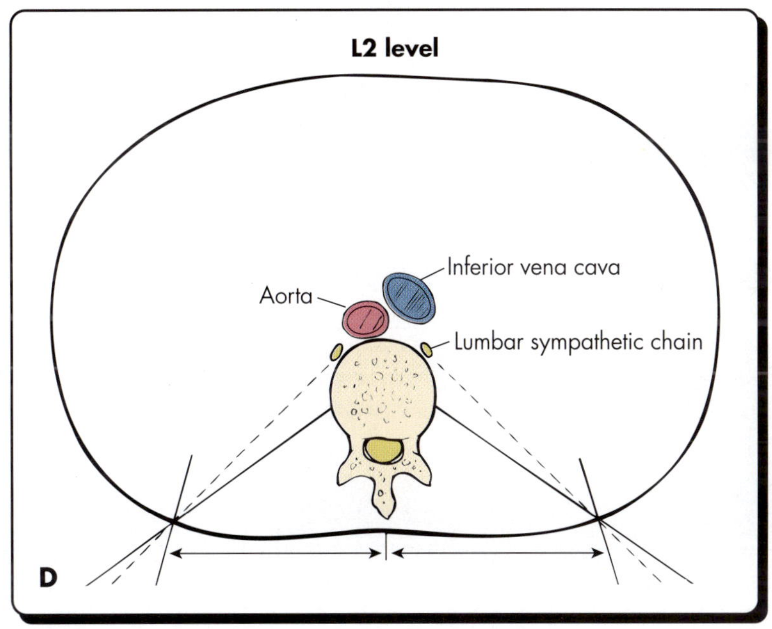

Figure 5-11. Lumbar sympathetic block. This nerve block is indicated to provide pain control and diagnosis of sympathetically maintained pain (SMP) syndromes of the lower extremity and to improve blood flow to the lower extremity. **A** and **B**, The major landmarks to be used as guides include line *A* at the midline, which connects the 12th thoracic vertebra to the fifth lumbar vertebra, and line *B*, which is 8 to 10 cm from the midline parallel to line *A* (this distance usually is determined by assessment of body size) [22]. "X" is the point at which line *B* crosses the last rib that can be palpated, usually the 12th rib. A straight line from point X will cross the body of L2 [23]. It has been recommended that the block be performed as a single-needle technique at the L3 level (upper third of the body of L3) [19,22,23]. This approach should prevent possible neuralgia in the distribution of the genitofemoral nerve and injury to the kidney. Insertion of the needle 8 to 10 cm from the midline enables the needle to reach the anterolateral angle of the vertebra body. This approach positions the needle closer to the sympathetic chain and away from the somatic nerve roots [23].

C and **D**, The technique for lumbar sympathetic block is as follows. The patient is placed in the prone position, with a pillow under his abdomen. A 6-inch (15-cm) 20-gauge needle is inserted on line *B* at the L3 level at an angle of 40° to 45° to the plane that is perpendicular to all planes of the skin. The needle is directed toward the upper half of the body of L3 [23a]. On contacting the body of the vertebra, the needle marker is placed 1 to 2 cm above the skin (depending on the patient's size). The needle is then withdrawn two thirds of the way out and reinserted at a 30° angle to the plane that is perpendicular to all planes of the skin. The needle is advanced until the needle marker touches the skin or until the needle reaches the anterolateral corner of L3. After confirmation by fluoroscopy, the anesthetic is injected with frequent aspiration. *The recommended local anesthetics include 0.5% lidocaine, 15 to 20 mL, or 0.25% bupivacaine, 15 to 20 mL.*

The anesthetist should keep in mind the following points while administering the block. (1) Properly drawn skin marking combined with fluoroscopy should eliminate the need for multiple attempts at needle insertion. (2) The single-needle injection technique is sufficient to cause adequate spread of the local anesthetic solution in both caudad and cephalad directions, eliminating the need for multiple needle techniques [22].

Complications of the lumbar sympathetic block include (1) subarachnoid block, (2) somatic nerve block, (3) kidney puncture, and (4) hypotension.

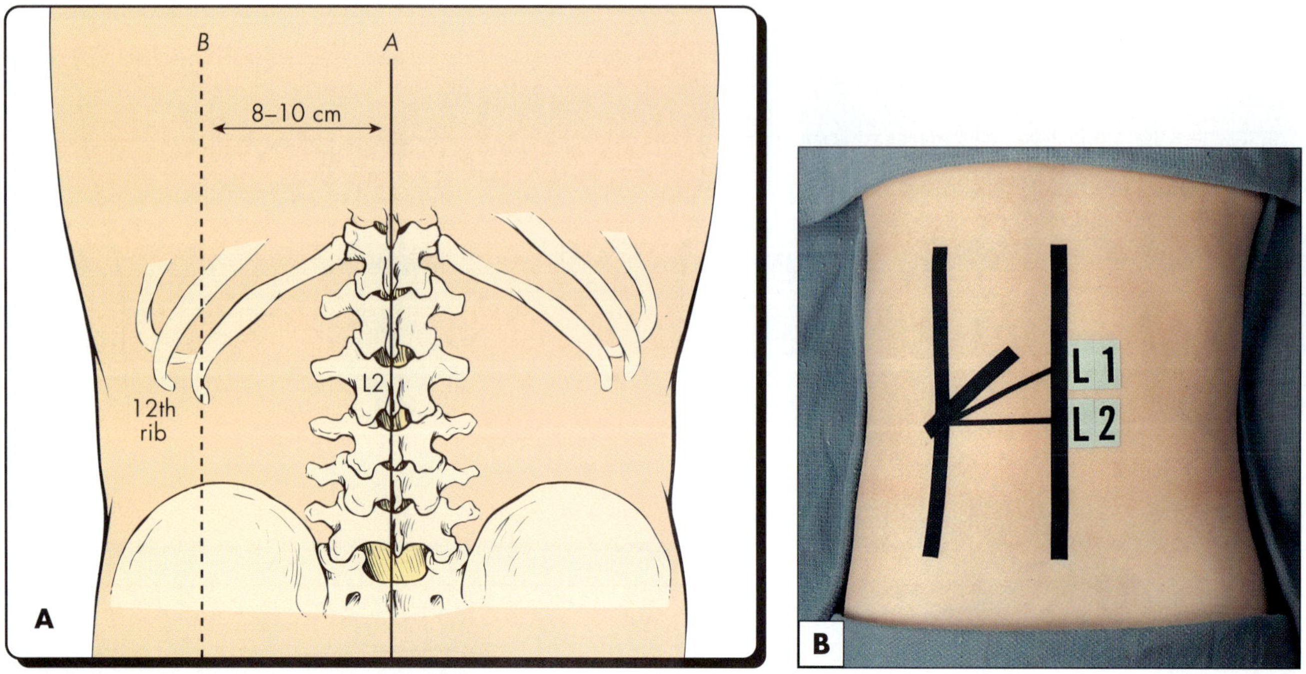

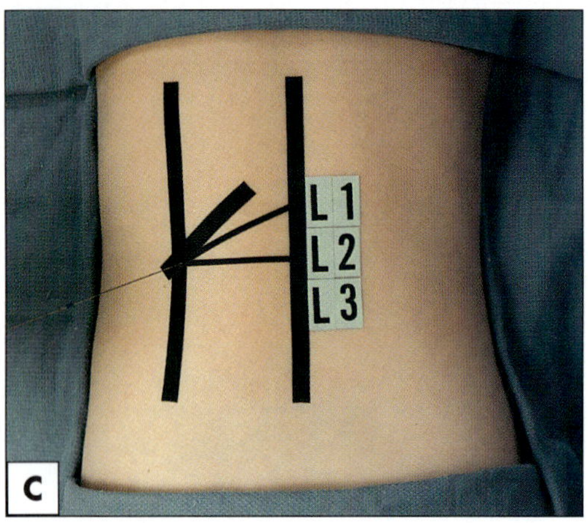

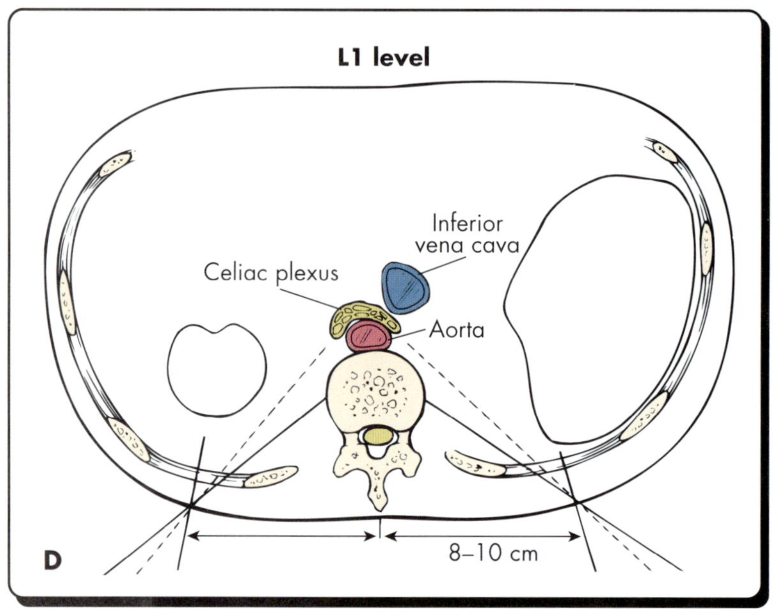

Figure 5-12. Celiac plexus block. This nerve block is usually administered to diagnose and control intractable pain caused by malignancy of the pancreas, liver, stomach, and gallbladder [24,25]. **A** and **B**, The landmarks to be used as guides include line *A* in the midline; line *B*, 10 to 8 cm from the midline; and "X," the point at which line *B* crosses the last rib, *ie*, the point at which the needle enters. A straight line from point X to the midline corresponds to the level of the second lumbar vertebra (L2). A line 30° cephalad to this line is directed toward the L1 vertebra.

C and D, The technique for a celiac plexus block is as follows. The patient is placed in the prone position, with a pillow under his abdomen to decrease the lumbar lordosis. The needle is inserted at point X and is directed toward the L1 vertebra which is approximately 30° cephalad to the line connecting point X to the side of the L2 vertebra. A 6-in (15-cm) 20-gauge needle should be inserted at an angle of 40° to 45° to the plane that is perpendicular to all planes of the skin. Once the needle contacts the body of the L1 vertebrae, the needle marker is adjusted 1 to 2 cm above the skin. The needle is then withdrawn two thirds of the way out and reinserted at a 30° angle to the plane that is perpendicular to all planes of the skin. The needle is advanced until the needle marker touches the skin or until the needle passes 1 to 2 cm beyond the vertebral body of the L1 vertebra [26]. After confirmation by fluoroscopy, the anesthetic is injected with frequent aspiration. There should be no resistance to the injection. *The recommended local anesthetics include 0.5% lidocaine, 40 to 50 mL, or 0.125% or 0.25% bupivacaine, 40 to 50 mL.*

The anesthetist should keep in mind the following points while administering the block. (1) The patient should be instructed not to breathe during needle insertion and advancement to prevent the needle from deviating from the target. (2) The patient's blood pressure must be monitored and hypotension treated vigorously.

Complications of celiac plexus block include the following. Hypotension may occur in over 50% of patients. Subarachnoid block, retroperitoneal hematoma, and kidney puncture are possible and usually occur with improper needle placement.

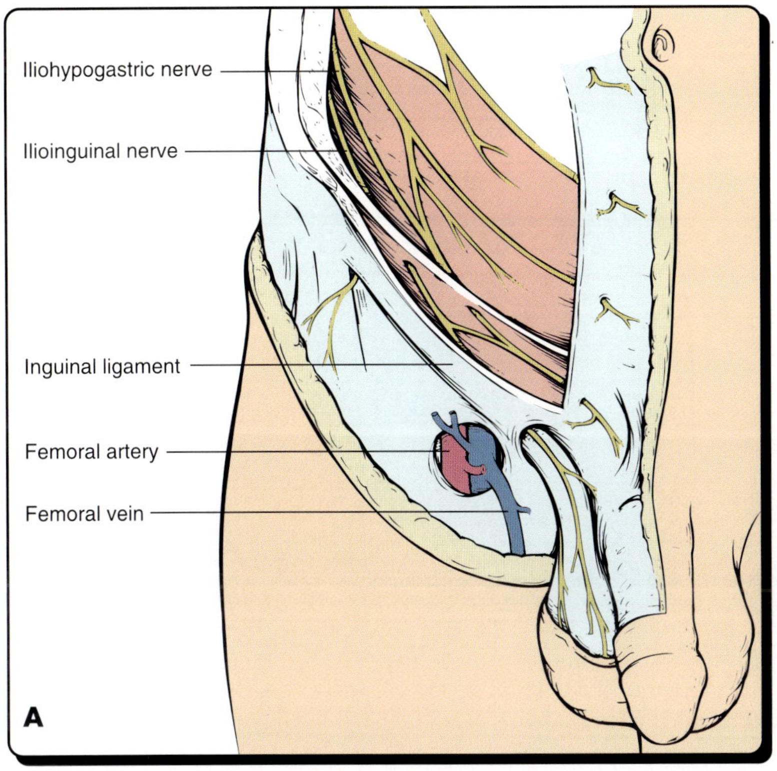

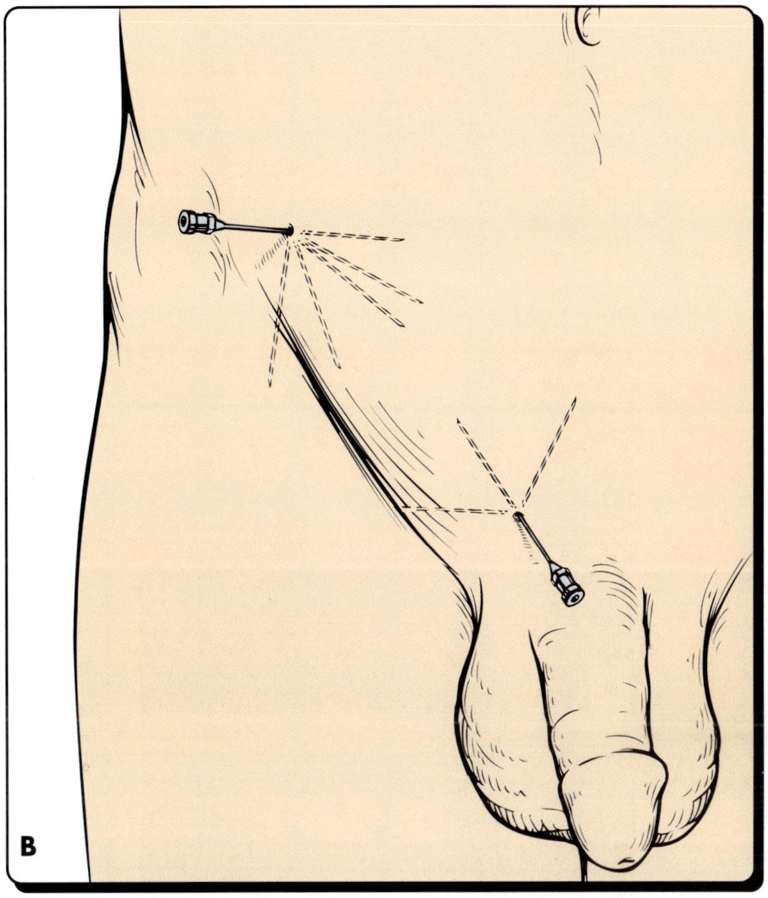

Figure 5-13. Field block for herniorrhaphy. This block in combination with skin infiltration along the line of the incision provides anesthesia for procedures located in the inguinal area. **A** and **B**, The technique for field block for herniorrhaphy is as follows. With the patient in the supine position, a 5-inch (10-cm) 22-gauge spinal needle is inserted 2.5 to 3 cm in the medial and caudad directions to the iliac spine and directed laterally to contact the ilium. Ten mL of local anesthetic solution is infiltrated through all layers of the abdominal wall. From the same point, additional local anesthetic is injected at the same depth and in a fan-like fashion in both cephalad and caudad directions. The ilioinguinal and iliohypogastric nerves are blocked. A second injection is made just distal and lateral to the pubic tubercle above the inguinal ligament. Injection of 10 ml of local anesthetic in fan-like fashion with penetration of the superficial fascia blocks the genitofemoral nerve [27]. *The recommended local anesthetics include 0.5% lidocaine, 20 to 30 mL, or 0.25% bupivacaine, 20 to 30 mL.*

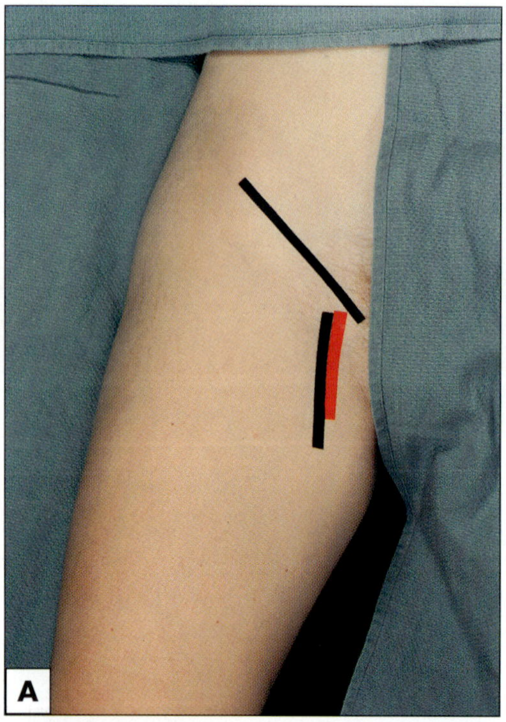

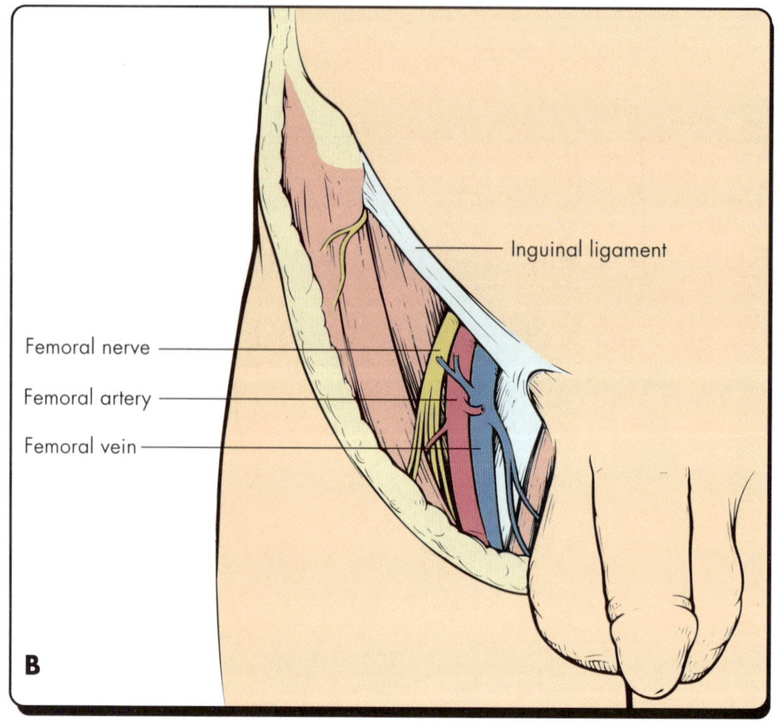

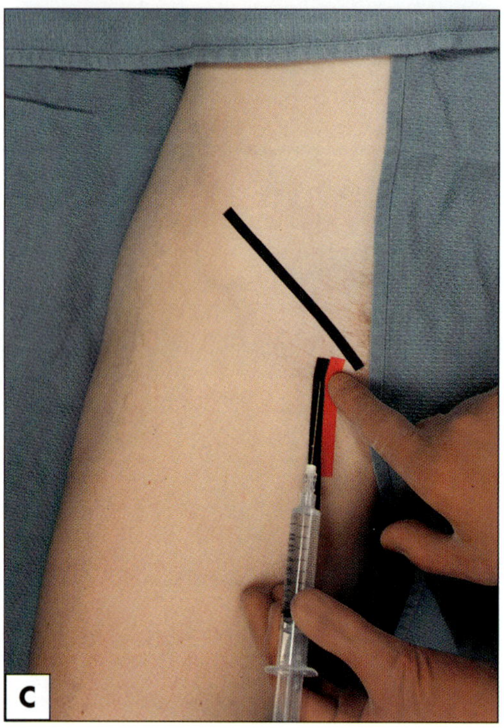

Figure 5-14. Femoral nerve block. This nerve block is indicated for operations of the leg and foot and to provide analgesia for fracture of the upper part of the femur [28]. **A** and **B**, The major landmarks to be used as guides include the femoral artery and inguinal ligament. **C**, The technique for femoral nerve block is as follows. The patient lies in the supine position. A line between the anterior superior iliac spine and the pubic tubercle represents the position of the inguinal ligament. The femoral artery is palpated, and a 5-cm 22-gauge needle is inserted just below the inguinal ligament approximately 0.5 to 1 cm lateral to the artery. The needle is inserted at a 45° angle to the skin in a cephalad direction and gently advanced until paresthesia is elicited. If no paresthesia is elicited at a depth of 3 to 4 cm, the needle is withdrawn to a subcutaneous position. The direction is then changed slightly before the needle is readvanced. On eliciting paresthesia, the needle is held firmly and the local anesthetic solution injected. *The recommended local anesthetics include 1% lidocaine, 10 to 15 mL, or 0.5% bupivacaine, 10 to 15 mL.*

The anesthetist should keep in mind the following points while administering the block. If a large volume of local anesthetic solutions is injected (20 to 30 mL), it may anesthetize the femoral nerve, obturator nerve, and femoral cutaneous nerve [29].

Complications of the femoral nerve block include neural injury and neuritis, which are rare.

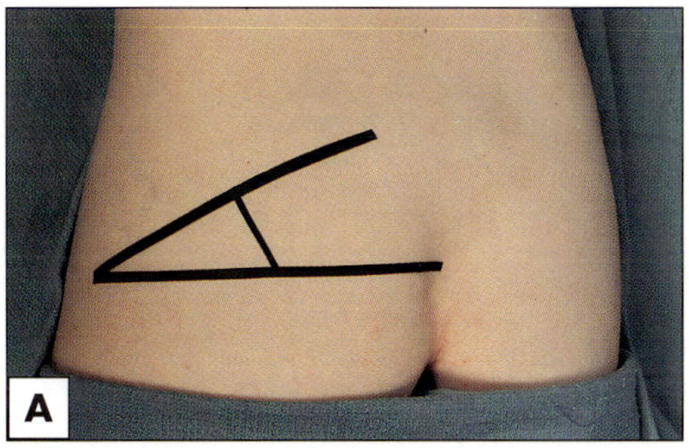

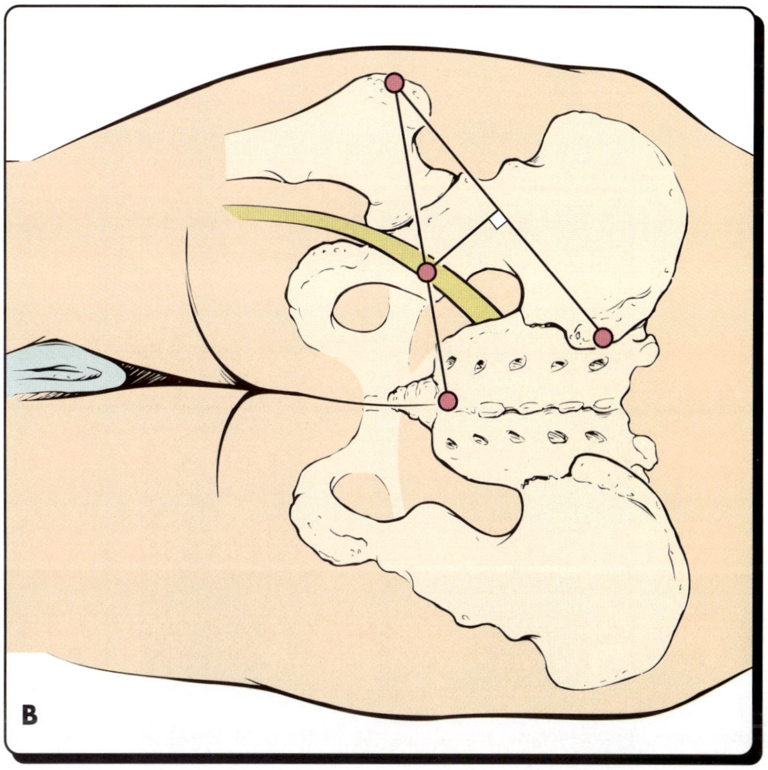

Figure 5-15. A and B, Sciatic nerve block. This nerve block is used in anesthesia for the back of the thigh, anterolateral part of the leg, and most of the foot. In combination with femoral or saphenous nerve block, it anesthetizes the entire leg below the knee. The major landmarks used as guides include the (1) greater trochanter, (2) posterior superior iliac spine, and (3) sacral hiatus.

There are several techniques for sciatic nerve block. We describe one here. Labat's posterior approach is the easiest to do and has the highest success rate [28]. The patient lies prone or on his side with the side to be blocked facing up. The patient's upper leg is flexed slightly. A line is drawn between the upper border of the greater trochanter and the posterior superior iliac spine. From the midpoint of this line, a perpendicular line is marked that extends 5 cm caudally. This is the point of needle insertion. A 3.5-in (9-cm) 22-gauge spinal needle is inserted perpendicular to all planes of the skin and advanced until paresthesia is obtained (usually at a depth of 6 to 8 cm for the average patient) or until the pelvic bone is encountered. If bone is encountered, the needle is withdrawn and redirected until paresthesia is obtained. Ideally paresthesia should radiate to the foot [30]. At this point the needle is held firmly and local anesthetic solution injected, with frequent aspiration. *The recommended local anesthetics include 1% lidocaine, 15 to 20 mL, or 0.5% bupivacaine, 15 to 20 mL.*

Complications of sciatic nerve block are extremely rare, with the exception of transient nerve injury [31].

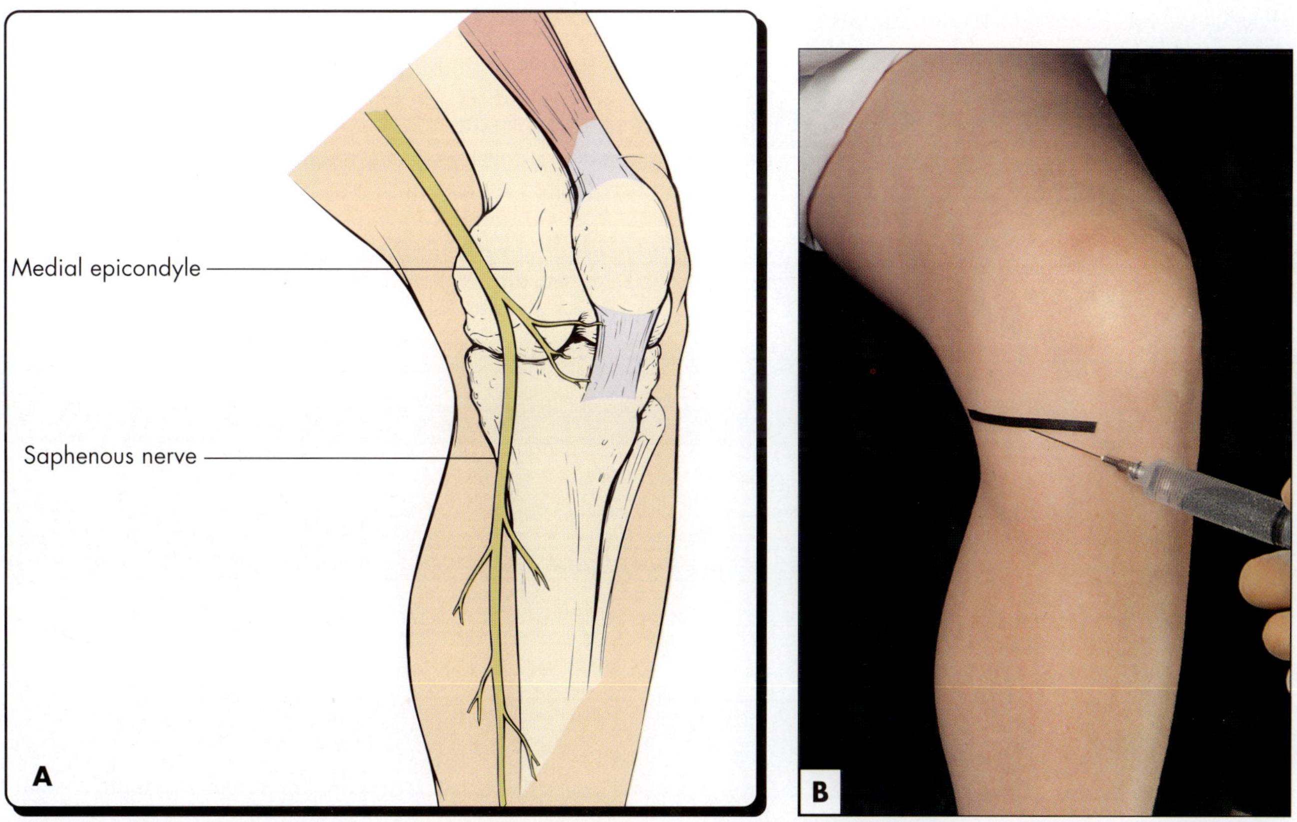

Figure 5-16. A saphenous nerve block is essential when a midcalf tourniquet is applied. The saphenous nerve is the terminal branch of the femoral nerve and carries sensation of the skin over the anterolateral aspect of the leg [1]. A, The landmarks to be used as guides include the head of the tibia and the lower border of the patella.

B, The technique for saphenous nerve block is as follows. The point of insertion of the needles is 2 cm below the lower border of the patella and medial to the head of the tibia. The nerve block is performed by subcutaneous infiltrations [28]. *The recommended local anesthetics include 1% lidocaine, 10 mL, or 0.5% bupivacaine, 10 mL.*

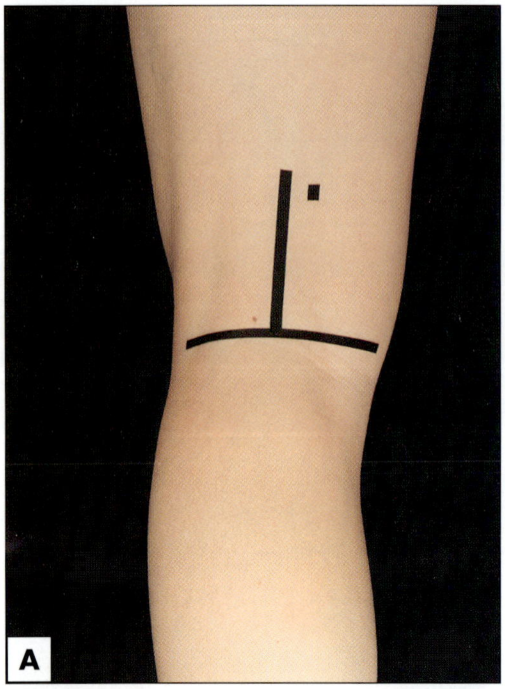

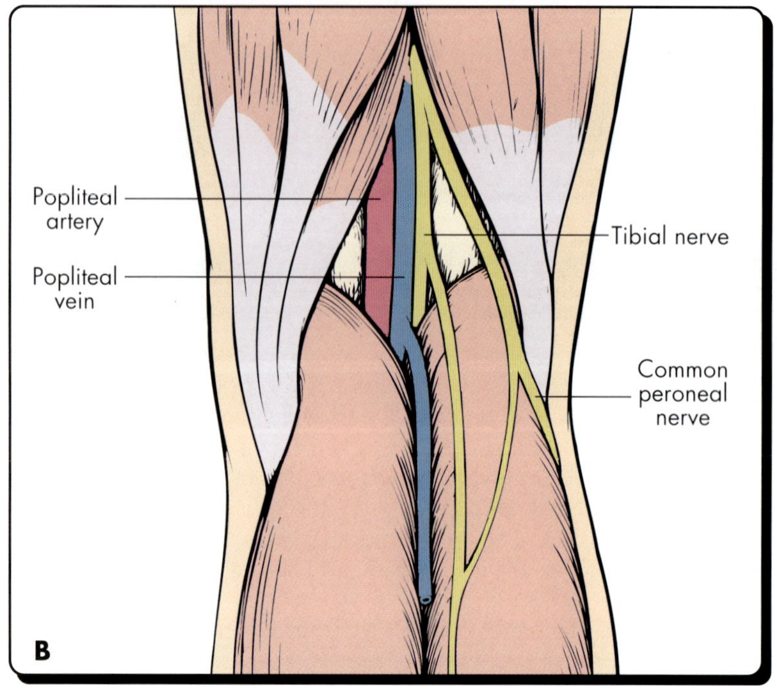

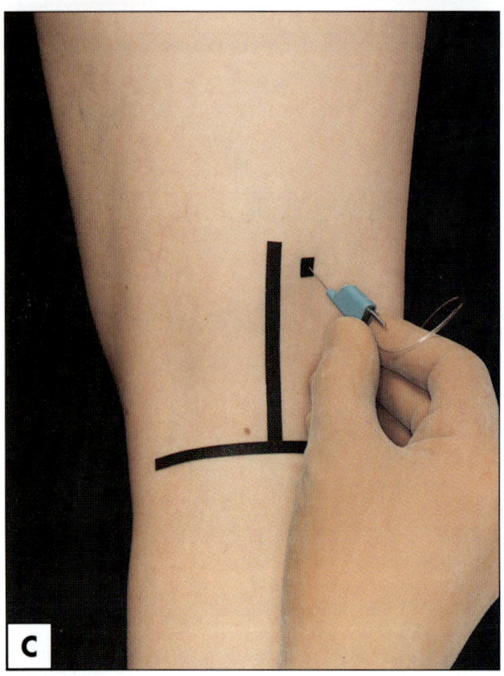

Figure 5-17. Sciatic nerve block at the popliteal fossa. This block, used in combination with the saphenous nerve block, is an ideal choice for operations on the ankle and foot [32]. **A** and **B**, The major landmarks to be used as guides include (with the leg flexed at the knee) (1) the tendons of the semimembranosus muscle medially and biceps femoris muscle laterally and (2) the skin crease formed by flexion of the knee. **C**, The technique for sciatic nerve block is as follows. With the patient in the prone position, a 7-cm-long line is drawn from the middle of the crease toward the femur. The needle is inserted 1 cm laterally to the superior part of this line. A 5-cm 22-gauge needle is inserted at about a 45° angle to the skin and advanced in a cephalad direction until the patient feels paresthesia in the foot. The nerve is usually 3 to 5 cm below the skin. If no paresthesia is obtained at a depth of 5 cm, the needle is withdrawn halfway and redirected slightly until paresthesia is elicited [28]. *The recommended local anesthetics include 1% lidocaine, 15 to 20 mL, or 0.5% bupivacaine, 15 to 20 mL.* A saphenous nerve block must be performed if a tourniquet is to be applied.

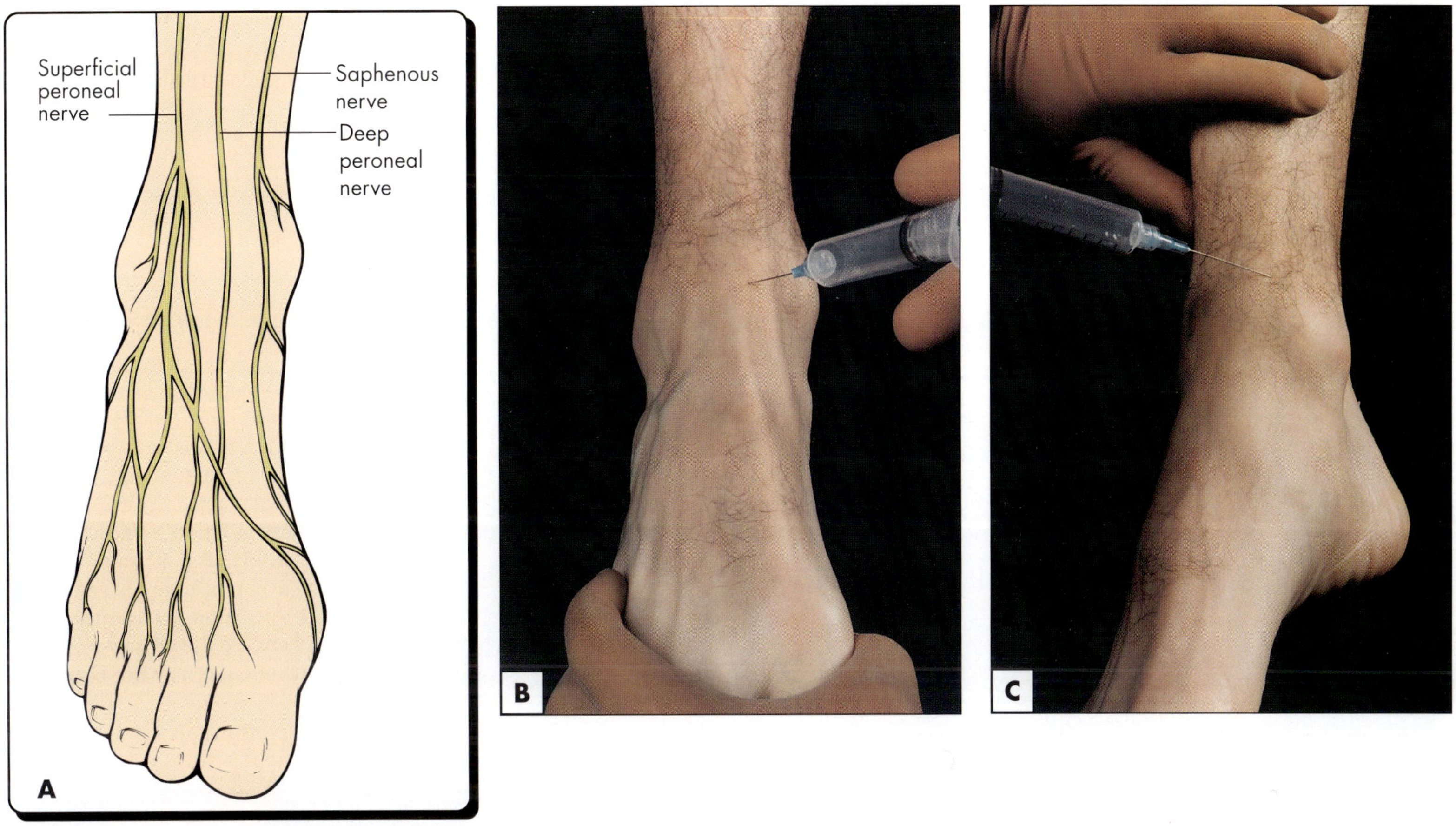

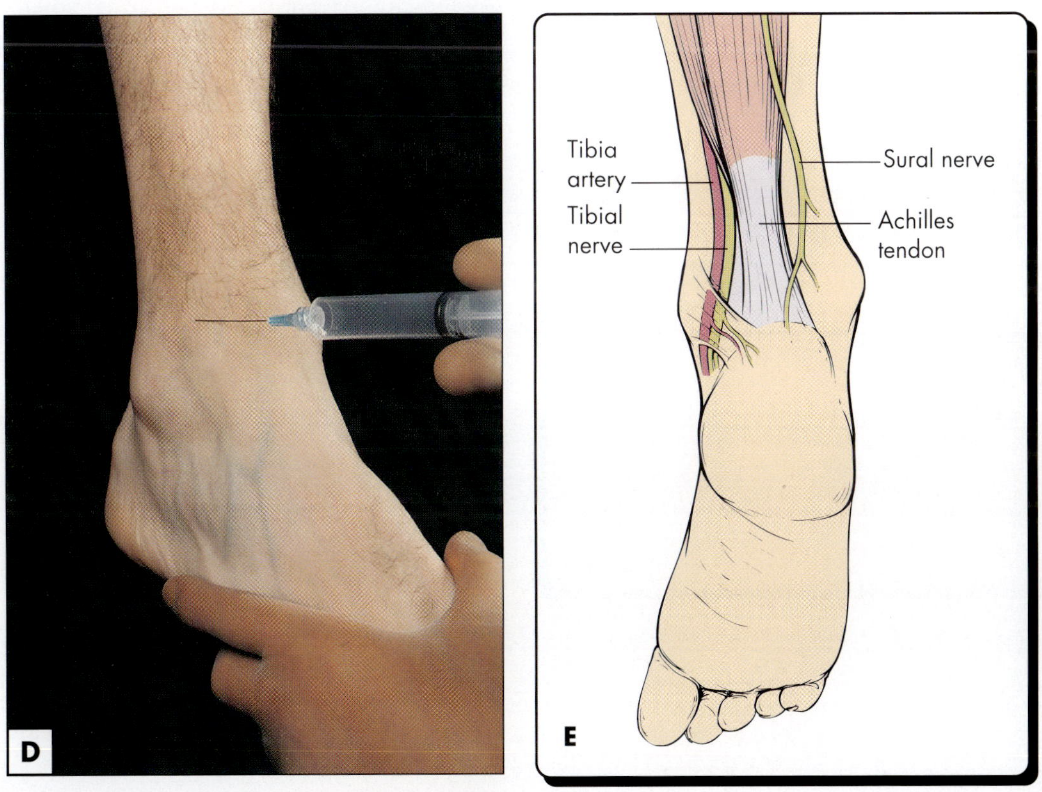

Figure 5-18. The ankle block is usually administered for surgical procedures on the foot that do not require a tourniquet. The recommended local anesthetics include 1% lidocaine, 20 to 25 mL, or 0.25% bupivacaine, 20 to 25 mL. Cutaneous innervation of the foot and ankle is shown in **A**. **B** and **C**, The technique for deep peroneal nerve block is as follows. Dorsiflexion of the patient's foot and toes makes the extensor hallucis longus and tibialis anterior muscles more prominent. At the level of the superior border of the medial or lateral malleolus, a 1.25-inch (4-cm) 25-gauge needle is inserted between these two tendons and advanced until it reaches the bone. At that point, 3 to 4 mL of local anesthetic solution is injected as the needle is gradually withdrawn to the subcutaneous tissue.

D and **E**, The technique for saphenous and superficial peroneal nerve block is as follows. As the needle is withdrawn to the subcutaneous level from the deep peroneal nerve block, it is directed to the upper border of each malleolus. A subcutaneous ring of local anesthetic is deposited, which should extend from the end of medial malleolus to the end of the lateral malleolus. A total of 10 to 15 mL of local anesthetic is injected.

(*Continued on next page*)

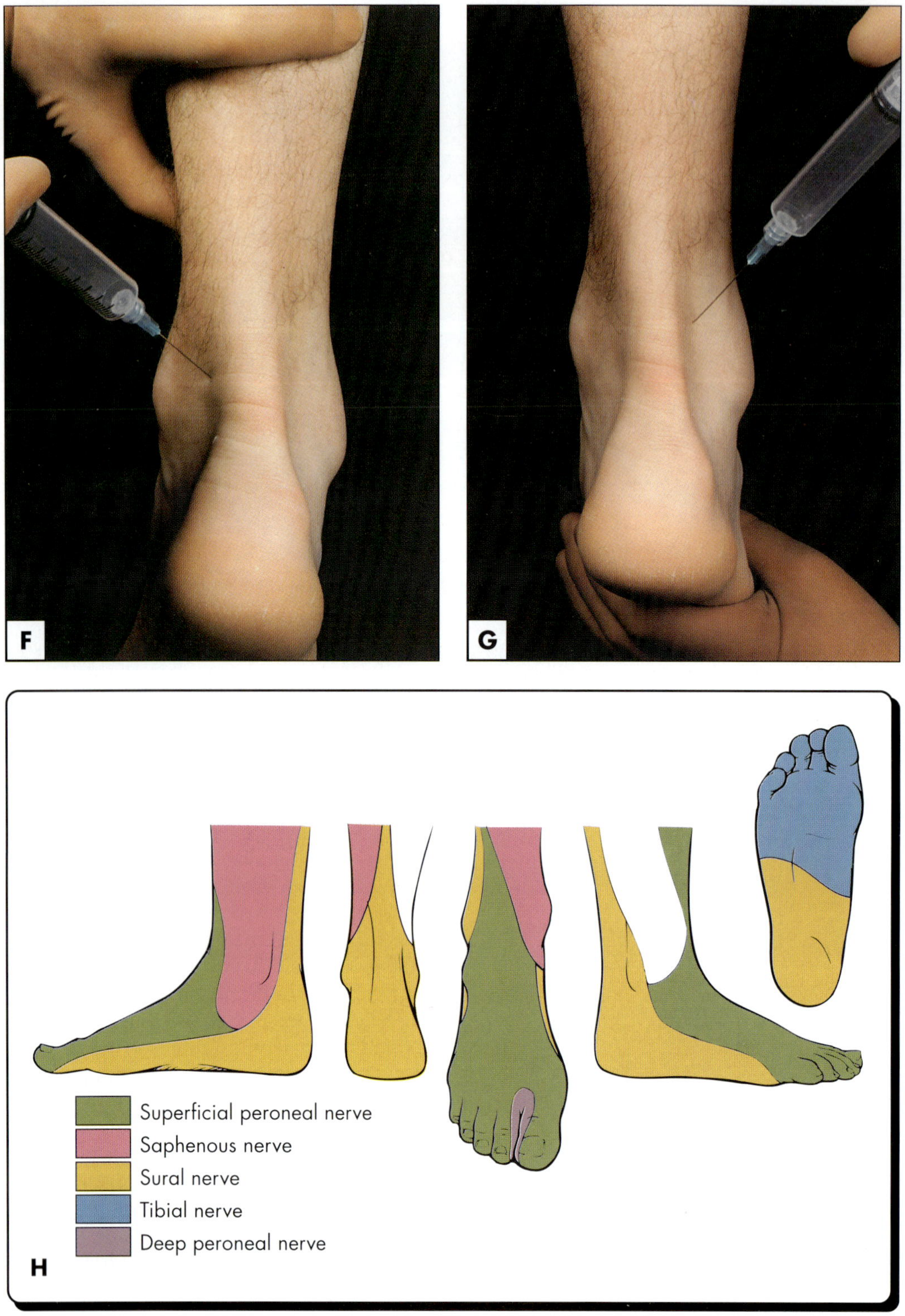

Figure 5-18. (*Continued*) F and G, The technique for tibial nerve block is as follows. A 1.5-in (4-cm) 25-gauge needle is inserted at the superior border of the medial malleolus between the malleolus and the Achilles tendon and is directed at the midpoint (if the tibial artery can be palpated, the needle is inserted just medial to the artery). The needle is advanced until paresthesia is produced or bone is contacted. At that point, 5 mL of local anesthetic solution is injected [30].

H, The technique for sural nerve block is as follows. A 1.5-in (4-cm) 25-gauge needle is inserted at the level of superior border of the lateral malleolus between the Achilles tendon and lateral malleolus. The needle is directed at the midpoint and advanced until paresthesia is produced or bone is contacted. At that point, 5 mL of local anesthetic solution is injected [30].

The anesthetist should keep in mind the following points while administering the ankle block. (1) The deep peroneal nerve innervates only a small area between the great toe and second toe, and therefore, it may not be essential in most surgical procedures. (2) With precise knowledge of anatomy, one can block individual nerves and achieve corresponding areas of anesthesia. Ankle blocks may require multiple injections and can be painful. In reality, by simplifying the technique and using small-gauge needles (25-gauge) most of the discomfort can be eliminated.

REFERENCES

1. Cavino GB: Clinical pharmacology of local anesthetic agents. In *Neural Blockade In Clinical Anesthesia and Management of Pain*. edn. 2. Edited by MJ Cousins and PO Bridenbough. Philadelphia: JB Lippincott; 1988:120–121.
2. Tulchinsky A: Nerve stimulator polarity and brachial plexus block. *Anesth Analg* 1993, 77:100–103.
3. Winnie AP: Interscalene cervical plexus block, a single injection technic: *Anesth Analg* 1975, 54:370–375.
4. Lauze E, Theiss D, Jankovic D: The extent of blockade following various techniques of brachial plexus block. *Anesthesia Analg* 1983, 65:55–58.
5. Winnie AP: Intra scalene brachial plexus block. *Anesth Analg* 1970, 49:455–466.
6. Winnie AP, Collins VJ: The subclavian perivascular technique of brachial plexus. *Anesthesia* 1964, 35:353–363.
7. Balas GI: Regional anesthesia for surgery on the shoulder. *Anesth Analg* 1971, 50:1036–1042.
8. Yasude I, Hirano T, Ojima T, *et al.*: Supraclavicular brachial plexus block using a nerve stimulator and insulated needle. *Br J Anaesth* 1980, 52:409–411.
9. Rock JJ, Sharrock NE, Neudochin L: Intra scalene brachial plexus block for shoulder surgery. *Anesth Analg* 1992, 75:386–388.
10. Lanz E, Theiss D, Jankovic D: The extent of blockade following various techniques of brachial plexus block. *Anesth Analg* 1983, 62:55–58.
11. Brockway MS, Wildsmith JAW: Axillary brachial plexus: method of choice? *Br J Anaeth* 1990, 64:224–231.
12. Dupre LJ, Danel V, Legrand JJ, *et al.*: Surface landmarks for supra clavicular block of the brachial plexus. *Anesth Analg* 1982, 61:28–31.
13 Hickey R, Garland TA, Ramonurthy S: Subclavian perivascular block: influence of location of paresthesia. *Anesth Analg* 1988, 68:767–771.
14. Hughes TS, Desgrand DA: Upper limb block. In *Principles and Practice of Regional Anesthesia*, Edited by JAW Wildsmith and EN Armitage. Edinburgh: Churchill Livingston; 1987:148–150.
15 Winnie, AP, Radonjic R, Akkineni SR, *et al.*: Factors influencing distribution of local anesthetic injected into the brachial plexus sheath. *Anesth Analg* 1979, 58:225–234.
16. Thompson GE, Rorie DK: Functional anatomy of the brachial plexus sheath. *Anesthesiology* 1983, 39:117–122.
17. Selander D, Edshage S, Wolff T: Paresthesia or no paresthesia? *Acta Anaesthesiol Scand* 1979, 23:27–33.
18. Carron H, Litwiller R: Stellate ganglion block. *Anesth Analg* 1975, 54:567– 570.
19 Lofstrom JB, Cousins MJ: Sympathetic neural blockade of upper and lower extremity. In *Neural Blockade in Clinical Anesthesia and Management of Pain*. edn. 2. Edited by MJ Cousins and PO Bridenbaugh. Philadelphia: JB Lippincott; 1988:474–479; 483–493.
20. Moore DC, Bush WH, Scurlock JE: Intercostal nerve block: A roentgenographic anatomic study of technique and absorption in humans. *Anesth Analg* 1980, 59:815–825.
21. Moore DC: Intercostal nerve block for post operative somatic pain following surgery of thorax and upper abdomen. *Br J Anaesth* 1975, 47:284–288.
22. Hatangdi VS, Boas RA; Lumbar sympathectomy. *Br J Anaesth* 1985, 57:285–289.
23. Cherry DA, Rao DM: Lumbar sympathetic and coeliac plexus blocks. *Br J Anaesth* 1982, 54:1037–1039.
23a. Umedas S, Arai T, Hatano Y, *et al.*: Cadaver anatomic analysis of the best side for lumber sympathectomy. *Anesth analg* 1987; 66:643–646.
24.Ischia S, Ischia A, Polati E, *et al.*: Three posterior percutaneous celiac plexus block techniques. *Anesthesiology* 1992, 76:534–540.
25. Thompson GC, Moore DC, Bridenbough LD, *et al.*: Abdominal pain and alcohol celiac plexus nerve block. *Anesth Analg* 1977, 56:1–5.
26. Ward EM, Rorie DK, Nauss LA, et al: The celiac ganglia in man: normal anatomic variations. *Anesth Analg* 1979, 58:461–465.
27. Littlewood DG: Regional anaesthesia of the trunk. In *Principles and Practice of Regional Anaesthesia*. Edited by JAW Wildsmith and EN Armitage. Edinburgh: Churchill Livingston; 1987:132–135.
28. Macrae WA: Lower limb blocks. In *Principles and Practice of Regional Anaesthesia*. Edited by JAW Wildsmith and EN Armitage. Edinburgh: Churchill Livingston; 1987:158–165.
29. Winnie AP, Ramamurthy S, Durrani Z: The inguinal paravascular technic of lumbar plexus anesthesia: the "3 in block." *Anesthe Analg* 1973, 52:989–996.
30. Carron H, Korbon GA, Rowlingson JC: *Regional Anesthesia Techniques and Clinical Applications* Orlando: Grune & Stratton; 1984:106–109; 116–121.
31. Gjessing J, Harley N: Sciatic and femoral nerve block with mepivacaine for surgery on the lower limb. *Anaesthesia* 1969, 24:213–218.
32. Rorie DK, Byer DE, Nelson DO, *et al.*: Assessment of block of sciatic nerve in the popliteal fossa. *Anesth Anal* 1980, 59:371–376.

6

Patient Positioning

Ronald J. Faust

Positioning is like much of the rest of anesthesia; it is expected to be perfect every time, and when a patient wakes up with a position-related complication many assume that appropriate care was not taken when the patient was positioned. Small details that are missed when a patient is positioned can lead to tragic outcomes. The complications can far overshadow the intended benefit of the surgical procedure. When a postoperative neurologic complication is noted immediately after surgery, usually no error in positioning is obvious. When the complication is not recognized until the patient has left the operating room, a mistake in positioning can almost never be recalled.

Recent work has shown, however, that neurologic complications might not always be position-related. In a series of over one million consecutive diagnostic and noncardiac surgical procedures, Warner *et al.* [1] have shown that 9% of patients with postoperative ulnar neuropathies have bilateral ulnar sensory or motor deficits. Preoperative neurologic conditions such as idiopathic brachial neuritis have been implicated as the cause of some postoperative neuropathies [2]. It has been suggested that automatic blood pressure cuffs can lead to postoperative neuropathy in patients with Charcot-Marie-Tooth disease, a hereditary degenerative neurologic disorder that causes demyelinization and fragmentation of axis cylinders of peripheral nerves. It is thought that the pressure produced by the cuff can accelerate the demyelinization process intraoperatively in these patients.

Nevertheless, anesthesiologists must continue to pay meticulous attention to detail during patient positioning. This chapter attempts to portray some of the critical details of the most commonly used surgical positions.

ULNAR NERVE INJURY

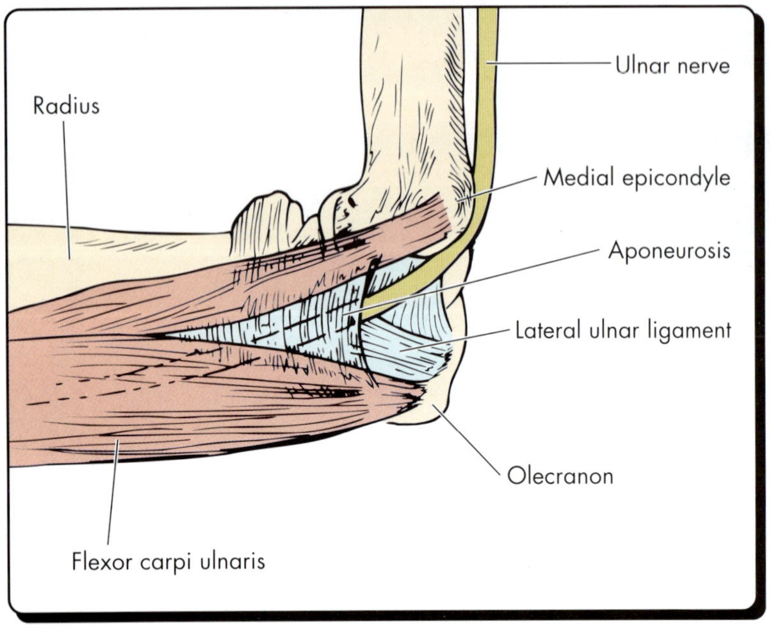

Figure 6-1. The ulnar nerve entering the cubital tunnel at the elbow. The ulnar nerve is most vulnerable at the elbow because of its position in the groove between the olecranon and the medial epicondyle of the humerus, where it is covered only by skin and fascia. Ulnar neuropathies occur at a rate of 1:2700 surgical patients and are bilateral in 9% of patients in whom they occur [1]. Although pressure is the mechanism usually suspected when a postoperative neuropathy occurs, stretching of the plexus, entrapment in the cubital tunnel, recurrent dislocation of the nerve, and pre-existing medical disorders such as diabetes mellitus and alcoholism are often implicated [3]. Charcot-Marie-Tooth disease, other hereditary neuropathies, and idiopathic brachial neuritis can also be responsible [2]. Postoperative ulnar neuropathy can occur without any apparent cause even when a patient's arms are carefully positioned and padded [3]. (*From* Nakata and Stoelting [4].)

SUPINE AND LITHOTOMY POSITIONS

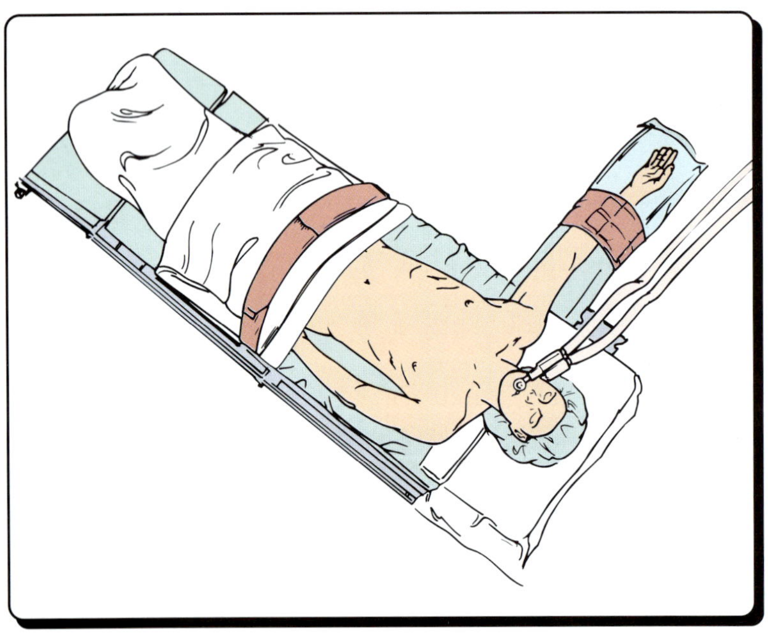

Figure 6-2. The supine position. To decrease the risk of compression injuries to the ulnar nerve, the patient's left arm has been tucked at the side and the elbows padded. The draw sheet is tucked under the patient's hip, not under the mattress. The right arm, which is on a padded arm board, is restrained and is not abducted more than 90%. Traction is avoided on both arms. Although supination of the hand offers a theoretic advantage in avoiding pressure on the ulnar nerve at the elbow, no data exist proving that it is advantageous to pronate the forearm. For surgeries of long duration, the use of extra padding on the entire table and slight flexion of the hips and knees may prevent pressure point sores and postoperative back pain.

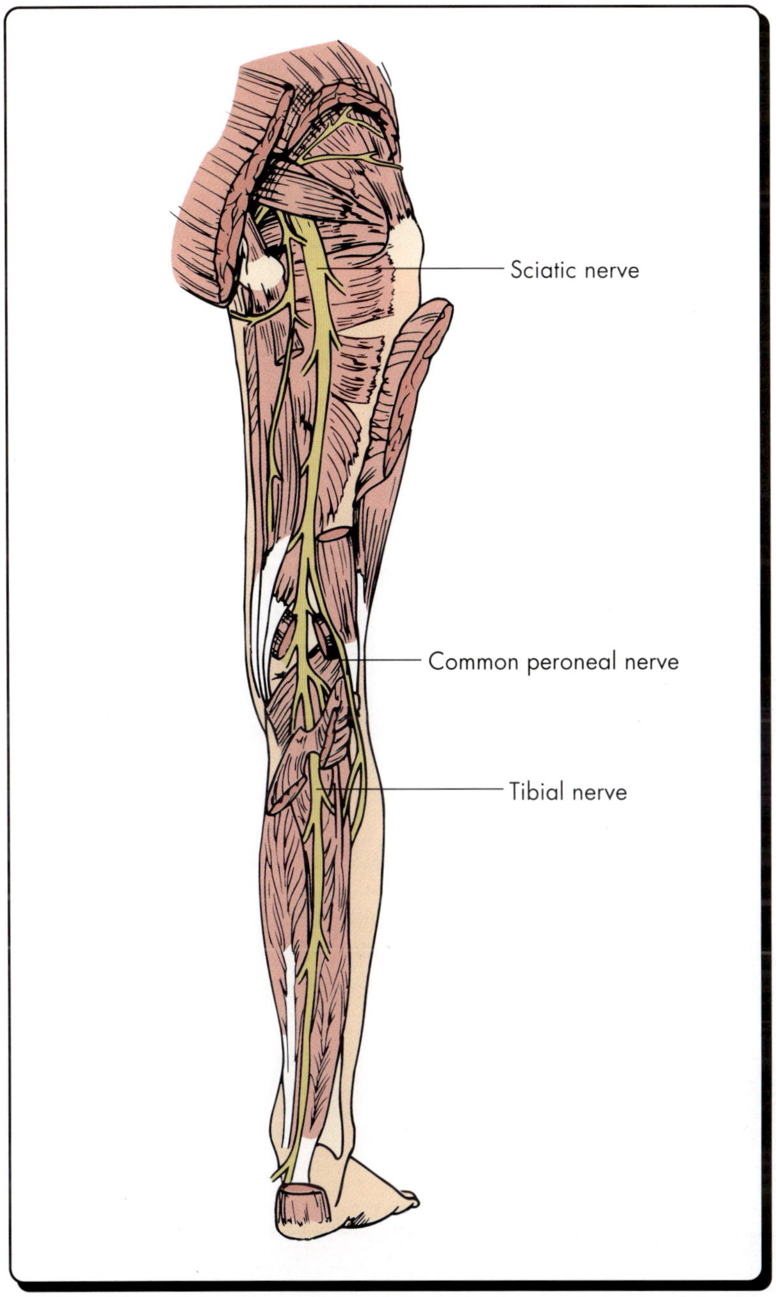

Figure 6-3. The common peroneal and sciatic nerves. The common peroneal nerve, a branch of the sciatic nerve, is depicted in its position lateral to the neck of the fibula. Neuropathy results in foot drop, inability to evert the foot, and loss of dorsal extension of the toes. Sciatic neuropathy is the second most common postoperative lower-extremity neuropathy [5]. Excessive external rotation can cause pressure on the sciatic nerve in the sciatic notch or distally. Neuropathy causes weakness or paralysis of all muscles below the knee and numbness of the lateral half of the calf and most of the foot. (*From* Gray [6].)

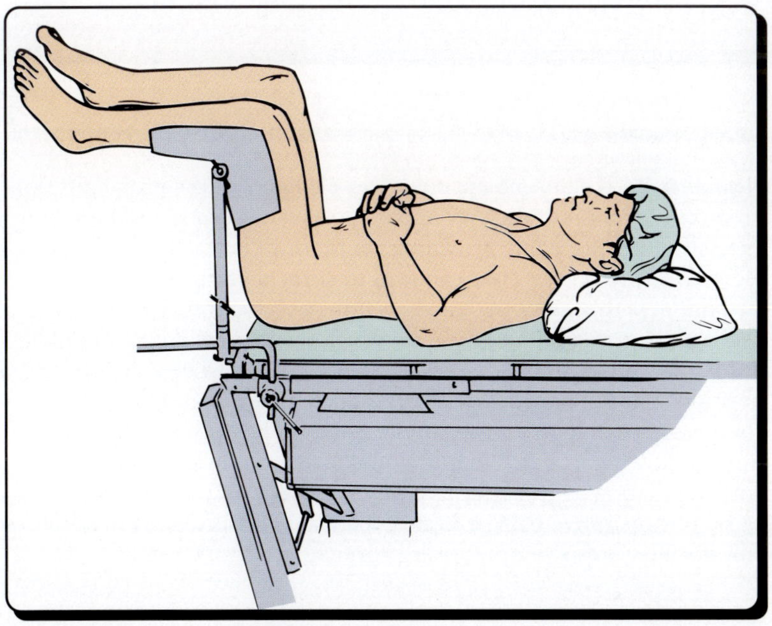

Figure 6-4. The lithotomy position. Both legs are supported in padded stirrups. Although lower extremity neuropathies are less common postoperatively than are those of the upper extremity, persistent neuropathies occurred in 1:3608 lithotomy patients in one series [5]. The common peroneal, sciatic, and femoral nerves were involved in 78%, 15%, and 7%, respectively, of 55 patients with motor deficits of at least 3 months' duration in this series of almost 200,000 consecutive lithotomy patients. The results of this series showed that a very thin body habitus, prolonged surgery, and recent cigarette smoking are strongly associated with the development of this complication. (*From* Kropp [7].)

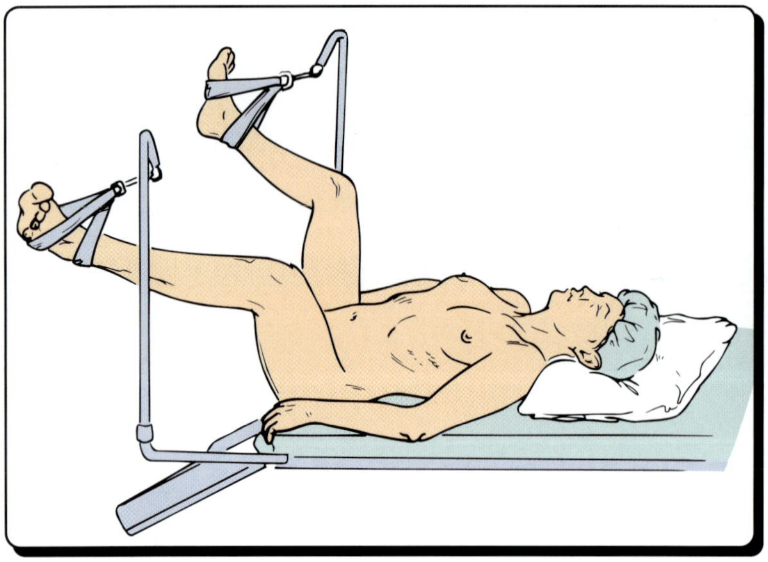

Figure 6-5. Lithotomy variation 2. Suspension of the legs from straps placed around the ankles enables the hips and knees to be flexed slightly more than 90°. Care must be taken to avoid serious hand injury at the break in the table. (*From* Welborn [8].)

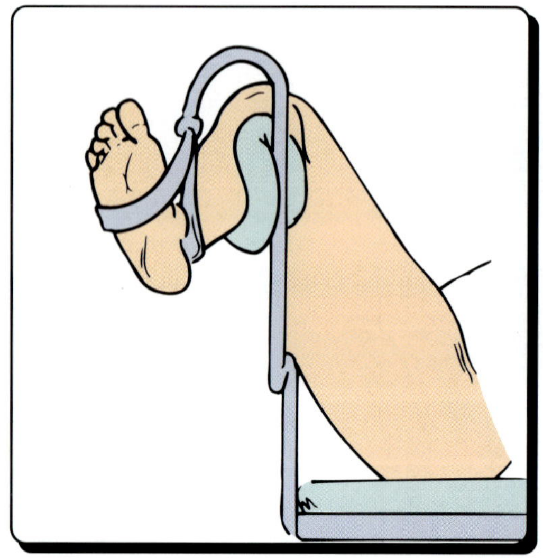

Figure 6-6. Lithotomy variation 3. Although it might be safer for the common peroneal nerve, this alternative lithotomy position can result in pressure on the saphenous nerve, while still risking a stretch injury to the sciatic nerve. (*From* Britt and Gordon [9].)

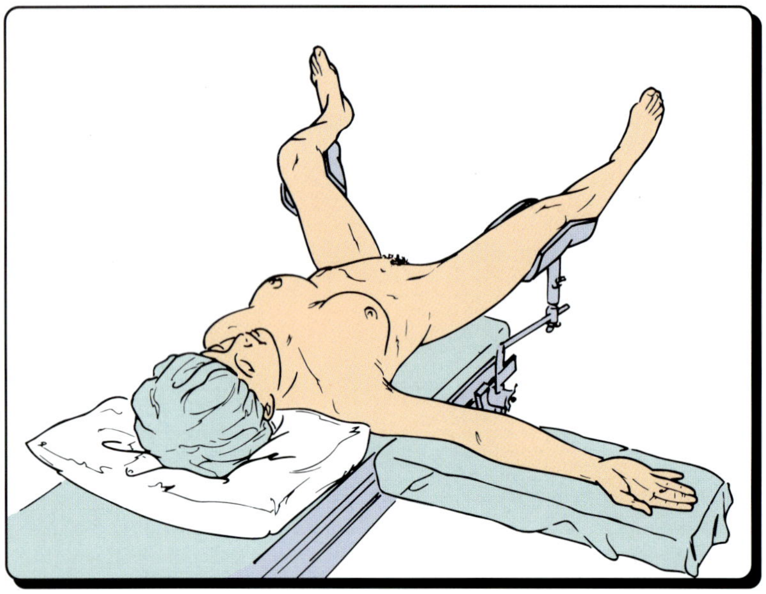

Figure 6-7. Lithotomy variation 4. Often referred to as the "low lithotomy" position, this variation allows simultaneous access to the perineum and the abdomen for combined procedures such as abdominoperineal resection. Although access by the anesthesiologist to the patient's head and face is usually limited, the position permits both parts of the procedure to be completed without repositioning, thereby reducing surgical time. (*From* Goldstein [10].)

THE PRONE POSITION

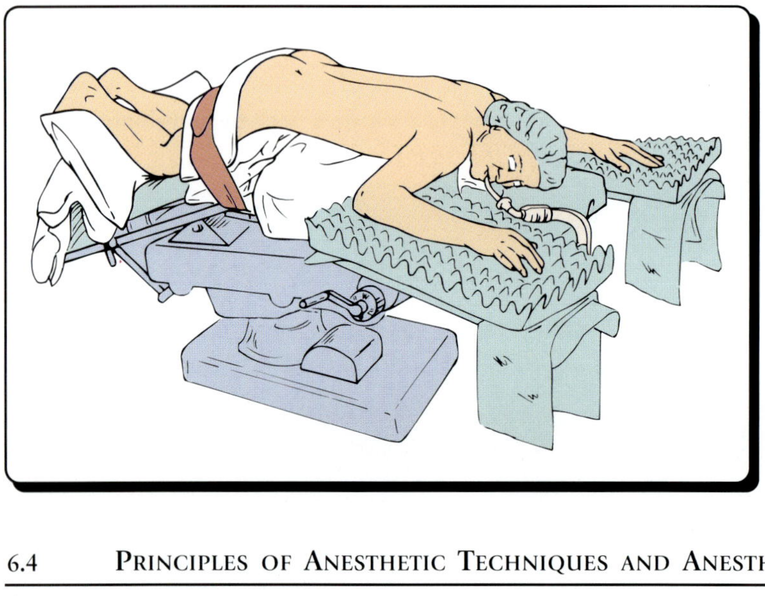

Figure 6-8. The prone position. Key elements of the prone position involve protection of the eye, upper extremity, breasts, and hips from excessive pressure while providing room for diaphragmatic movement. Pressure on the orbit can lead to corneal abrasion or monocular blindness through ophthalmic venous obstruction. The head and neck can be turned to one side; however, the head and neck should not be flexed or extended excessively. The arms can be padded and positioned at the patient's sides or abducted no more than 90°. The chest is supported on long cushions or on a longitudinal support frame, allowing as much diaphragmatic and abdominal movement with ventilation as possible. Excessive pressure on the breasts could cause postoperative pain or nipple necrosis. Pressure sores over the anterior iliac crests or anterior leg surfaces are another risk.

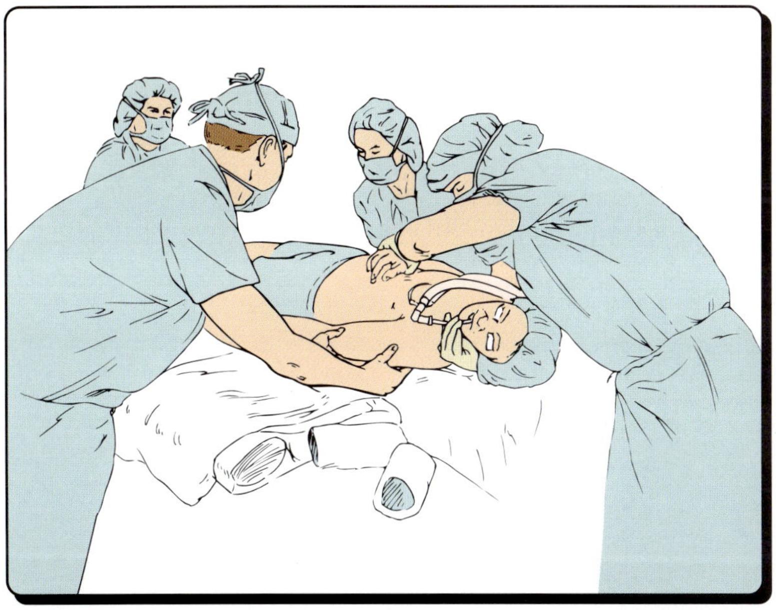

Figure 6-9. Moving the patient into the prone position A. Nonobese patients can be turned from supine to prone smoothly with only four operating room personnel in addition to the anesthesiologist when using the maneuver depicted. The head is first turned in the direction it will eventually face. The head is cradled in the anesthesiologist's forearm, the endotracheal tube being stabilized with his fingers. The patient's left arm can be grasped after the endotracheal tube is disconnected.

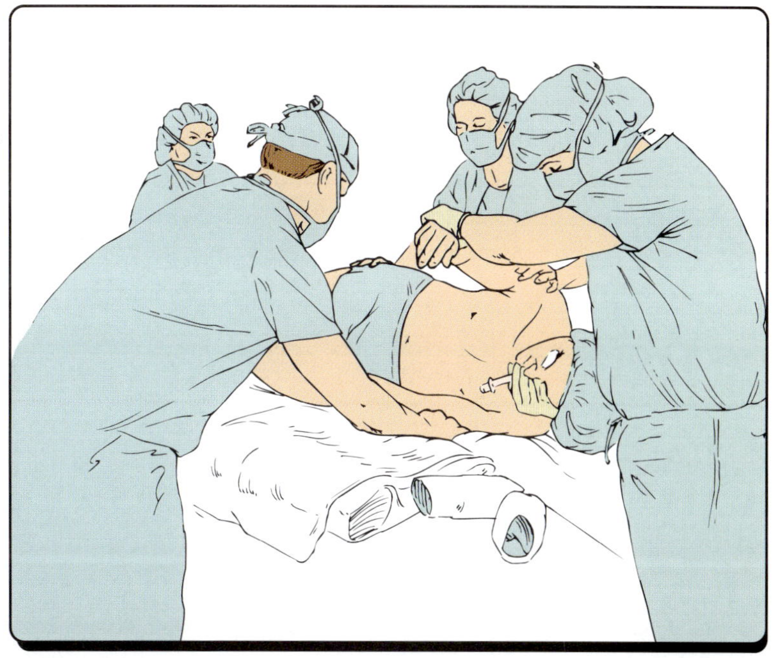

Figure 6-10. Moving the patient into the prone position B. One person on the patient's side pushes the patient up into the lateral position, while operating room personnel prepare to support the torso. A third person guides the feet and legs. Coordination is necessary; Martin [11] discusses dropping the patient as a possible complication of changing position from prone to supine. More likely risks are accidental extubation, loss of vascular access lines, catheters, and monitors; and accentuation of multiple trauma.

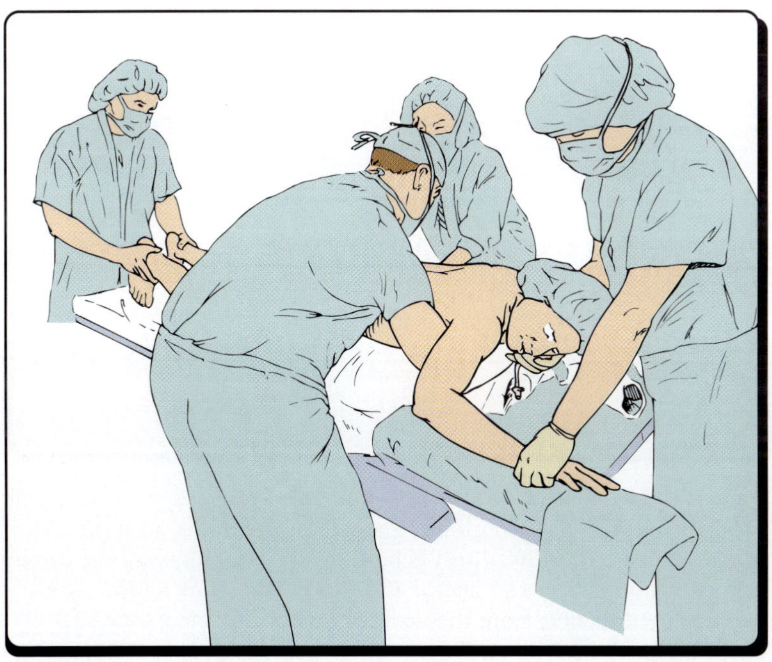

Figure 6-11. Moving the patient into the prone position C. The anesthesiologist supports the patient's head in his right arm, while the patient's arm is controlled with the anesthesiologist's other hand. The person supporting the torso adjusts the patient's position on the bed up or down, as necessary, before sliding his arms from under the patient. Large patients require two operating room personnel to support the torso, abdomen, and hips. Care is taken that the patient's arms are not allowed to fall before being supported on arm boards or at the patient's sides. When cervical pathology or injury is present in a patient having elective or emergency surgery, caution should be used to keep the patient's neck in a neutral position before and after the turn. A pinion headrest can be used to ensure that the patient's cervical spine remains in a neutral position during the surgery.

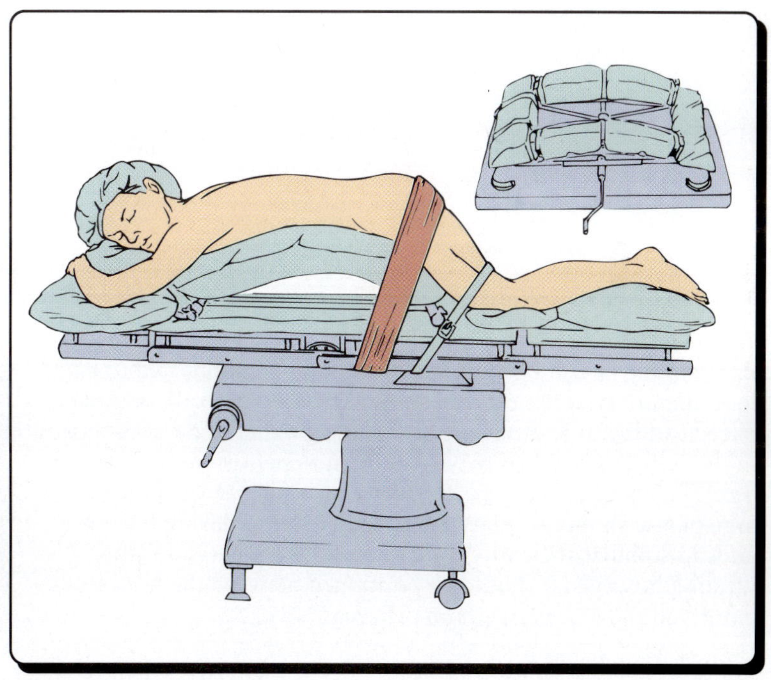

Figure 6-12. The Wilson frame. The Wilson frame is a longitudinal support device that can be used to support patients in the prone position. The curvature of the two sides of the device easily can be adjusted to increase lumbar flexion of the patient. (*From* Elliott [12].)

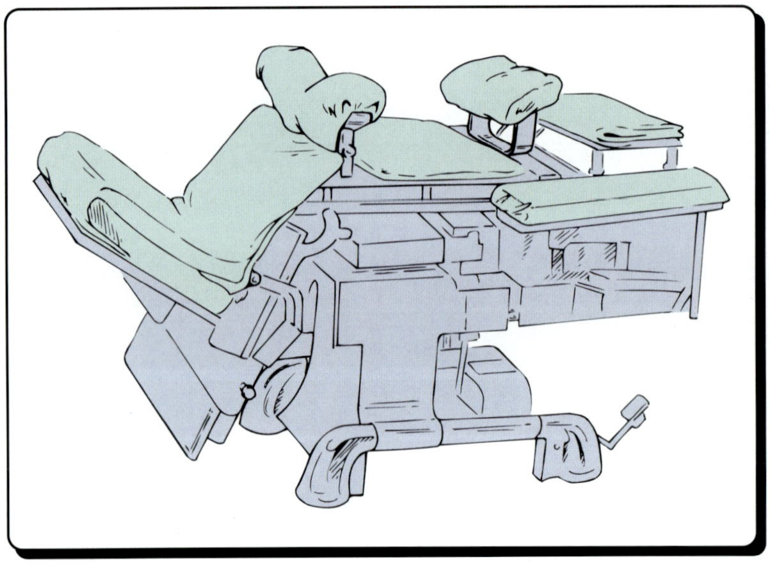

Figure 6-13. The Tower table. The Tower table can also be used to position patients prone when lumbar and hip flexion are necessary. This pedestal support device bears most of the patient's weight on adjustable padded supports under the patient's chest and iliac crests. Weight-bearing should be equally divided between the patient's knees and iliac crests. The arms of thin patients can be positioned under the abdomen; however, this should not be attempted with an obese patient with a pendulous abdomen [12]. (*From* Elliott [12].)

LATERAL POSITIONS

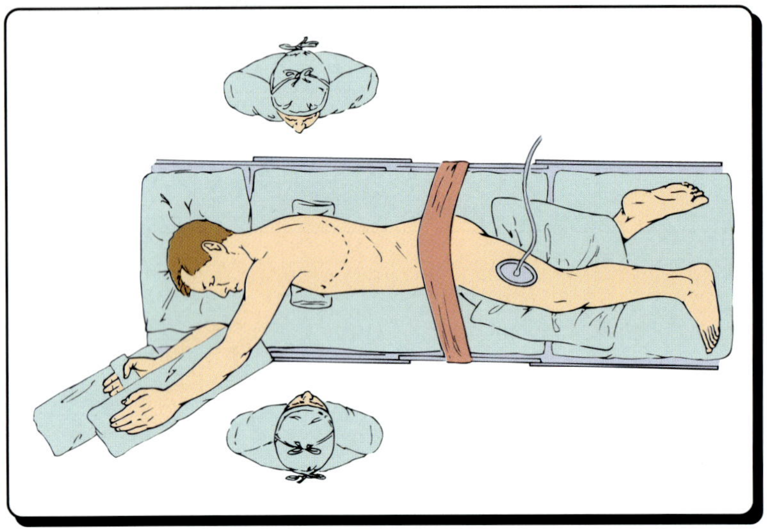

Figure 6-14. The lateral decubitus position. When patients are placed in the lateral position, the head must be supported to avoid poor alignment of the cervical spine. An "axillary roll" or pad is placed caudad to and outside of the lower axilla to decrease pressure on the patient's brachial plexus and ensure perfusion of the lower arm. The upper arm can be supported in a sling or on a pillow. A large pillow should be placed between the legs. Flexing one knee tends to stabilize the entire torso. A strap is also used for this purpose; however, it should be positioned between the head of the femur and the iliac crest. (*From* Thomas [13].)

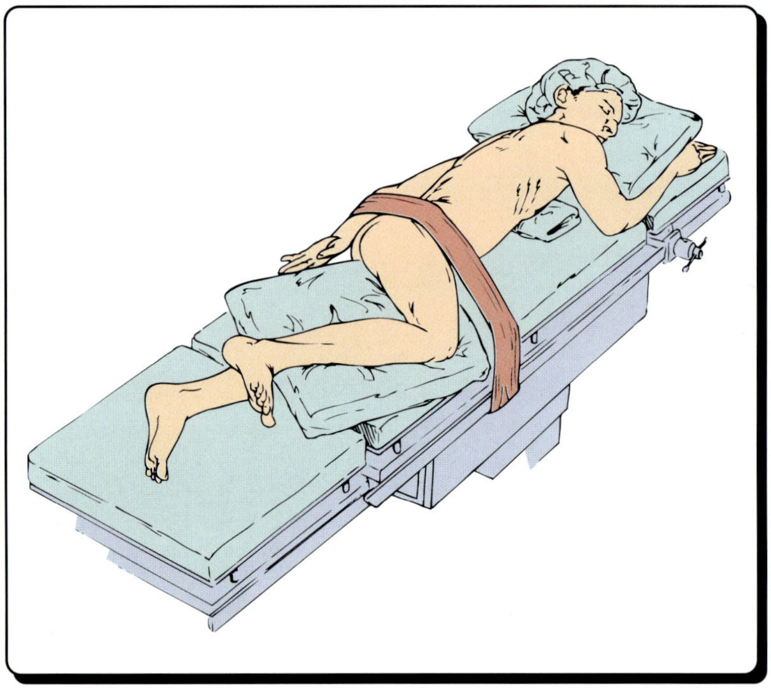

Figure 6-15. The park bench position, also referred to as the semi-prone position. This variation of the lateral decubitus position moves the patient's lower arm behind the thorax, allowing the torso to be positioned between lateral and prone and allowing the patient to face any direction from the wall to the floor for neurosurgical procedures. The park bench position is used most often in neurosurgery and for some procedures in the posterolateral thoracic area. Care must be taken to avoid the loss of venous and arterial catheters in the lower arm while the patient is being placed in this position. (*From* Lawson [14].)

THE SITTING POSITION

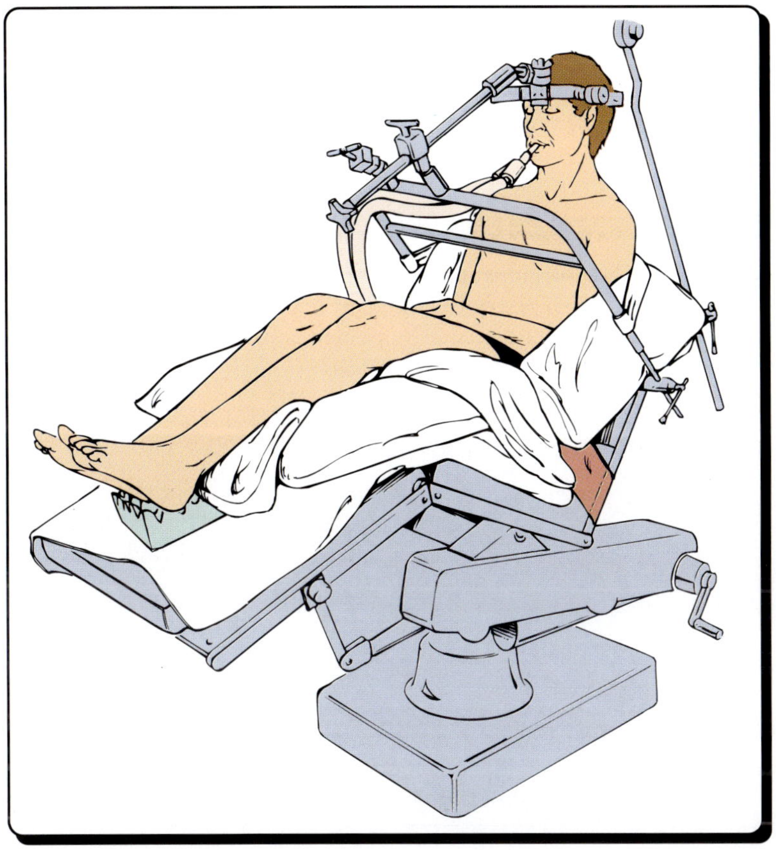

Figure 6-16. The sitting position. This position gives access to the posterior neck and occipital areas for cervical and posterior fossa surgery. Proponents say the surgical exposure is greatly improved when patients are in the sitting position instead of the prone position because blood drains out of the field, allowing easier visualization of the sources of bleeding. The risk of air embolism is increased; however, the safety of the position has been documented in a large clinical series [15]. Key points on positioning involve the neck, arms, and buttocks. The range of motion of the neck should be checked before the patient is anesthetized, and cervical flexion in the sitting position should not exceed the range of motion the patient has while awake. Excessive cervical flexion can cause obstruction of venous drainage of the head, stretching of the cervical spinal cord or roots, and pressure sores of the chin and sternum. The arms hang beside the torso once the patient is sitting; they should be carefully padded to prevent pressure from the frame that supports the head. The buttocks should be supported on a soft flotation pad to protect the patient's sciatic nerves. The buttocks must be squarely positioned in the break in the table; if the patient is too far down on the table and a space can be palpated behind the buttocks, he will be sitting in a slouched position and the operating field will be too close to the top of the back of the table. Both the hips and knees are flexed less than 90° to decrease stretch on the sciatic nerves and prevent postoperative back pain.

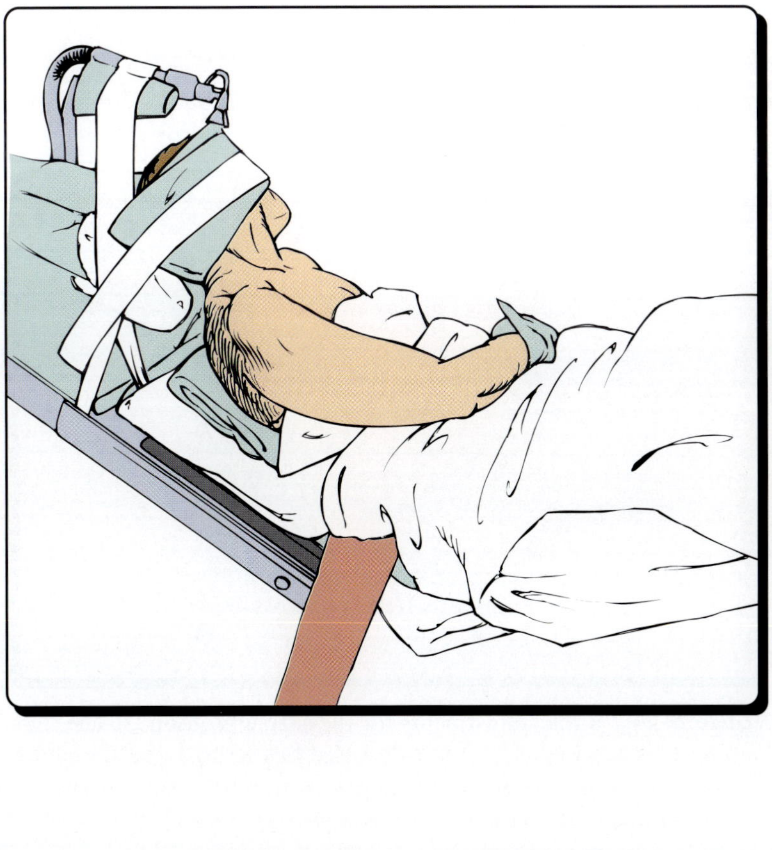

Figure 6-17. The shoulder position. This position is a variation of the sitting position in which the surgeon's access is to the front and side of the patient instead of the posterior aspects of the patient's head and neck. The head is usually secured against a horseshoe headrest with tape. The risk of air embolus, although certainly present, is probably not as great as it is during posterior fossa surgery, because the wound is not as far above the heart and the patient is usually not as upright as is necessary for posterior fossa surgery. Special care must be taken to make certain that the hoses for the anesthesia circle are secured. (*From* Elliott [12].)

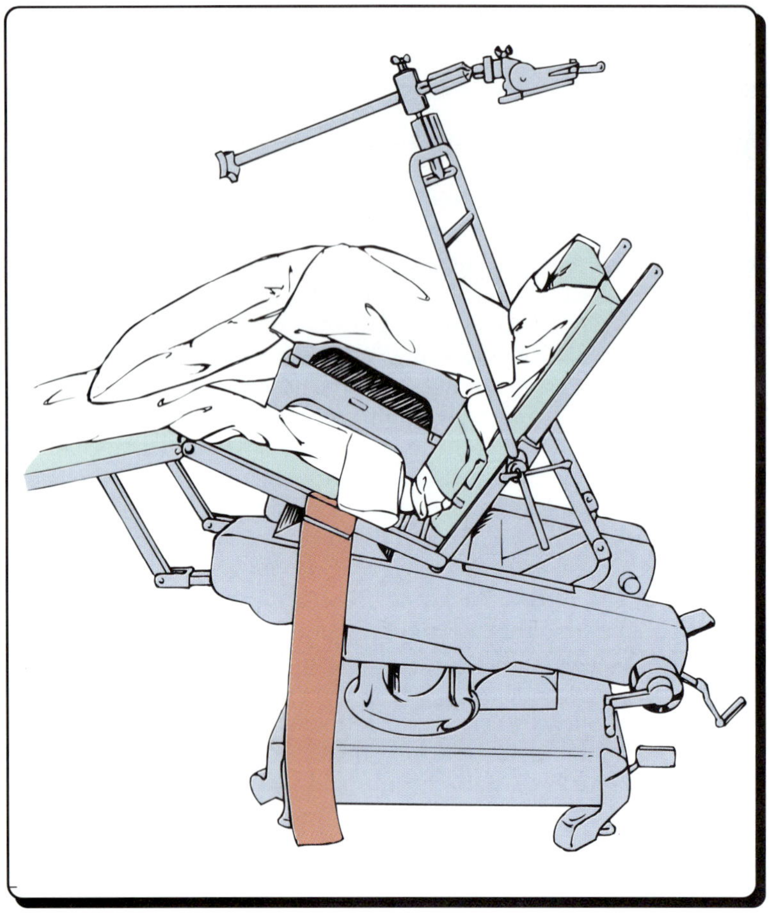

Figure 6-18. Table setup for the sitting position for a pediatric patient. When pediatric patients or very short adults undergo procedures in the sitting position, step blocks can be used to elevate the patient to a proper surgical height. As with adults, the pinion head frame is placed on the patient in the supine position after vascular access lines are placed. The table is then adjusted to the sitting position, and the frame that supports the head is locked into position.

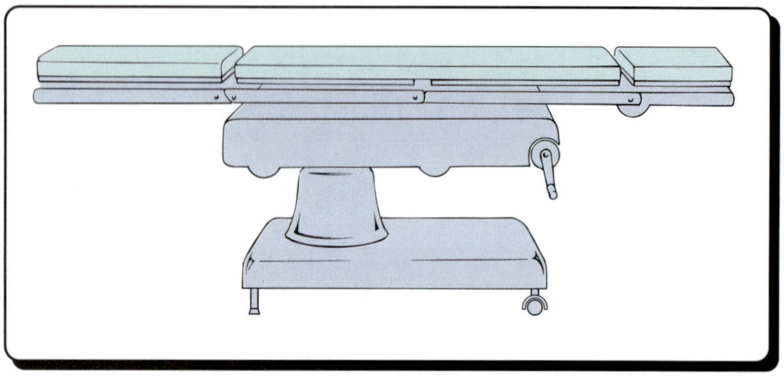

Figure 6-19. Table adjustments for the sitting position A. The sequence of steps necessary to adjust an operating table into the sitting position are illustrated. The patient starts in the supine position on a flat table. (*From* Martin [16].)

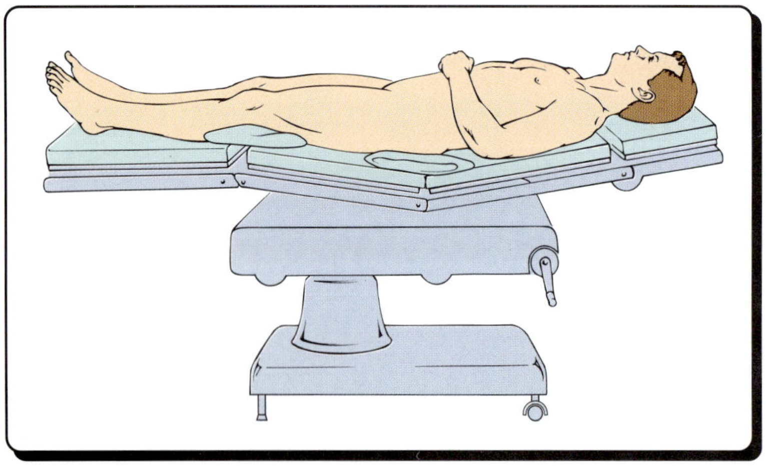

Figure 6-20. Table adjustments for the sitting position B. The table is flexed slightly and the foot depressed. If flexion is excessive on some tables, it will be impossible to subsequently raise the back as far as necessary. (*From* Martin [16].)

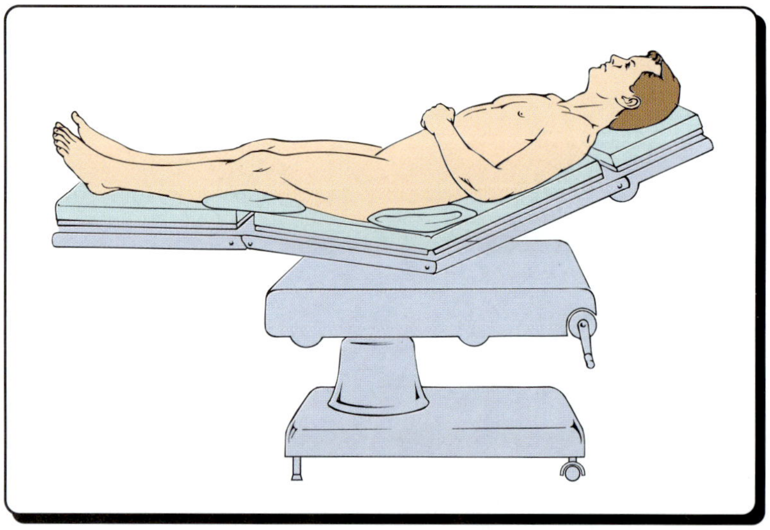

Figure 6-21. Table adjustments for the sitting position C. The back section is raised. The foot is lowered further to avoid stretch of the sciatic nerve and postoperative back pain. (*From* Martin [16].)

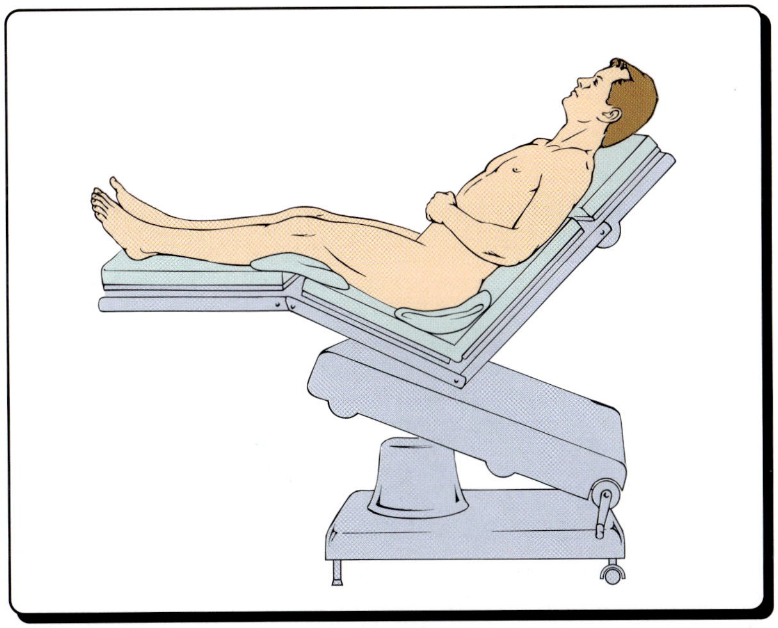

Figure 6-22. Table adjustments for the sitting position D. The head of the table chassis is rotated back to raise the level of the lower limbs with respect to the heart level. This also brings the operating field closer to the surgeon. (*From* Martin [16].)

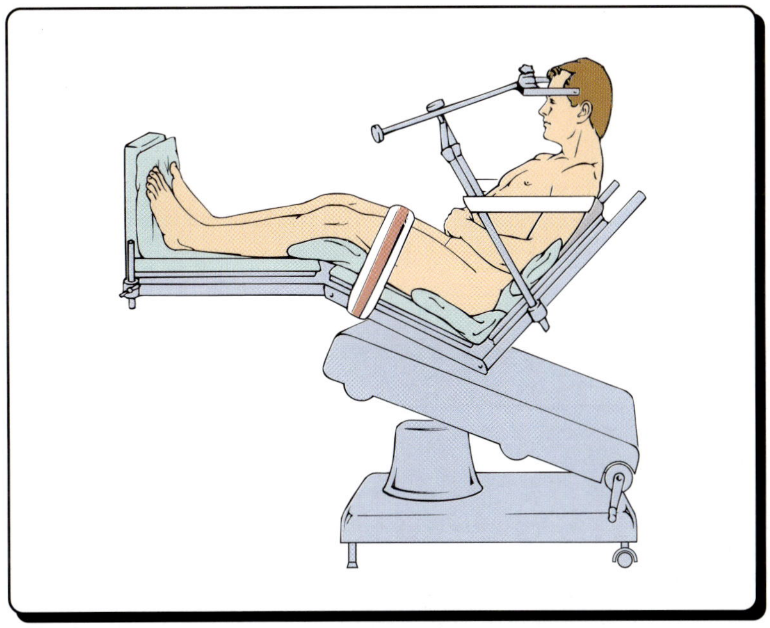

Figure 6-23. Table adjustments for the sitting position E. The head frame holding brace is attached and the head and neck are precisely positioned and locked into place. Shoulder-restraining tapes can be added to pull the shoulders forward. (*From* Martin [16].)

REFERENCES

1. Warner MA, Warner ME, Martin JT: Ulnar neuropathy. Incidence, outcome, and risk factors in sedated or anesthetized patients. *Anesthesiology* 1994, 81:1332–1340.
2. Fibuch EE, Mertz J, Geller B: Postoperative onset of idiopathic brachial neuritis. *Anesthesiology* 1996, 84:455–458.
3. Stoelting RK: Postoperative ulnar nerve palsy: is it a preventable complication? *Anesth Analg* 1993, 76:7–9.
4. Nakata DA, Stoelting RK: Positioning the Extremities.In *Positioning in Anesthesia and Surgery*, edn. 3. Philadelphia: WB Saunders; 1997:211.
5. Warner MA, Martin JT, Schroeder DR, *et al.*: Lower-extremity motor neuropathy associated with surgery performed on patients in lithotomy position. *Anesthesiology* 1994, 81:6–12.
6. Gray H: *Anatomy of the Human Body*, edn 26. Edited by Goss CM. Lea & Febiger; Philadelphia, PA: 1959:1049.
7. Kropp KA: The lithotomy position. Surgical aspects: urology. In *Positioning in Anesthesia and Surgery*, edn 2. Edited by Martin JT. Philadelphia, PA: WB Saunders; 1987:53–56.
8. Welborn SG: The lithotomy position. Anesthetic considerations. In *Positioning in Anesthesia and Surgery*, edn2. Edited by Martin JT. Philadelphia, PA: WB Saunders; 1987:57–62.
9. Britt BA, Gordon RA: Peripheral nerve injuries associated with anesthesia. *Can Anaesth Soc J* 1964, 11:514.
10. Goldstein PJ: The lithotomy position. Surgical aspects: obstetrics and gynecology. In *Positioning in Anesthesia and Surgery*, edn 2. Edited by Martin JT. Philadelphia, PA: WB Saunders; 1987:53–62.
11. Martin JT: The Ventral Decubitus (Prone) Position. In *Positioning in Anesthesia and Surgery*, edn 3. Edited by Martin JT, Warner MA. Philadelphia, PA: WB Saunders; 1987:191–222.
12. Elliott BA: Positioning and monitoring. *Orthopedic Anesthesia*. Edited by Wedel DJ. New York: Churchill Livingstone; 1993:99–128.
13. Thomas AN: The lateral decubitus position. Surgical aspects. In *Positioning in Anesthesia and Surgery*, edn 2. Edited by Martin JT. Philadelphia, PA: WB Saunders; 1987:147–154.
14. Lawson NW: The lateral decubitus position. Anesthesiologic considerations. In *Positioning in Anesthesia and Surgery*, edn 2. Edited by Martin JT. Philadelphia, PA: WB Saunders; 1987:155–180.
15. Black S, Ockert DB, Oliver WC, Jr, Cucchiara RF: Outcome following posterior fossa craniectomy in patients in the sitting or horizontal positions. *Anesthesiology* 1988, 69:49–56.
16. Martin JT: The head-elevated positions. Anesthesiologic considerations. In *Positioning in Anesthesia and Surgery*, edn 2. Edited by Martin JT. Philadelphia, PA: WB Saunders; 1987:79–116.

7

Transfusion Therapy in the Perioperative Period

Paul E. Kazanjian

Over 12 million units of red blood cells are transfused annually in the United States and approximately two thirds of these are given in the perioperative period [1]. At one time or another, every practicing anesthesiologist is involved in the administration of blood and blood products. Like any other medication, the beneficial effects of blood products must be weighed against the risks of adverse effects and complications. Current thinking about the risks and benefits of transfusion is undergoing constant evolution and refinement. For instance, the hemoglobin concentration at which red blood cell (RBC) transfusion improves clinical outcome has not been established. There is consensus, however, that red blood cell transfusions should **not** be based on a single indicator, such as a predetermined hemoglobin level [2]. There has been considerable enthusiasm for preoperative autologous blood donation, acute normovolemic hemodilution (ANH) and directed donation as means of reducing the risks of disease transmission. Yet, there is controversy whether preoperative autologous blood donation and ANH are cost-effective [3–6]. Nevertheless, the anesthesiologist will remain one of the primary physicians responsible for the transfusion of blood products.

In order to maximize the benefit and reduce the risk of blood transfusions, it is important for the anesthesiologist to be familiar with the basic elements of blood component processing, storage, and administration. This chapter presents background information on the use of blood components in the hospital and the nature of blood component procurement and storage. Modern transfusion practice is characterized by "component therapy," which is based on transfusing only the specific portion of blood that is necessary. Several groups have published guidelines that define indications for the use of these various components. These practice guidelines have been incorporated into algorithmic decision aids to illustrate the multiple factors the practitioner must consider before the transfusion of each unit of blood product. All components share certain risks especially risks due to the transmission of infectious agents. Packed red blood cells (PRBCs) are much more likely than other components to cause hemolytic transfusion reactions but this complication is extremely rare. Finally, it is important to be familiar with blood delivery systems, blood conservation methods, and alternatives to homologous blood transfusions.

OVERVIEW OF BLOOD PRODUCT USAGE

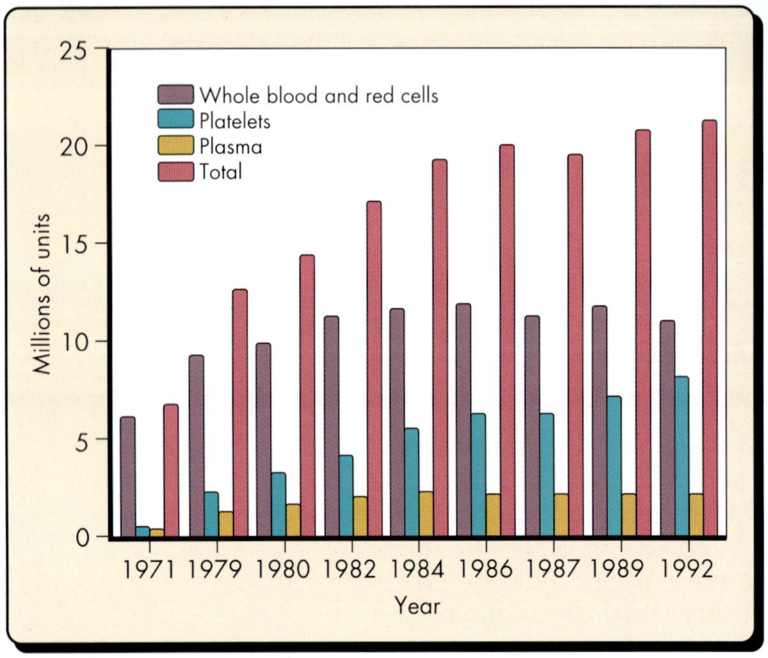

Figure 7-1. Transfusion patterns in the United States. Between 1971 and 1980, total blood utilization in the United States doubled from 6.91 million units to 14.72 million units. In contrast, total blood utilization has begun to level off and red blood cell (RBC) transfusion has declined in the ten year period between 1982 and 1992. This change in the pattern of transfusion has coincided with the emergence of AIDS and the increased concern over the risk of disease transmission due to blood transfusion [7]. Data are from multiple sources [7–10].

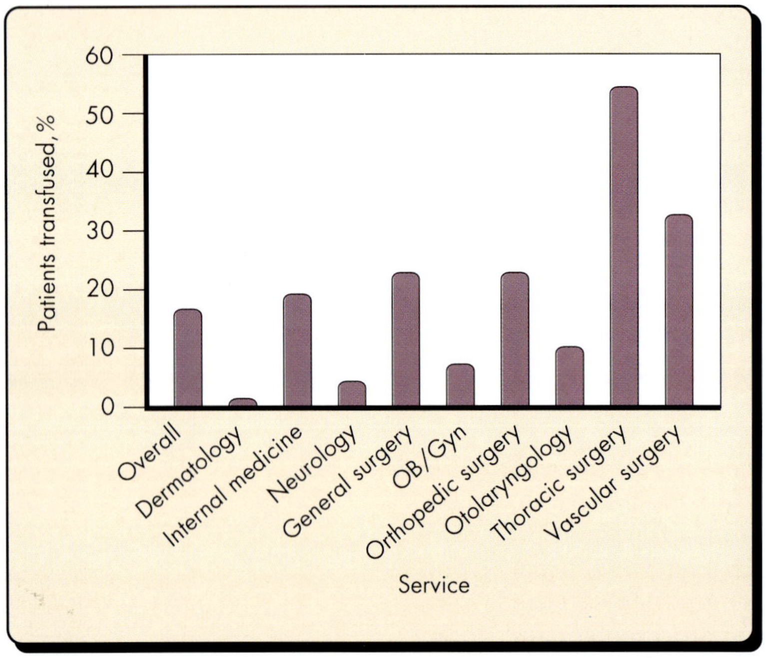

Figure 7-2. Blood component usage in hospitalized patients by service. These figures represent unpublished data from a large teaching hospital and are intended to provide a rough estimate of the percentage of patients admitted to the hospital who receive blood products. The data are averaged over a three-year period, 1991–1994. Overall, approximately 15.6% of patients admitted to this hospital received one or more transfusions of blood products. Patients on surgical services were more likely to receive a blood transfusion, and most of this blood was administered intraoperatively or in the first 24 hours following an operation. In patients undergoing operations in this hospital, those having cardiac operations and liver transplants were most likely to receive a transfusion.

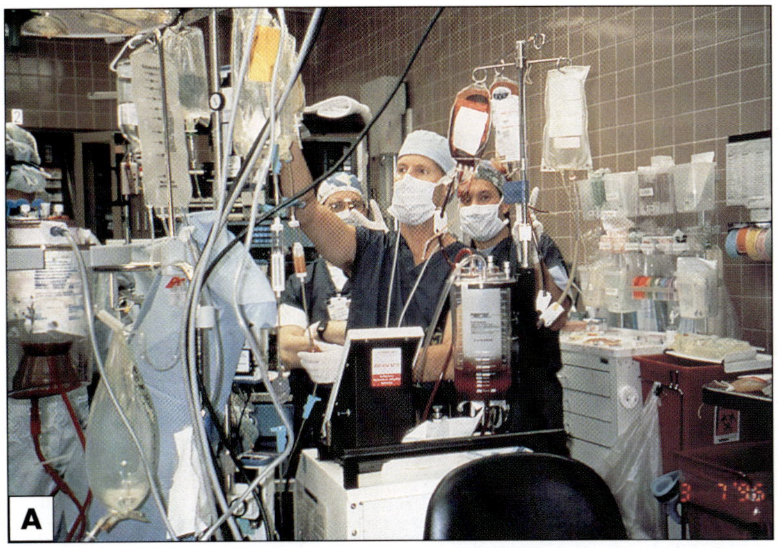

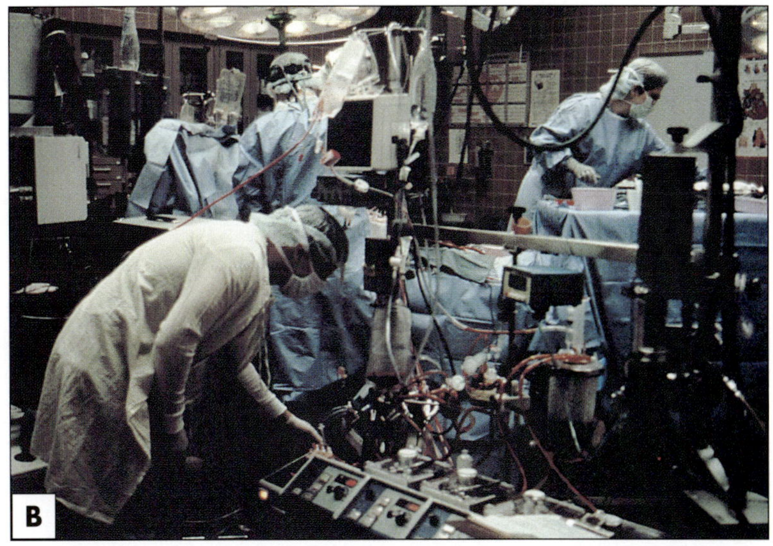

Figure 7-3. Operations with significant blood loss. Several operations typically invoke significant blood loss requiring transfusion therapy. Over the last decade, the use of blood components has increased partly because of the rise in the number of "bloody" operations such as liver transplant (**A**), repair of ruptured abdominal aneurysm, aortic arch replacement (**B**) with circulatory arrest, and operation for trauma [11]. Likewise, many operations that usually have low blood loss (*eg*, hysterectomy) have the potential to incur significant blood loss. Complex operations have placed an increasing burden on the donor pool, blood banks, and transfusion services to provide ever increasing amounts of blood products. The anesthesiologist involved with cases known to incur significant blood loss should be prepared to rapidly and safely transfuse blood products.

Published data confirm that certain operations invoke significant blood loss, but transfusion requirements vary. In a multicenter review of transfusion practices for solid organ transplantation, an average of 17.3 units of red cells was transfused during liver transplant surgery but less than one unit was needed for renal allograft surgery [11]. Liver transplants also required significant amounts of platelets, cryoprecipitate, and plasma. There is considerable variation in transfusion practices among institutions as indicated by multicenter audits [12,13]. In one study, adult patients undergoing first-time coronary artery bypass grafting were transfused a mean of 2.9 ± 0.1 red cell units, but the range was from a low of 0.4 ± 0.2 to a high of 6.3 ± 0.6 red cell units [13].

REVIEW OF BLOOD BANKING PROCEDURES

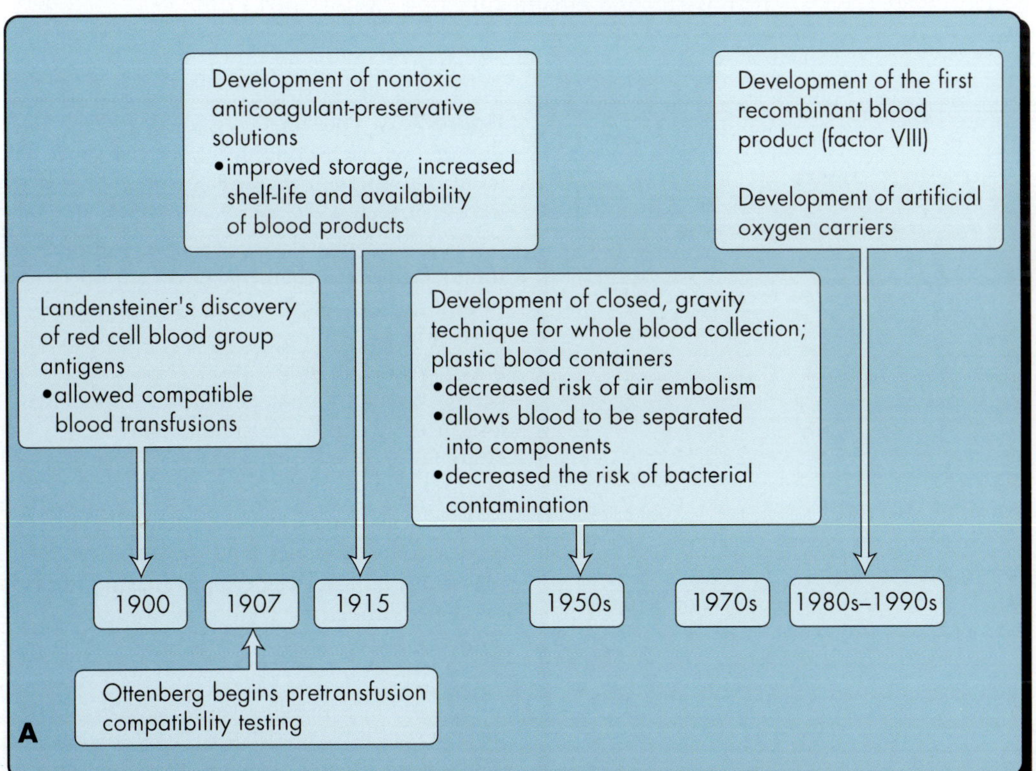

Figure 7-4. Technological advances and quality assurance. During the 20th century, numerous technologic advances, as shown in the timeline in **A**, have made transfusion medicine extremely safe. Modern transfusion therapy was made possible by the discovery of blood groups, the implementation of compatibility testing, and the development of efficacious methods to store and transfuse blood. In the early 1900s, Karl Landsteiner made the truly landmark discovery of blood groups. Reuben Ottenberg demonstrated the relationship between fatal transfusion reactions and blood groups, emphasizing the importance of pre-transfusion compatibility testing. The development of citrate anticoagulants was instrumental to the success of indirect transfusions. Nonreusable, chemically inert, plastic, closed-collection systems and plasma fractionation techniques were refined during World War II.

(*Continued on next page*)

B. RELIANCE ON VOLUNTEER DONATION AND IMPROVED DONOR SCREENING

Ensuring the Safety of the Blood Supply: Donor Screening

Donors are provided with information to encourage "self-deferral" and are given an opportunity for confidential self-exclusion

- Allows donors who feel obligated, or coerced, to give blood an opportunity to have their blood excluded

An interview is performed to eliminate high risk donors

- Screens for donors whose lifestyle, behaviors or medical history places them at risk of contracting transfusion related diseases

Donors are examined for evidence of infection or illicit drug use.

Donors who are excluded by the above process are placed on a deferral list.

- limits future donation

Donors who live in or travel to areas of the world where transfusion transmitted diseases are endemic are excluded

- Reduces the risk of malaria
- Reduces the risk of HIV from Haitians

Figure 7-4. (*Continued*) B and C, while infectious complications remain one of the more frequent significant risks of blood transfusions, improved screening of donors and donor blood testing have reduced the risk of acquiring virally transmitted diseases such as AIDS and hepatitis [7,14]. (Part B and C *from* Sayers [14a].)

C. DEVELOPMENT OF RELIABLE TESTS FOR THE PRESENCE OF VIRAL AND BACTERIAL MICROORGANISMS

Transmissible Agent	Test	Date Test Instituted
Treponema pallidum	Antibody to the agent	1939-1941
Hepatitis B	Viral antigen (hepatitis B surface antigen)	1971
Human immunodeficiency virus 1	Antibody to the virus	1985
Cytomegalovirus	Antibody to the virus	1985-1988
Non-A, non-B hepatitis	Hepatitis B core antibody and alanine aminotransferase	1986-1988
Human T-lymphotropic virus	Antibody to the virus	1989
Hepatitis C	Antibody to viral protein	1990
Human immunodeficiency virus 1 and 2	A combination test for antibodies to both viruses	1992
Human immunodeficiency virus 1	HIV p24 antigen	1996

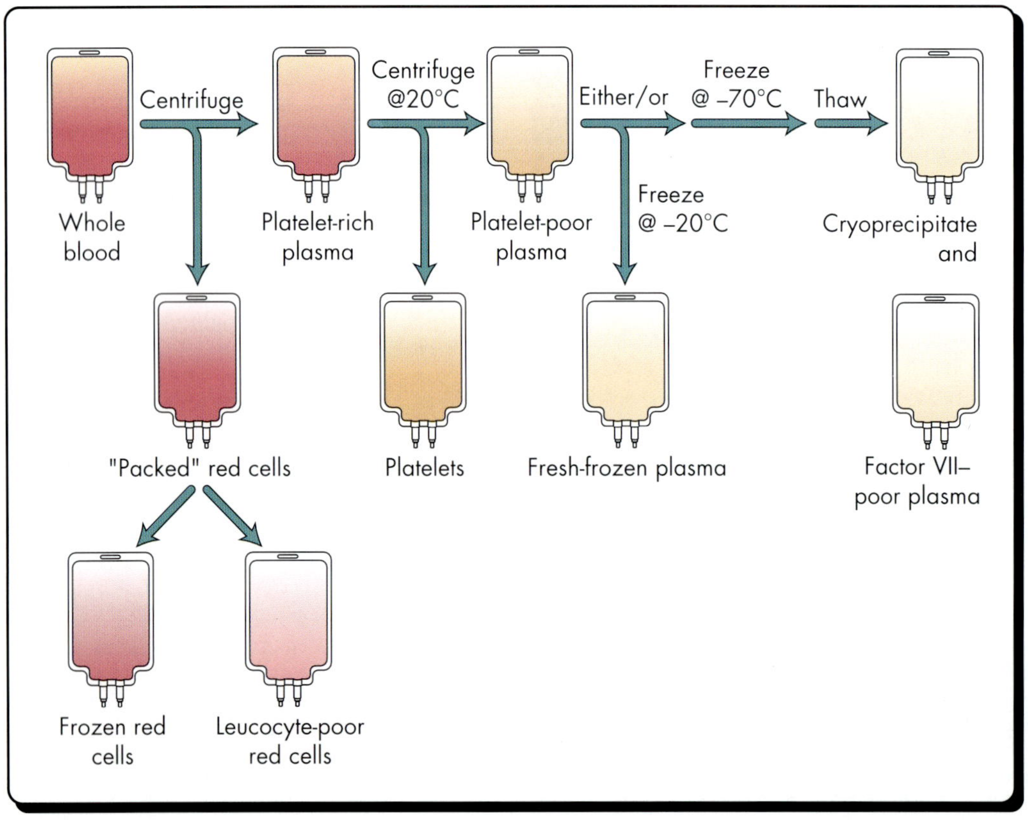

Figure 7-5. The steps used in separating donated whole blood into various components. Component therapy is a major advance in transfusion medicine whereby several discrete products are derived from one donor unit. Component therapy allows administration of the specific fraction of blood that a patient lacks. After appropriate donor screening and skin site preparation, the donor blood is harvested into a bag containing anticoagulant, usually citrate phosphate dextrose. Whole blood is centrifuged to yield packed red blood cells (PRBCs) and platelet rich plasma. The latter is centrifuged again and separated into platelets and platelet poor plasma. A unit of platelet poor plasma can be processed into *either* fresh frozen plasma or cryoprecipitate.

If the platelet poor plasma is frozen to –20°C, then the product is called fresh frozen plasma (FFP). Plasma that is "fresh frozen" contains all plasma proteins, including the labile factors V and VIII. Cryoprecipitate (CRYO) is formed when platelet poor plasma is frozen to –70°C and then thawed. (*Adapted from* Miller [15]; with permission.)

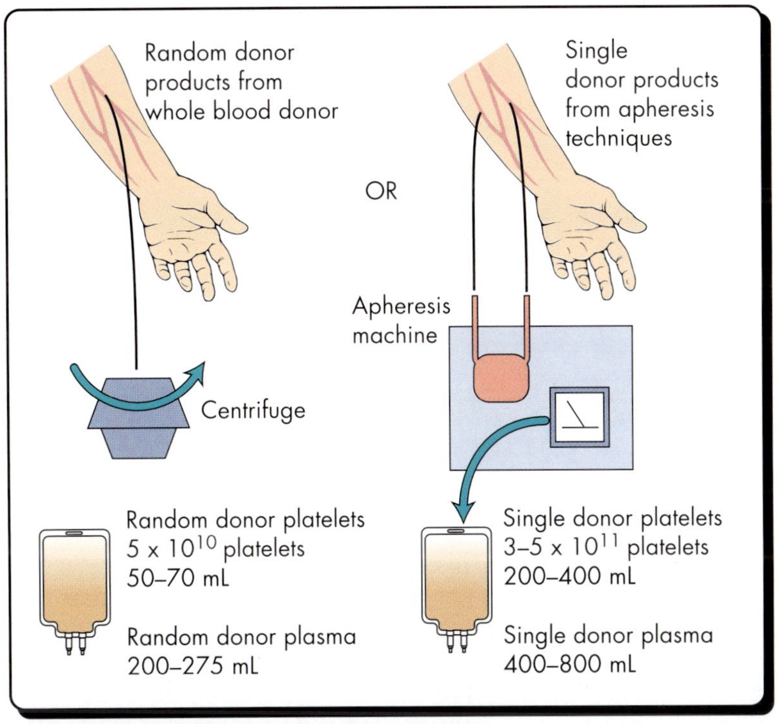

Figure 7-6. Platelet collection. There are two types of platelet products and two types of plasma products. *Random donor* products are derived from the centrifugation and separation process described in Figure 7-5. *Single donor* products are derived from apheresis techniques, which collect the equivalent of 4 to 8 random donor platelet units or two units of plasma from a single donor. These products are preserved with citrated anticoagulant solutions.

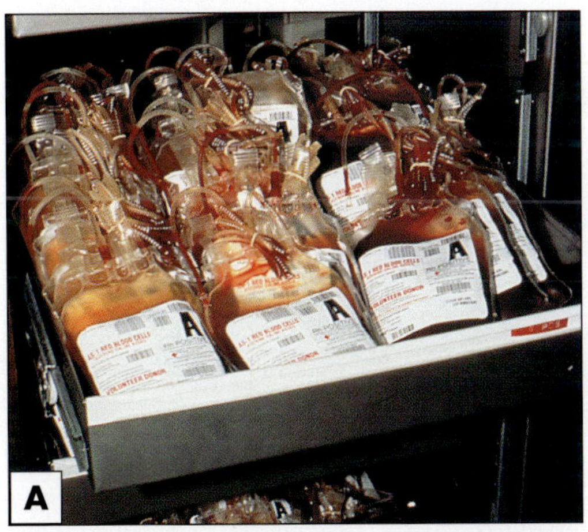

Figure 7-7. Red blood cell composition and storage. Red blood cells require energy for a variety of cellular functions including: maintenance of shape and flexibility, maintenance of iron in hemoglobin in the ferrous state, and maintenance of transmembrane electrolyte concentrations. Refrigeration (**A** and **B**) and modern anticoagulant-preservative solutions (**C**) allow stored PRBCs to remain viable for at least 35 days. Citrate phosphate dextrose (CPD) is the basic anticoagulant preservative used most frequently. Normal coagulation mechanisms require calcium as a cofactor. Citrate acts as an anticoagulant by chelating calcium thus preventing clotting of blood. Dextrose provides the cells with an energy source, while refrigeration reduces the metabolic activity of the red cells. Phosphate is added as a buffer. The addition of adenine (CPDA-1) allows the red cells to resynthesize adenosine triphosphate (ATP), extending the storage from 21 to 35 days. The storage time can be extended even further by the addition of special preservative solutions containing a variety of chemicals such as adenine, mannitol, additional glucose, and sodium chloride.

B. RED BLOOD CELLS: COMPOSITION AND STORAGE CONDITIONS

	CPDA-1*	AS-1, AS-3*
Contents per unit	Red blood cells suspended in a small amount of anticoagulant solution and plasma Hematocrit 70–80%	Red blood cells suspended in a small amount of anticoagulant solution and plasma Hematocrit 55%–65%
Long-term storage conditions	Refrigerated at 1°–6°C	Refrigerated at 1°–6°C
Shelf life	Refrigerated: 35 days	Refrigerated: 42 days

*See: Fig.7-7 C: Anticoagulant solutions.

C. COMMON ANTICOAGULANT SOLUTIONS*

	CDPA-1	CPD	ADSOL AS-1	Nutricel AS-3
Sodium Citrate	1.66 g	1.66 g		588 mg
Citric acid	206 mg	206 mg		42 mg
Sodium Phosphate	140 mg	140 mg		276 mg
Dextrose	2.0 g	3.22 g	2.2 g	1.1 g
Sodium chloride			900 mg	400 mg
Mannitol			750 mg	
Adenine	17.3 mg		27 mg	30 mg

*Typical composition of 1 unit of PRBCs.

Despite preservative solutions, a number of biochemical changes occur in stored blood (referred to as "the storage lesion"). The plasma pH falls and PCO_2 rises as red cells metabolize glucose (dextrose) to lactate. Plasma potassium concentrations rise, while red cell 2,3 diphosphoglycerate levels fall. The osmotic fragility of red cells increases, which may account for the tendency of older PRBCs to sludge in the microvasculature [16].

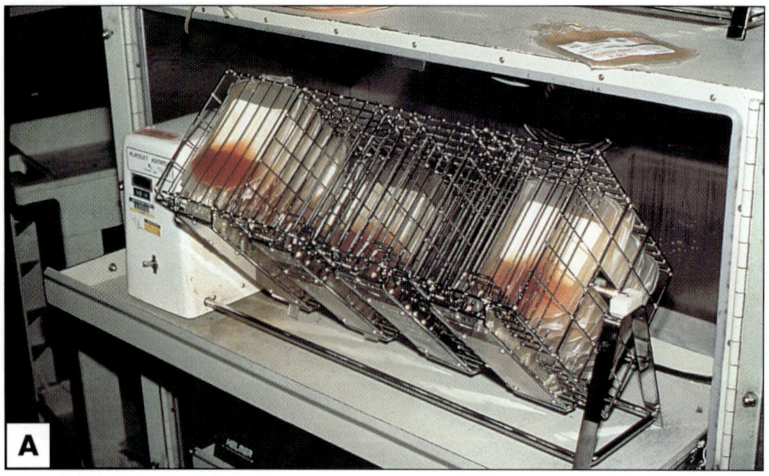

B. PLATELETS: COMPOSITION AND STORAGE CONDITIONS

Contents per unit
- 5.5 *times* 10^{10} platelets suspended in 50 mL of donor plasma

Long-term storage conditions
- Room temperature
- Constant, gentle agitation

Shelf life
- Unpooled units: 5 days
- Pooled: 4 hours; Do not refrigerate

Figure 7-8. Platelet storage and composition (A and B). Random donor and single donor platelets are suspended in a small amount of anticoagulant solution and donor plasma. A and B, Platelets are constantly agitated at room temperature in plastic containers and can be safely stored for up to five days. The metabolically active platelet concentrates are kept in semipermeable plastic containers that allow carbon dioxide to escape and oxygen to enter.

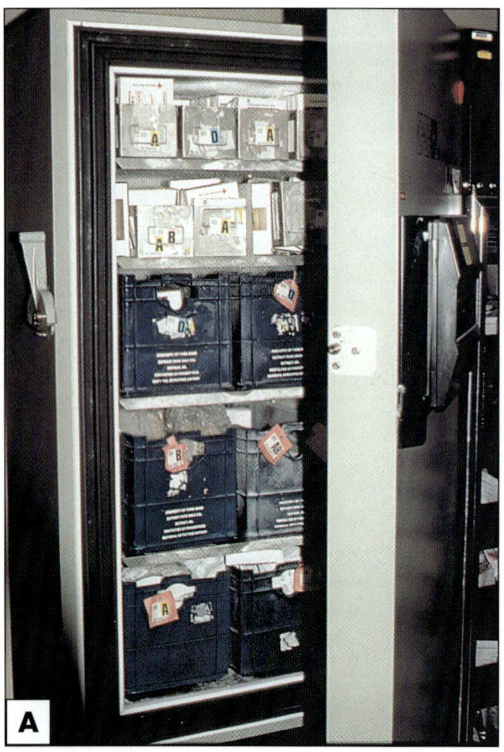

B. PLASMA PRODUCTS: COMPOSITION AND STORAGE CONDITIONS

	FFP	Cryoprecipitate
Contents per unit	All of the plasma proteins Labile factor V Labile factor VIII	≈100 Units of Factor VIII activity 170–250 mg fibrinogen von Willebrand factor Fibronectin
Long-term storage conditions	Frozen at < – 18°C	Frozen at < –18°C
Shelf life	Frozen: one year Thawed: 24 hours Refrigerate at 1°-6°C	Frozen: one year Thawed: transfuse immediately; do not refrigerate

Figure 7-9. Storage and composition of plasma and cryoprecipitate (A and B). Fresh frozen plasma (FFP) is plasma that has been collected either by component separation or by apheresis techniques and is frozen within 6 hours of collection. It is kept frozen at –18°C or lower to preserve the activity of labile coagulation factors. Single donor plasma (SDP) is comparable to FFP except that it is relatively deficient in Factor V. SDP comes from several sources: it can be separated from whole blood any time during storage up to 5 days after expiration or prepared from outdated FFP. Cryoprecipitate contains large quantities of factor VIII, von Willebrand factor, fibrinogen, fibronectin and factor XIII. Each unit of cryoprecipitate contains approximately 70-100 units of factor VIII activity and 250 mg of fibrinogen. Cryoprecipitate and FFP are stored frozen and can be kept frozen up to one year. Once thawed, FFP and cryoprecipitate should be transfused as soon as possible. FFP can be kept stored at 1–6°C up to 24 hours, but pooled cryoprecipitate should not be refrigerated and is outdated in four hours.

PHYSIOLOGY OF BLOOD COMPONENTS

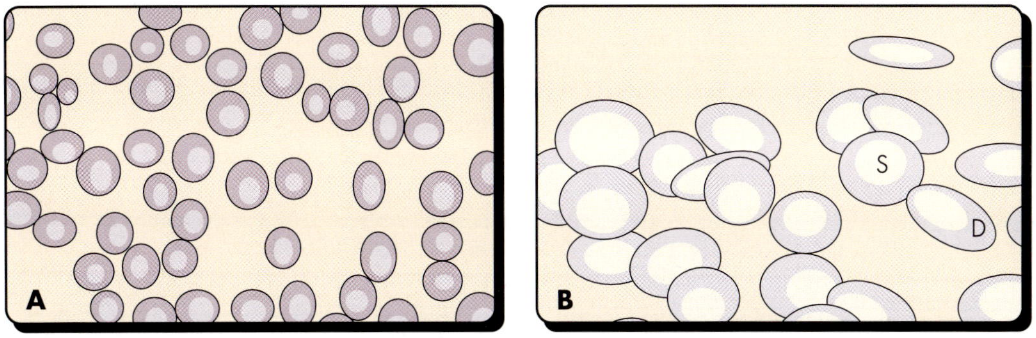

Figure 7-10. Physiology of blood components. Red blood cells (**A**) in transfused blood are the simplest cells of the body. Circulating PRBCs normally do not have nuclei, ribosomes, mitochondria, or Golgi aperta. Thus, they are unable to synthesize new proteins. Ninety-five percent of the protein in PRBCs is hemoglobin, an extremely efficient oxygen carrier. The intracellular location of hemoglobin allows adequate oxygen carrying capacity without the significant plasma oncotic effect it would otherwise have as a free plasma protein.

Normal circulating PRBCs are shaped as biconcave discs and are remarkably plastic. PRBCs can fit through capillaries 1/2 the diameter of the cell. RBC membranes can stiffen and become less deformable with age or storage. Thus, older transfused cells may be more prone to sludging in the microcirculation.

Plasma contains a large assortment of proteins and macromolecules, low molecular weight electrolytes, and uncharged solutes in a complex aqueous solution. Besides the labile and stable coagulation factors, it contains fibrinolytic factors, immunoglobulins, complement components, and transport proteins such as albumin. Albumin plays an important role in the maintenance of plasma oncotic pressure and blood volume. It also serves as a transport protein for small organic molecules including many drugs and toxins. The immunoglobulins and complement proteins function together to clear antigenic material. The coagulation and fibrinolytic factors are responsible for the production and destruction of fibrin. Serine protease inhibitors, like antithrombin III and C1 inhibitor, are involved in the regulation of other coagulation enzymes [17].

Platelets (**B**) are membrane-encapsulated cytoplasmic fragments derived from megakaryocytes in the bone marrow. The platelet lacks a nucleus and is unable to synthesize new proteins but can support metabolic activity such as arachidonate metabolism, phospholipid metabolism, and secretion of granule contents. The nonactivated platelet is disc shaped. Platelets adhere to subendothelium exposed by vascular injury and play a pivotal role in forming the initial hemostatic plug. Adhered platelets change their shape from discoid to spheroid, release the contents of their granules, and aggregate or cohere. The procoagulant surface of activated platelets initiates and promotes a number of steps in the coagulation cascade [18]. D—disk-shaped platelet, S—Spheroid platelets.

COMPONENT THERAPY

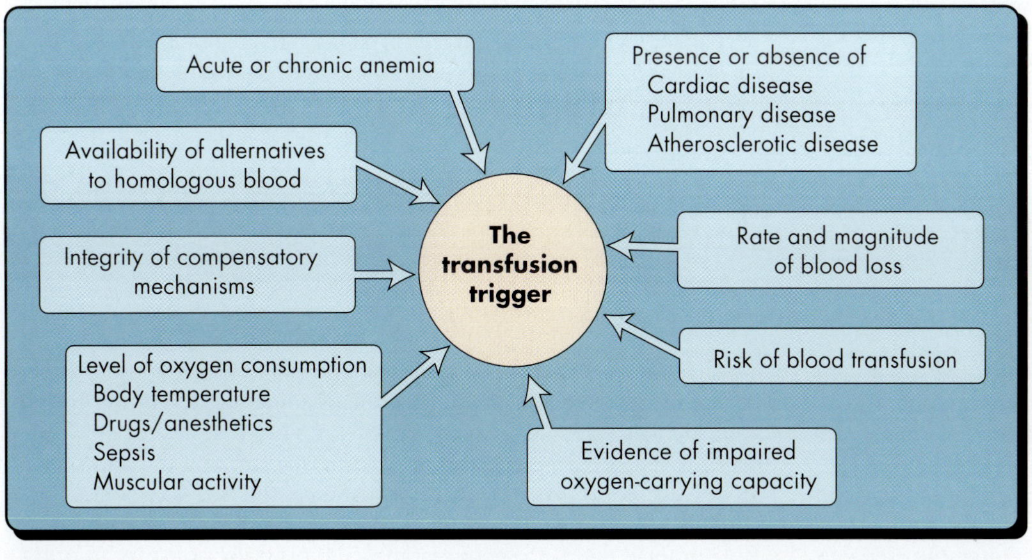

Figure 7-11. The transfusion "trigger." Multiple factors must be considered prior to transfusing blood products. For instance, the decision to transfuse *red blood cells* is based on evidence of inadequate oxygen delivery due to impaired oxygen carrying capacity. The primary adverse clinical effect of decreased oxygenation is potential ischemia of the brain, myocardium and other vital organs. Determining whether anemia is contributing to inadequate oxygen delivery requires evaluation of multiple variables. Use of a 'transfusion trigger' based only on a hemoglobin level is no longer acceptable. Chronic anemia is better tolerated than acute anemia because of increases in 2,3 diphosphoglycerate levels. The normal compensation for anemia is increased cardiac output, and there are many factors that can limit or impair the patient's ability to compensate for anemia (cardiopulmonary reserve). Older patients may be less able to increase stroke volume and cardiac output in response to exercise [19]. The presence of coexisting diseases such as peripheral vascular occlusive disease or coronary artery disease may impair compensatory mechanisms or change the hemoglobin level at which organ ischemia is likely to occur. The adequacy of oxygen delivery depends on the oxygen consumption. The mixed venous oxygen saturation (SVO_2) is a rough indicator of the balance between whole body oxygen consumption and delivery. Multiple factors including anesthesia can increase or decrease the level of oxygen consumption. Finally, the anesthesiologist must take into account the dynamic nature of surgical hemorrhage. Many of these considerations apply not only to the transfusion of PRBCs but also to the transfusion of other blood components as well. Fortunately, there are several published guidelines establishing criteria and indications for blood transfusion [1,20–22].

ASA PRACTICE GUIDELINES FOR BLOOD COMPONENT THERAPY

Recommendations: RBC

The task force concludes that

(1) transfusion is rarely indicated when the hemoglobin concentration is greater than 10 g/dL and is almost always indicated when it is less than 6 g/dL, especially when the anemia is acute.

(2) the determination of whether intermediate hemoglobin concentrations (6-10 g/dL) justify or require RBC transfusion should he based on the patient's risk for complications of inadequate oxygenation.

(3) the use of a single hemoglobin "trigger" for all patients and other approaches that fail to consider all important physiologic and surgical factors affecting oxygenation are not recommended.

(4) when appropriate, preoperative autologous blood donation, intraoperative and postoperative blood recovery, acute normovolemic hemodilution, and measures to decrease blood loss (deliberate hypotension and pharmacologic agents) may be beneficial.

(5) the indications for transfusion of autologous RBCs may be more liberal than for allogeneic RBCs because of the lower (but still significant) risks associated with the former.

Recommendations: Platelets

The task force concludes that

(1) prophylactic platelet transfusion is ineffective and rarely indicated when thrombocytopenia is due to increased platelet destruction (*e.g.*, idiopathic thrombocytopenic purpura).

(2) prophylactic platelet transfusion is rarely indicated in surgical patients with thrombocytopenia due to decreased platelet production when the platelet count is greater than 100×10^9/L and is usually indicated when the count is below 50×10^9/L. the determination of whether patients with intermediate platelet counts ($50–100 \times 10^9$/L) require therapy should be based on the risk of bleeding.

(3) surgical and obstetric patients with microvascular bleeding usually require platelet transfusion if the platelet count is less than 50×10^9l and rarely require therapy if it is greater than $100/10^9$/L. With intermediate platelet counts ($50–100 \times 10^9$/L), the determination should be based on the patient's risk for more significant bleeding.

(4) vaginal deliveries or operative procedures ordinarily associated with insignificant blood loss may be undertaken in patients with platelet counts less than 50×10^9/L.

(5) platelet transfusion may be indicated despite an apparently adequate platelet count if there is known platelet dysfunction and microvascular bleeding.

Recommendations: FFP

The task force recommends the administration of FFP with the following guidelines:

(1) for urgent reversal of warfarin therapy.

(2) for correction of known coagulation factor deficiencies for specific concentrates are unavailable.

(3) for correction of microvascular bleeding in the presence of elevated (> 1.5 times normal) PT or PIT.

(4) for correction of microvascular bleeding secondary to coagulation factor deficiency in patients transfused with more than one blood volume and when PT and PIT cannot be obtained in a timely fashion.

(5) FFP should be given in doses calculated to achieve a minimum of 30% of plasma factor concentration (usually achieved with administration of 10–15 mL/kg of FFP), except for urgent reversal of warfarin anticoagulation, for which 5-8 ml/kg of FFP usually will suffice. Four to five platelet concentrates, on unit of single donor apheresis platelets, or one unit o whole blood provide a quantity of coagulation factors similar to that contained in one unit of FFP (except for decreased, but still hemostatic, concentrations of factors V and VIII in whole blood).

(6) FFP is contraindicated for augmentation of plasma volume or albumin concentration.

Recommendations: Cryoprecipitate

The task force recommends considering the administration of cryoprecipitate for

(1) prophylaxis in nonbleeding perioperative or peripartum patients with congenital fibrinogen deficiencies or von Willebrand's disease unresponsive to DDAVP (whenever possible, these decisions should be made in consultation with the patient's hematologist).

(2) bleeding patients with von Willebrand's disease.

(3) correction of microvascular bleeding in massively transfused patients with fibrinogen concentrations less than 80–100 mg/dL (or when fibrinogen concentrations cannot be measured in a timely fashion).

Figure 7-12. Indications for transfusion. Recently, the American Society of Anesthesiologist Task Force on Blood Component Therapy published practice guidelines for transfusing red blood cells, platelets, fresh-frozen plasma and cryoprecipitate [2]. The ASA guidelines focused on the effectiveness of perioperative and peripartum blood component therapy. The task force reviewed the published scientific evidence and expert opinion regarding the effectiveness of transfusion therapy. They then considered the potential clinical benefits, adverse effects, and costs of blood component therapy in their determination of effectiveness. Other groups, including the National Institutes of Health and the College of American Pathologists, have issued similar clinical guidelines for blood component therapy [1,20,21]. Practice guidelines are helpful but not foolproof in assisting the anesthesiologist in determining the appropriateness of blood transfusions. For instance, the ASA task force guidelines recommend the use of cryoprecipitate in patients with von Willebrand's disease. These recommendations are contrary to other authorities who advocate the use of virally inactivated factor VIII concentrates in this setting [23]. (*From* American Society of Anesthesiologists [24]; with permission.)

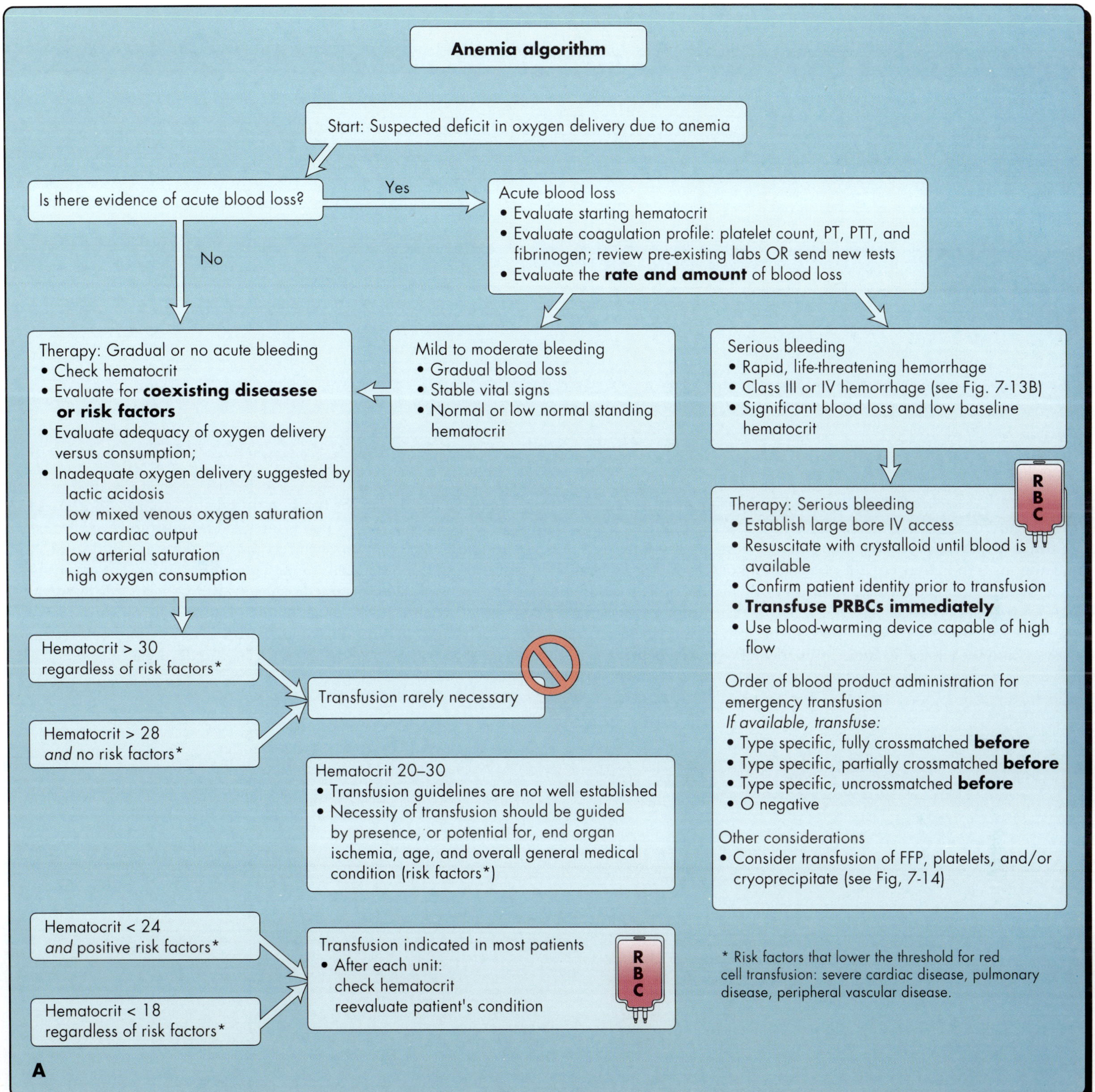

Figure 7-13. Suspected deficit in oxygen delivery due to anemia. A, Anemia algorithm. Initial steps should include evaluation of the airway, breathing, and circulation and administration of supplemental oxygen, if indicated. Established intravenous access and administer crystalloid if the patient shows signs of hypovolemia. Positively identify the patient according to hospital guidelines, and check if the patient has a current blood type and screen sample in the blood bank. If none is available, draw a blood sample, label properly, and deliver to the blood bank.

(Continued on next page)

B. AMERICAN COLLEGE OF SURGEONS CLASSES OF ACUTE HEMORRHAGE

Factors	Class I	Class II	Class III	Class IV
Blood loss, *ml**	Up to 750	750–1500	1500–2000	2000 or more
Blood loss, %*BV**	Up to 15	15–30	30–40	40 or more
Pulse, *BPM*	> 100	> 100	> 120	140 or higher
Blood pressure	Normal	Normal	Decreased	Decreased
Pulse pressure (mm Hg)	Normal or increased	Decreased	Decreased	Decreased
Capillary refill test	Normal	Positive	Positive	Positive
Respiration *per min*	14–20	20–30	30–40	> 35
Urine output, *ml/hr*	30 or more	20–30	5–15	Negligible
CNS (mental status)	Slightly anxious	Mildly anxious	Anxious confused	Confused lethargic
Fluid replacement (3:1 rule)	Crystalloid	Crystalloid	Crystalloid + blood	Crystalloid + blood

*For a 70-kg male.

Figure 7-13. (*Continued*) Early on, determine whether acute bleeding is present and if so, determine the rate and degree of hemorrhage (**B**). Significant hemorrhage (*eg*, hypotension that does not respond to rapid administration of up to 2 L of crystalloid or Class III or IV hemorrhage) may require immediate infusion of PRBCs. In other cases, the practitioner should *check a hematocrit* before transfusion. Besides the hematocrit, other factors such as the patient's pre-existing medical condition and the clinical evidence of inadequate oxygen delivery should be factored in to the decision to transfuse. This algorithm is for instructional purposes only and is intended to illustrate possible decision making based on published recommendations and indications for transfusion of red blood cells to patients with anemia. The algorithm has not been validated or tested clinically. BPM—beats per minute; BV—blood volume; FFP—fresh frozen plasma; PT—prothrombin time; PTT—partial thrombin time. (Part B Courtesy of the American College of Surgeons, 55 Eque Street, Chicago, IL 60611.)

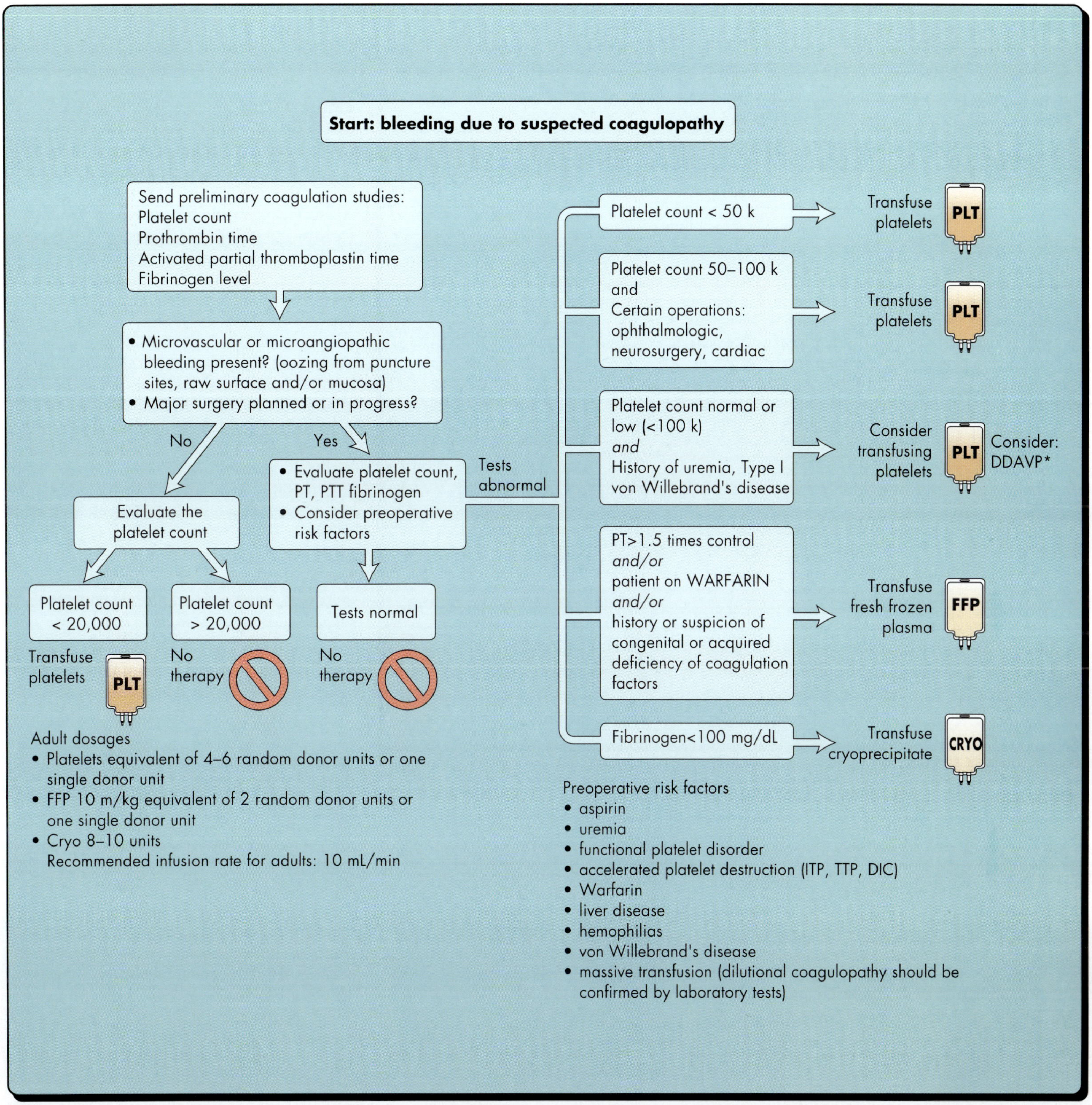

Figure 7-14. Coagulopathy algorithm. Initial steps should include evaluation of the airway, breathing, and circulation and administration of supplemental oxygen, if indicated. Establish intravenous access and administer crystalloid if the patient shows signs of hypovolemia. Positively identify the patient according to hospital guidelines and check if the patient has a current blood type and screen sample in the blood bank. If none is available, draw a blood sample, label it properly and deliver it to the blood bank. *Platelet transfusions* are indicated where either decreased platelet numbers or abnormal platelet function impair the patient's ability to form platelet plugs at bleeding sites. Regardless of evidence of bleeding or plans for surgery, most patients with a platelet count less than 20,000/mm^3 are at risk of bleeding and should be transfused platelets prophylactically. Otherwise, the transfusion is based on the clinical abnormality of microvascular bleeding or plans for surgery in the presence of laboratory abnormalities such as a low platelet count. Microvascular bleeding that does not respond to platelet transfusion or other abnormal laboratory values such as elevated prothrombin time, elevated partial thromboplastin time or low fibrinogen level may indicate the need for plasma products. Microvascular bleeding is evidenced by oozing from raw wounds, puncture sites, and mucosal surfaces. This algorithm is for instructional purposes only and is intended to illustrate possible decision making based on published recommendations and indications for transfusion of plasma products and platelets to patients with a coagulopathy. This algorithm has not been validated or tested clinically. Cryo—cryoprecipitate; DIC—disseminated intravascular coagulation; FFP—fresh frozen plasma; ITP—idiopathic thrombocytopenic purpura; PLT—platelets; PT—prothrombin time; PTT—partial thrombin time; TTP—thrombotic thrombocytopenic purpura.

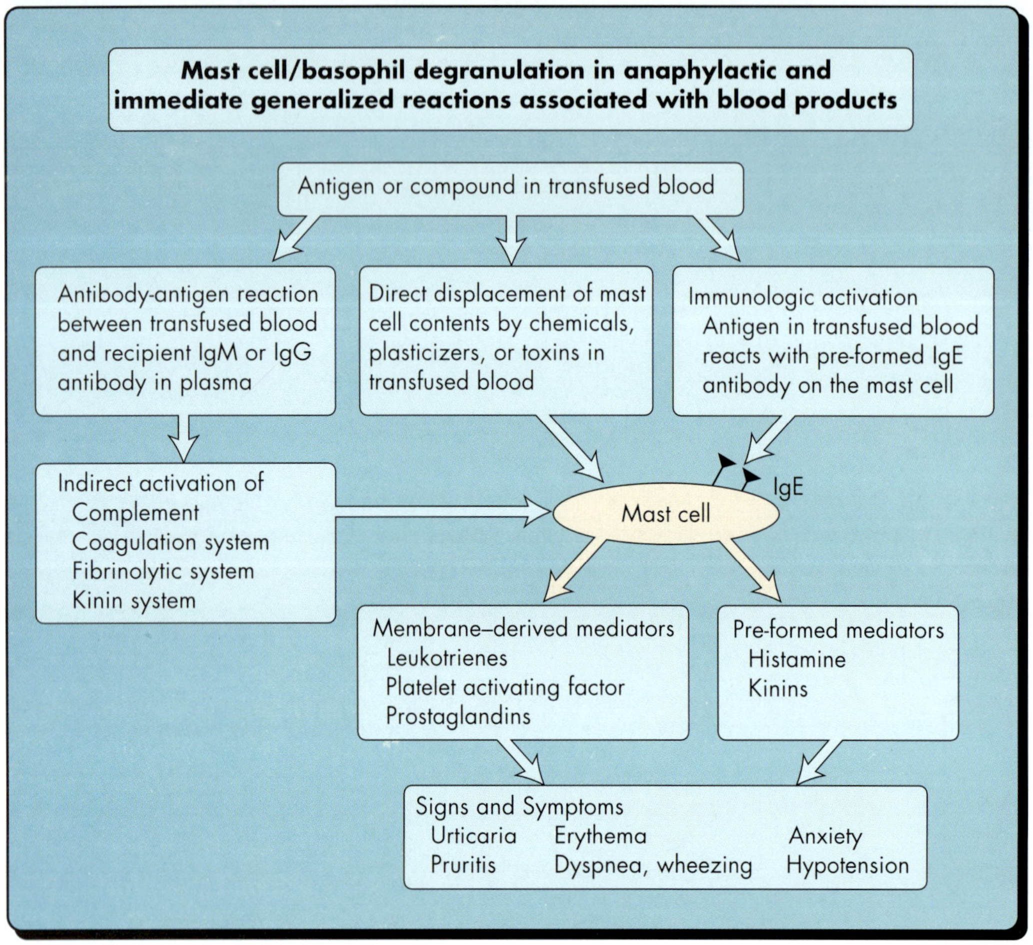

Figure 7-15. Allergic reactions. Allergic reactions are immune-complex–mediated hypersensitivity reactions that can range in severity from minor urticarial reactions to fulminant anaphylactic shock and death. Mast cell activation, through nonimmunologic or immunologic mechanisms, is central to allergic reactions. Antigens in donor blood can react directly with preformed IgE antibodies on the mast cell leading to direct activation. There are several mechanisms for nonimmunologic activation including antigen-IgG or antigen IgM activation of the complement cascade, activation via the coagulation, fibrinolytic or kinin cascades, or direct activation by chemicals, plasticizers, or toxins. Once activated, mast cells degranulate, discharging preformed mediators such as histamine. Activated mast cells also synthesize and release secondary mediators such as leukotrienes. These compounds cause bronchial smooth muscle contraction, increased vascular permeability, and increased glandular secretion leading to typical signs and symptoms [25].

A. ADVERSE REACTIONS TO TRANSFUSION

Type of reaction	Incidence
Febrile reactions	1% of PRBC transfusions; 20% of PLT transfusions
Allergic (urticarial) reactions	1/1000 transfusions
Acute hemolytic transfusion reactions	≈ 1/33,000 U PRBCs
Delayed hemolytic transfusion reactions	≈ 1/2,500 U PRBCs
Transfusion related acute lung injury (TRALI)	1/10,000 U PRBCs

Figure 7-16. Complications of transfusion reactions. **A**, Adverse reactions to transfusion. *Febrile nonhemolytic reactions* are common but are usually self-limited and almost never life-threatening. They are related to the infusion of passenger leukocytes and elevated recipient levels of pyrogenic cytokines (IL-1*beta*, IL-6, TNF-*alpha*). Allergic reactions and acute hemolytic reactions are discussed in separate figures. *Delayed hemolytic reactions* are secondary immune responses that are often difficult to diagnose due to nonspecific signs of low-grade fever, anemia, and hyperbilirubinemia. *Graft vs. host disease* (GVHD) is a rare complication where donor lymphocytes engraft in the recipient leading to a syndrome of chronic rejection affecting the skin, lung, and kidneys. Patients at risk for GVHD include HLA-matched relatives of the donor (as in directed donation), bone marrow transplant recipients, patients with immunodeficiency syndromes or Hodgkin's disease, and neonates. These patients should receive irradiated blood products. The postulated mechanism of *transfusion-related acute lung injury* involves a reaction between donor leukoagglutinating antibodies and the recipient's white cells. This reaction leads to neutrophil sequestration, complement activation, macrophage aggregation, and the release of cytokines and the metabolites of the arachidonic acid cascade within the lung. Transfusion-related lung injury due to inflammation is one of the numerous precipitant events that can result in the adult respiratory distress syndrome [26–28].

B, Infections. Overall, the risk of transmitting viral diseases through blood transfusions continues to decline and is usually smaller than the risks from the underlying disease process [29]. The risk of transmitting HIV through transfusion of properly screened blood has been estimated by several groups and this risk appears to be very small, approximately 1 case in every 493,000 to 660,000 donations [14,30]. Effective screening tests have reduced the risk of acquiring hepatitis C or hepatitis B to *approximately*1 in 34,000 [14]. Cytomegalovirus is probably the most common viral agent transmitted by blood transfusions. Fortunately, transfusion associated CMV infection is subclinical, but it can be a significant threat to immunocompromised patients. Clinically significant disease or death due to bacterial contamination of blood products is extremely rare. A detailed discussion of infectious complications is beyond the scope of this monograph but more information is available in several reviews [31–33].

(*Continued on next page*)

B. INFECTIONS

Type of Infection	Incidence
Viral	
Hepatitis B	1/63,000
Hepatitis C	1/103,000
Hepatitis NA, NB	
CMV	
HIV	1/600,000
Bacterial	1/2,500,000 U PRBCs

C. METABOLIC CONSEQUENCES OF MASSIVE TRANSFUSION

- Storage lesion
- Citrate toxicity
- Derangements in acid-Base balance
- Changes in potassium
- Changes in 2,3-diphosphoglycerate
- Disseminated intravascular coagulation, coagulopathy, and bleeding
- Platelet abnormalities
- Hypothermia

Figure 7-16. (*Continued*) C, Metabolic Consequences of Massive Transfusion. The metabolic consequences of massive transfusion are usually transient and not life-threatening. The "storage lesion" is described in Figure 7-7. Citrate in blood is rapidly metabolized by the liver to bicarbonate unless the rate of transfusion exceeds one unit every 5 minutes or the patient has impaired hepatic function. If citrate metabolism is exceeded, circulating citrate can bind ionized calcium leading to depressed myocardial function and hypotension from hypocalcemia. Transient hyperkalemia can develop during massive transfusion but occasionally the alkalosis from citrate metabolism causes hypokalemia. As stored blood ages, citric acid and lactic acid accumulate. Both of these organic acids are rapidly metabolized. Citrate metabolism can generate an alkalosis that promotes hypokalemia. Hypothermia is a significant problem and should be prevented or treated by active warming of all IV fluids and blood. The vigilant anesthesiologist can avoid many of these potential problems by standard safe transfusion practices and careful monitoring of patient temperature, electrolytes, and coagulation profile [34,35].

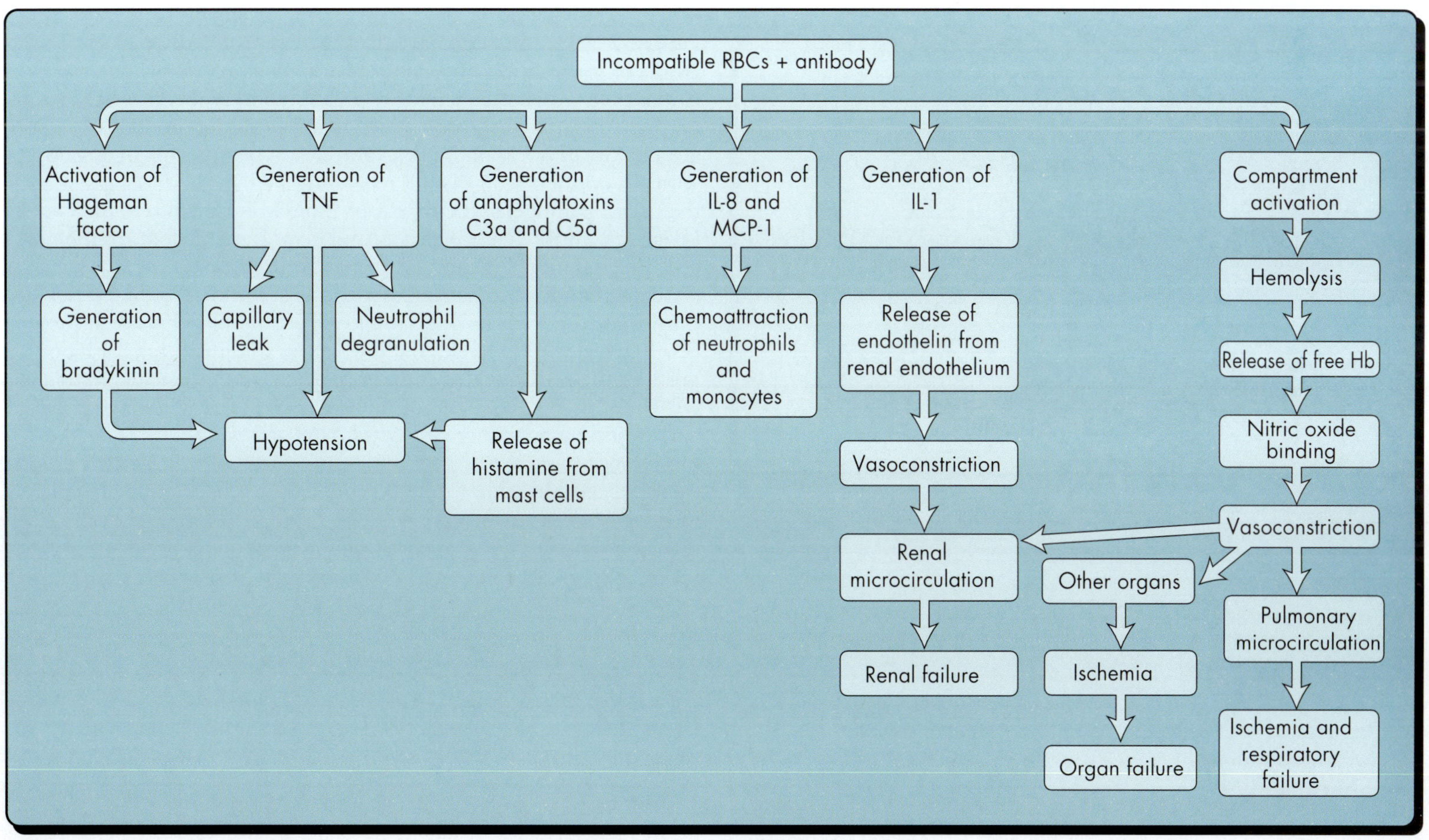

Figure 7-17. Acute hemolytic transfusion reactions. These reactions occur when ABO-incompatible blood is administered to a recipient. Preformed antibodies in the recipient blood react with antigens on the donor red cell. The antigen-antibody complex binds complement leading to donor red cell lysis and a cascade of inflammatory responses. Acute hemolytic transfusion reactions (HTR) are characterized by tachycardia, hypotension, and shock, disseminated intravascular coagulation (DIC), hemoglobinuria, renal failure, and respiratory failure. General anesthesia may mask many of the symptoms and signs of HTRs.

Recent insights into the pathogenetic mechanism of the systemic inflammatory response syndrome (SIRS) and HTRs have allowed investigators to propose various mechanisms to explain the clinical manifestations of HTRs. The clinical similarity between SIRS, sepsis, and HTRs suggests a *common pathway*. In vitro models of antibody-mediated red blood cell incompatibility demonstrate that the administration of incompatible PRBCs with plasma containing antibodies precipitates the release of cytokines, inflammatory mediators, and complement [25]. (Adapted from Capon and Goldfinger [36]; with permission.)

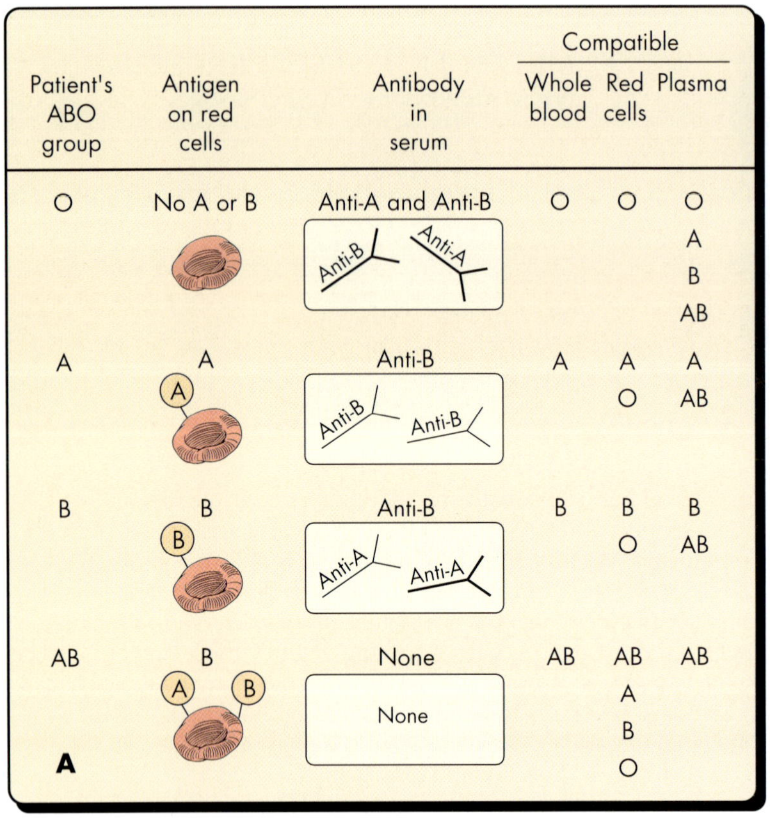

B. POTENTIAL CAUSES OF HEMOLYTIC TRANSFUSION REACTIONS DUE TO ABO ERRORS

Collection of the Recipient Blood Sample 12%–17%

Blood sample drawn from the *wrong* patient*
Misidentification of the blood specimen*
Error in the blood release form

Processing in the Blood Bank 14%–29%

Blood samples misidentified in the blood bank
Recording error or mislabeled blood bag
The wrong donor unit is released from the blood bank
Error made in serologic testing process
Serologic testing failed to identify an antibody < 5%

Administration of Blood Products

Blood given to the wrong patient*

Anesthesiologist needs to take special care to avoid errors in these areas

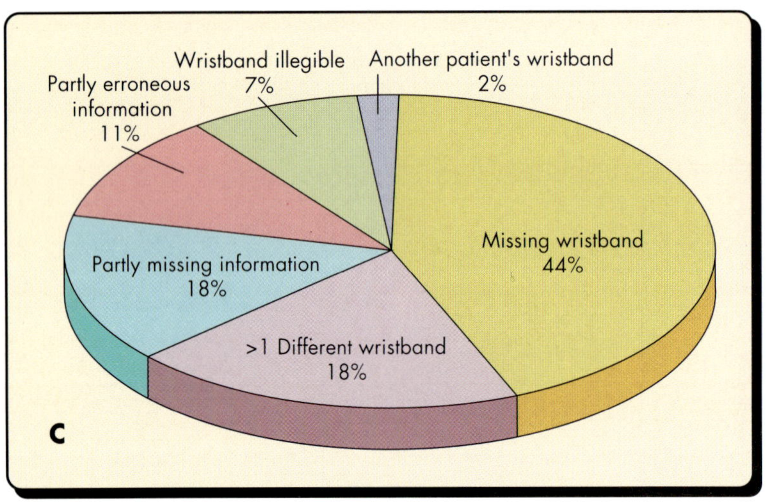

Figure 7-18. ABO compatibility and causes of ABO errors. The ABO compatibility chart demonstrates which blood products are compatible with a recipient of a certain blood type (**A**). ABO incompatibility occurs when pre-formed recipient antibodies react to antigens on the donor blood. For example, a type O recipient has no antigens on their red cells but has preformed antibodies against both the A and B antigens. If either A or B blood is transfused, the O recipient's antibodies will attack and hemolyze the donor red blood cells precipitating a hemolytic transfusion reaction.

Acute hemolytic transfusion reactions are primarily due to human error that can occur during sample collection, blood product processing in the blood bank, and during the administration of blood products (**B**). Misidentification of patients is often attributed to wristband errors (**C**). The graph displays types of wristband errors and their frequency (not related to ABO errors) [37,38]. The anesthesiologist must exercise extreme care when collecting patient blood samples, checking donor blood products and checking the recipient's identity before transfusion.

MANAGEMENT OF A SUSPECTED TRANSFUSION REACTION

Primary Treatment

1. Stop the transfusion immediately
2. Administer oxygen and intubate airway, if necessary.
3. Request assistance immediately. If the patient is suffering from cardiopulmonary collapse, initiate CPR.
4. Disconnect the intravenous line form the intravenous catheter. Attach a new IV tubing set and prime with saline. Open the line to a slow drip. In certain cases, such as a mild urticarial reaction or a repeated chill fever reaction, it maybe possible to restart the blood transfusion after evaluation and initial treatment of the patient.
5. Administer epinephrine for treatment of *cardiopulmonary collapse* and/or *bronchoconstriction.*
6. Consider secondary treatment measures depending on the nature of the transfusion reaction. (See Anaphylactic Reactions in this chapter)
7. Check to ensure that the patient name and registration number on the blood bag label corresponds exactly with information on the patients wristband
8. Save the unit of blood for subsequent investigation of the suspected blood transfusion

Secondary Treatment

1. Administer antihistamines, diphenphydramine 1 mg/kg and ranitidine 1 mg/kg.
2. For persistent bronchospasm: aminophylline 6 mg/kg AND/OR inhaled β agonists.
3. Hydrocortisone 5 mg/kg initially, then 2.5 mg/kg q 4–6 h OR methylprednisolone 1 mg/kg initially, then 0.8 mg/kg q 4–6 h.
4. For persistent hypotension, continue catecholamines by continuous infusion
   - Epinephrine
   - Norepinephrine
   - Dopamine 5–15 μg/kg/min
5. Check arterial blood gases, adjust ventilation as needed and administer bicarbonate as indicated.

Figure 7-19. Management of a suspected transfusion reaction. CPR—cardiopulmonary resuscitation; IV—intravenous.

BLOOD CONSERVATION METHODS

A. COST-EFFECTIVENESS OF VARIOUS MEDICAL INTERVENTIONS

Intervention	Cost per QALY
CABG for "left main" disease, compared with medical therapy	$6,000
Pap smear every 4 y	$11,000
Propranolol for hypertension compared to no therapy	$12,000
Kidney transplantation	$18,000
Heart transplantation	$30,000
Hemodialysis for end-stage renal disease	$48,000
Captopril for hypertension, compared to no therapy	$79,000
Preoperative autologous blood donation	$200,000

Figure 7-20. Alternatives to homologous blood transfusion. Several strategies have been advocated as methods to reduce or eliminate the use of homologous blood and decrease the risk of transfusion related morbidity and mortality. Preoperative autologous donation (PAD) is considered a safe, effective method in most patients. The amount of blood collected is determined by anticipated use of allogeneic blood and is limited by the time available before the operation. While PAD is effective in reducing the use of homologous blood, the cost per quality-adjusted year of life saved may be very high. Several groups have used complex cost-benefit analyses to evaluate the cost of medical interventions relative to years of life saved (adjusted for quality) by implementing the interventions (**A**).

(*Continued on next page*)

B. THE COST EFFECTIVENESS OF AUTOLOGOUS BLOOD DONATION IN FOUR SURGICAL PROCEDURES

Variable	Total Hip Replacement	Coronary Artery Bypass Grafting	Abdominal Hysterectomy	Transurethral Prostatectomy
Units transfused/units donated	0.84	0.072	0.026	0.04
Added cost per unit transfused, $*	68	107	594	4783
Incremental effectiveness per unit transfused (QALY)*	0.00029	0.00022	0.00044	0.0002
Cost effectiveness, *$/QALY*	235,000	494,000	1,358,000	23,643,000

*As compared with a unit of allogeneic blood

Figure 7-20. (*Continued*) Examples of these interventions are treatment of hypertension, coronary artery bypass grafting surgery, and kidney transplantation. One group estimated the societal cost-effectiveness of preoperative autologous blood donation for four different operations (**B**). They found the cost of each autologous unit to range from $235,000 to over $23 million per quality-adjusted year of life (QALY) saved depending on the operation [6]. Another group estimated that PAD in CABG surgery costs $508,000 to 909,000 per quality-adjusted year of life saved [39].In acute normovolemic hemodilution (ANH), blood is collected from the patient immediately before surgery and replaced with an equal or greater amount of crystalloid. The collected blood is kept fresh and reinfused once major bleeding has stopped. The red cell savings depend on the starting hematocrit, the amount of blood removed during the hemodilution process, and the amount of surgical blood loss. The amount of blood saved by ANH is controversial and there are few if any carefully controlled, randomized clinical studies of ANH. Two separate mathematical models of ANH suggested that the theoretic savings in red cell volume attributable to ANH is less than purported by clinical trials [3,5].

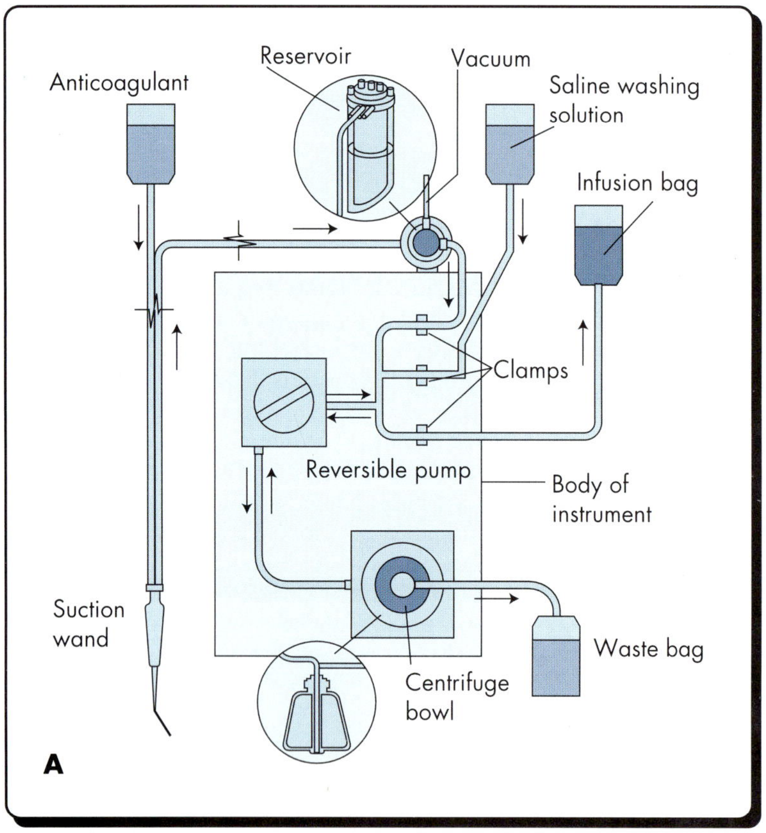

Figure 7-21. Blood cell salvage equipment and methods (**A–C**). Development of a safe, practical method of intraoperative blood salvage can be attributed to Wilson and Taswell at the Mayo Clinic. The "cell-saver" uses a semi-continuous flow, centrifuge-based device that provides washed, saline-suspended red cells for transfusion. **A**, Blood is aspirated from the surgical field and mixed with an anticoagulant. The anticoagulated blood is collected in a cardiotomy reservoir, and when a sufficient amount of blood has been collected, it is pumped into the bottom of the centrifuge bowl. **B**, As the bowl spins, supernatant and waste overflow from the top of the bowl. The PRBCs are washed with normal saline, which circulates through the red blood cell layer and displaces the waste. Eventually, the overflow runs clear and almost all of the free hemoglobin and anticoagulant are washed into the waste bag [40]. (Parts B and C *from* Haemonetics Corporation; with permission; part A *from* Williamson and coworkers [41]; with permission.)

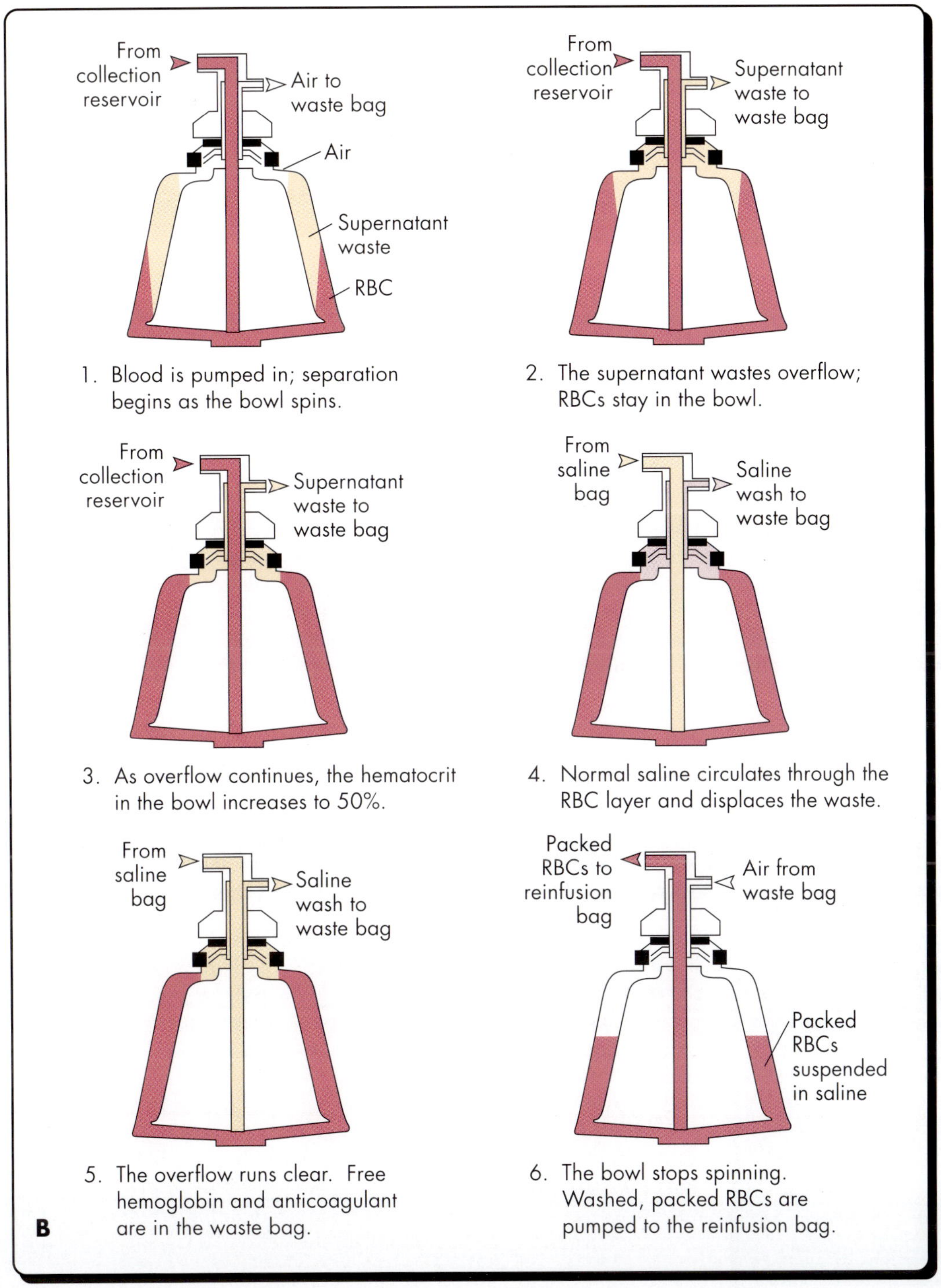

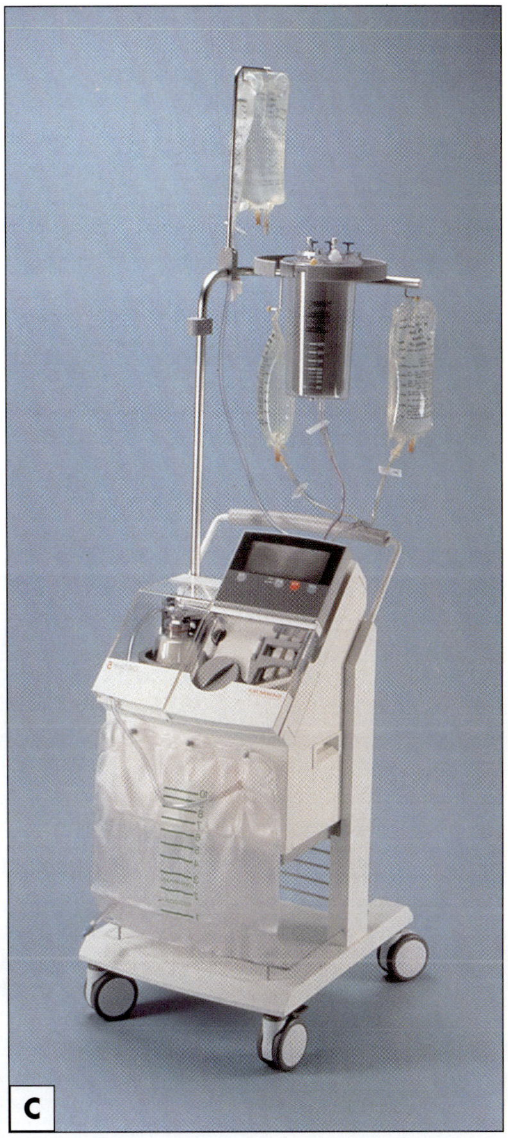

Figure 7-21. *(Continued)*

INDICATIONS, CONTRAINDICATIONS, AND COMPLICATIONS OF INTRAOPERATIVE BLOOD SALVAGE

Indications (approximate recovery)	Contraindications	Complications
Cardiac surgery (50%)	Malignancy controversial	Air embolism
Vascular surgery (60%)	Infection	Coagulopathy
Orthopedic surgery (50%–60%	Microfibrillar collagen hemostatic materials	Infection
Liver transplants (32%–45%)		Miscellaneous
Trauma (28%–60%)		Infusion of toxic antibiotics from irrigants
Neurosurgery?		Removal of therapeutic drugs
Religious reasons		Fat embolism
		Infusion of microaggregates
		Infusion of methyl methacrylate

Figure 7-22. The indications, contraindications, and complications of intraoperative cell salvage. There are very few absolute contraindications to intraoperative cell salvage. Blood salvage should be discontinued once microfibrillar collagen hemostats are used. One of the more dangerous complications is air embolism but the potential for this complication can be reduced by draining the washed blood into a separate "transfer pack" before reinfusion. Salvaged blood is deficient in coagulation factors and platelets and the transfusion of large amounts of washed, salvaged blood may result in a dilutional coagulopathy. A theoretical coagulopathy due to the release of thromboplastic materials from the processed product has been proposed. Despite concerns regarding the potential for septic complications, according to one review: "...there are no reports of infectious complications associated with the routine use of intraoperatively salvaged blood that has been washed and concentrated." [40]. Determination of the cost effectiveness of cell salvage is very complex and depends on multiple factors including the cost of providing homologous blood, the cost of the potential morbidity and mortality of homologous blood, and the amount of blood salvaged versus the capital cost of the equipment and disposables. In certain operations with low blood loss, cell salvage techniques may not be cost effective [40].

INTRAVENOUS ACCESS, TRANSFUSION PROCEDURES AND METHODS

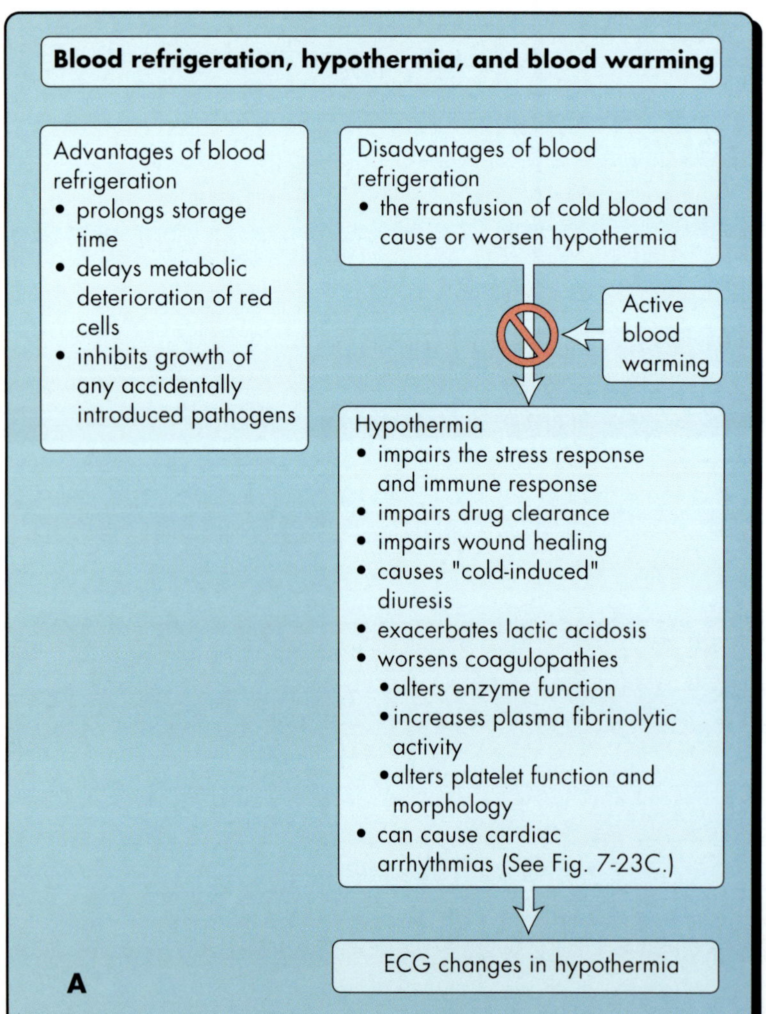

Figure 7-23. Blood refrigeration, hypothermia, and blood warming techniques. Modern preservation technology is based on the effective refrigeration of certain blood components. Refrigeration prolongs the storage time of PRBCs by decreasing metabolic activity (**A**). Refrigeration or freezing of flesh, fruz on plasma (FFP), plasma, cryoprecipitate and PRBCs inhibits growth of any accidentally introduced pathogens. Slow, elective transfusion of one or two units of cold blood is usually well tolerated and active warming is not required. On the other hand, rapid transfusion of cold blood can cause hypothermia.

(*Continued on next page*)

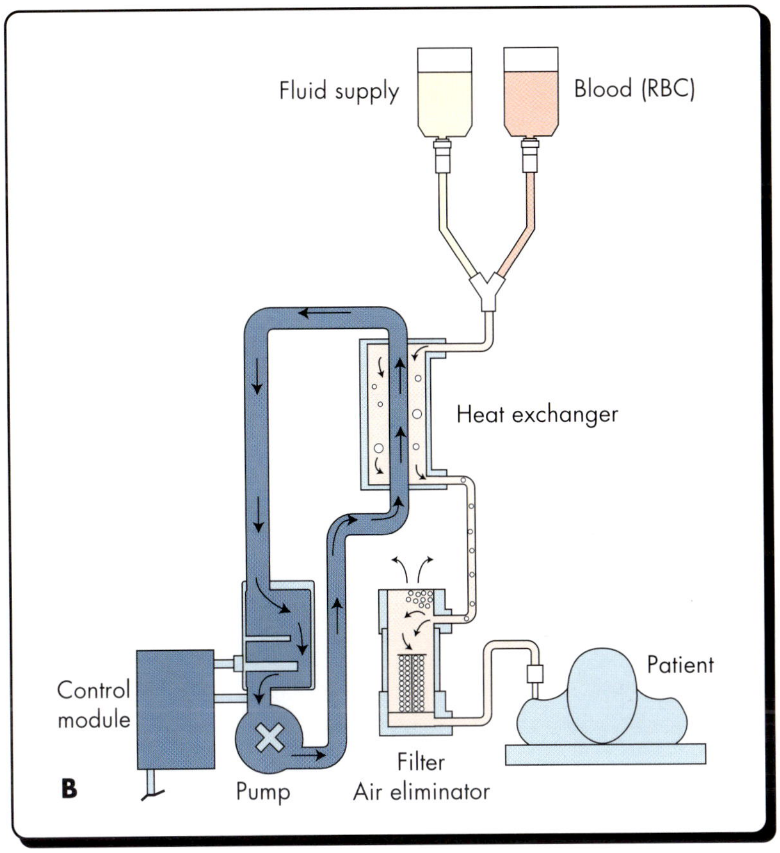

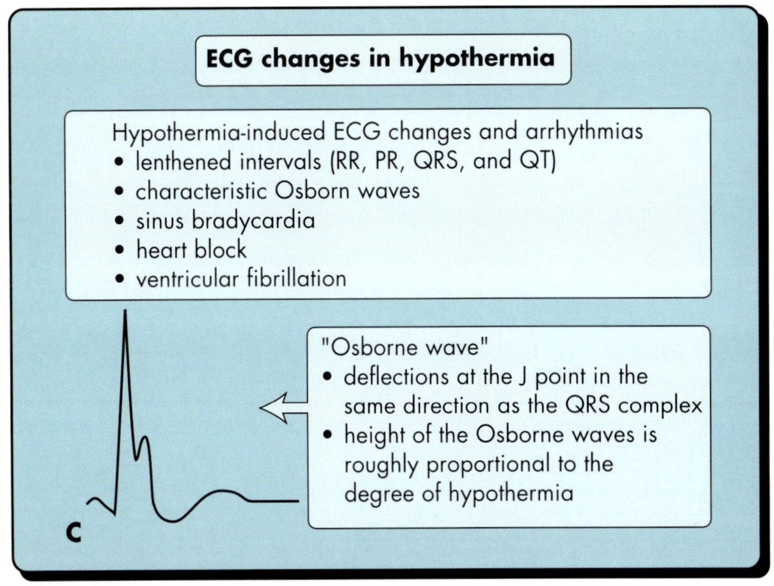

Figure 7-23. (*Continued*) Active measures, such as blood warming (**B**), to prevent intraoperative hypothermia, can significantly decrease morbidity and possibly mortality (**C**) [42]. Effective, active warming is advantageous in *rapid massive transfusion* (patients total blood volume replaced within 24 hours), trauma and infants. The most common method of warming is in-line warming. With in-line warming, the blood is passed through IV tubing that is immersed in a water bath or which passes through dry heaters. Newer water bath warmers make use of the countercurrent heat exchangers. Flow rates can reach up to 750 ml/min and are primarily limited by the flow capacity of the intravenous catheter [43].

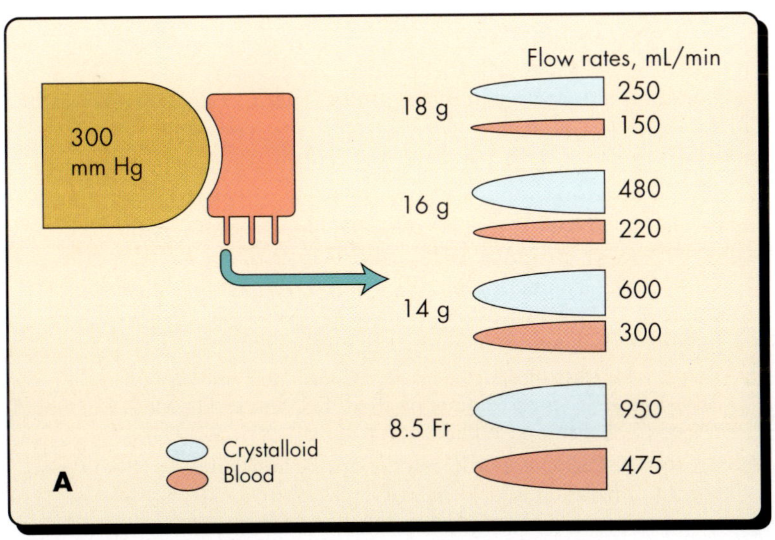

B. FLOW RATE THROUGH LEVEL ONE FLUID WARMER

Cannula size*	Crystalloid	Packed RBCs
Flow rates (mL/min with constant 300 mm Hg pressure)		
18 g	250	150
18 g (2)	440	200
16 g	480	220
16 g (2)	620	260
14 g	600	300
14 g (2)	750	380
8.5 Fr	950	475
Flow rates (mL/min) with gravity (39-in drop)		
18 g	110	40
18 g (2)	185	60
16 g	150	50
16 g (2)	275	60
14 g	260	70
14 g (2)	310	85
8.5 Fr	345	90

*18 g × 1.25 inch long; 16 g × 1.25 inch long; all by Jelco.
8.5 FR × 4 inch long, by Argon.

Figure 7-24. Fluid flow through catheters of different sizes. The resistance to flow of a fluid is directly proportional to the length of the tube, the viscosity of the fluid and the pressure gradient (**A** and **B**). The resistance is inversely proportional to the fourth power of the radius. Thus, small increases in the diameter of infusion catheters result in large decreases in resistance to flow and increases in flow rate. Longer catheters of the same diameter have lower flow rates for a constant driving pressure. Finally, blood is more viscous than crystalloid and flows less rapidly than intravenous (IV) fluid. When massive transfusion is anticipated, the anesthesiologist should insert at least two, large-gauge venous catheters. All blood products and intravenous fluids should be passed through a device capable of efficiently warming fluids at high flow rates. The pressure gradient driving flow can be increased through the use of pressure bags, specialized pumps (Haemonetics Rapid Infuser, Haemontics Corporation, Braintree, MA), or infusion devices (Level One, Level One Technologies, Inc., Rockland, MA) [34]. (Part A *Adapted from* Ping and coworkers [44], with permission; Part B data *from* Level One Technologies, Inc., Rockland, MA; with permission.)

EMERGENCY TRANSFUSION OF BLOOD COMPONENTS

Management of life-threatening hemorrhage requiring urgent blood replacement

1. Infuse available volume expanders until blood products arrive.
   cyrstalloid, hetastarch
2. Draw a blood sample for typing and cross-matching.
   Do not circumvent standard patient identification procedures.
   If feasible, actively warm intravenous fluids and blood products using an in-line warming device.
3. Transfuse group O PRBCs when available.
   Usually does not preclude subsequent transfusion with type specific blood.
4. Transfuse type specific, uncrossmatched blood when available
   Time required for type specific, uncrossmatched blood to be available varies with the blood bank but usually ≈ 10 to 15 min.
   The blood is released prior to the completion of all testing, but complete testing will be carried out.
5. Transfuse type-specific, partially crossmatched blood.
6. Transfuse type specific, crossmatched blood.

Note: If a type and screen is available or the patient but there is no current crossmatch, approximately 20 min are need to crossmatch blood.

Figure 7-25. Management of life-threatening hemorrhage requiring urgent blood replacement.

REFERENCES

1. Office of Medical Applications of Research. National Institutes of Health: Perioperative red blood cell transfusion. *JAMA* 1988, 260:2700–2703.
2. Practice guidelines for blood component therapy: A report by the American Society of Anesthesiologists Task Force on Blood Component Therapy. *Anesthesiology* 1996, 84:732–747.
3. Feldman JM, Roth JV, Bjoraker DG: Maximum blood savings by acute normovolemic hemodilution. *Anesth Analg* 1995, 80:108–113.
4. Monk TG, Goodnough LT, Birkmeyer JD, Brecher ME, Catalona WJ: Acute normovolemic hemodilution is a cost-effective alternative to preoperative autologous blood donation by patients undergoing radical retropubic prostatectomy. *Transfusion* 1995, 35:559–565.
5. Brecher ME, Rosenfeld M: Mathematical and computer modeling of acute normovolemic hemodilution. *Transfusion* 1994, 34:176–179.
6. Etchason J, Petz L, Keeler E, *et al.*: The cost effectiveness of preoperative autologous blood donations. *N Engl J Med* 1995, 332:719–724.
7. Rossi EC, Simon TL, Moss GS, Gould SA: Transfusion into the Next Millennium. In *Principles of Transfusion Medicine*. Edited by Rossi EC, Simon TL, Moss GS, Gould SA, edn 2. Baltimore: Williams & Wilkins; 1995:1–11.
8. Surgenor DM, Wallace EL, Hao SH, Chapman RH: Collection and transfusion of blood in the United States, 1982–1988. *N Engl J Med* 1990, 322:1646–1651.
9. Wallace EL, Surgenor DM, Hao HS, An J, Chapman RH, Churchill WH: Collection and transfusion of blood and blood components in the United States, 1989. *Transfusion* 1993, 33:139–144.
10. Wallace EL, Churchill WH, Surgenor DM, *et al.*: Collection and transfusion of blood and blood components in the United States, 1992. *Transfusion* 1995, 35:802–812.
11. Danielson CF, Filo RS, O'Donnell JA, McCarthy LJ: Institutional variation in hemotherapy for solid organ transplantation. *Transfusion* 1996, 36:263–267.
12. Surgenor DM, Wallace EL, Churchill WH, *et al.*: Red cell transfusions in coronary artery bypass surgery (DRGs 106 and 107). *Transfusion* 1992, 32:458–464.
13. Goodnough LT, Despotis GJ, Hogue C Jr, Ferguson T Jr: On the need for improved transfusion indicators in cardiac surgery. *Ann Thorac Surg* 1995, 60:473–480.
14. Schreiber GB, Busch MP, Kleinman SH, Korelitz JJ: The risk of transfusion-transmitted viral infections. *N Engl J Med* 1996, 334:1685–1690.

14a. Sayers MH: *Arch Pathol Lab Med* 1994, 118:346–349.

15. Miller RD: Transfusion Therapy. In *Anesthesia*. Edited by Miller RD, edn 4. New York: Churchill Livingstone Inc.; 1994:1638.
16. Marik PE, Sibbald WJ: Effect of stored-blood transfusion on oxygen delivery in sepsis. *JAMA* 1993, 269:3024–3029.
17. Carlson TH: Composition of Plasma. In *Principles of Transfusion Medicine*. Edited by Rossi EC, Simon TL, Moss GS, Gould SA, edn 2. Baltimore: Williams & Wilkins; 1995:383–392.
18. Kunicki TJ: Role of Platelets in Hemostasis. In *Principles of Transfusion Medicine*. Edited by Rossi EC, Simon TL, Moss GS, Gould SA, edn 2. Baltimore: Williams & Wilkins; 1995:221–230.
19. Crosby ET: Perioperative haemotherapy: I. Indications for blood component transfusion. *Can J Anaesth* 1992, 39:695–707.
20. Office of Medical Applications of Research. National Institutes of Health. Fresh-frozen plasma: indications and risks. *JAMA* 1985, 253:551–553.
21. Office of Medical Applications of Research. National Institutes of Health. Platelet transfusion therapy. *JAMA* 1987, 257:1777–1780.
22. Stehling L, Zauder HL: Controversies in transfusion medicine. Perioperative hemodilution: pro. *Transfusion* 1994, 34:265–268.
23. Slaughter TF, Greenburg CS: Practice guidelines and treatment of patients with von Willebrand's Disease [letter]. *Anesthesiology* 1996, 85:441–442.
24. American Society of Anesthesiologists: Practice guidelines for blood component therapy. *Anesthesiology* 1996, 84:732–747.
25. Jeter EK, Spivey MA: Noninfectious complications of blood transfusion. *Hematol Oncol Clin North Am* 1995, 9:187–204.
26. Sloop GD, Friedberg RC: Complications of blood transfusion. How to recognize and respond to noninfectious reactions. *Postgrad Med* 1995, 98:159–162, 166, 169–172.

27. Stack G, Judge JV, Snyder EL: Febrile and Nonimmune Transfusion Reactions. In *Principles of Transfusion Medicine*. Edited by Rossi EC, Simon TL, Moss GS, Gould SA, edn 2. Baltimore: Williams & Wilkins; 1995:773–784.
28. Malouf M, Glanville AR: Blood transfusion related adult respiratory distress syndrome. *Anaesth Intensive Care* 1993, 21:44–49.
29. Holland PV: Viral infections and the blood supply. *N Engl J Med* 1996, 334:1734–1735.
30. Lackritz EM, Satten GA, Aberle-Grasse J, *et al.*: Estimated risk of transmission of the human immunodeficiency virus by screened blood in the United States. *N Engl J Med* 1995, 333:1721–1725.
31. Wylie BR: Transfusion transmitted infection: viral and exotic diseases. *Anaesth Intensive Care* 1993, 21:24–30.
32. Crosby ET: Perioperative haemotherapy: II. Risks and complications of blood transfusion. *Can J Anaesth* 1992, 39:822–837.
33. Sazama K: Bacteria in blood for transfusion: a review. *Arch Pathol Lab Med* 1994, 118:350–365.
34. Donaldson MD, Seaman MJ, Park GR: Massive blood transfusion. *Br J Anaesth* 1992, 69:621–630.
35. Labadie LL: Transfusion therapy in the emergency department. *Emerg Med Clin North Am* 1993, 11:379–406.
36. Capon SM, Goldfinger D: Acute hemolytic transfusion reaction, a paradigm of the systemic inflammatory response: new insights into pathophysiology and treatment. *Transfusion* 1995, 35:513–520.
37. Sazama K: Analysis of causes of blood transfusion fatalities. *ASCP Fall 1992 Teleconference Series*: American Society of Clinical Pathologists; 1992.
38. Murray DJ: Blood Component Therapy: Indications and Risks. In *Principles and Practice of Anesthesiology*. Edited by Rogers MC, Tinker JH, Covino BG, Longnecker DE, edn. 2. St. Louis: Mosby-Year Book, Inc.; 1993:2492.
39. Birkmeyer JD, AuBuchon JP, Littenberg B, *et al.*: Cost-effectiveness of preoperative autologous donation in coronary artery bypass grafting. *Ann Thor Surg* 1994, 57:167–169.
40. Williamson KR, Taswell HF: Intraoperative blood salvage: a review. *Transfusion* 1991, 31:662–675.
41. Williamson KR, Taswell HF, Rettke SR, Krom RA: Intraoperative transfusion: its role in orthotopic liver transplantation. *Mayo Clin Proc* 1989, 64:340–345.
42. Kurz A, Sessler DI, Lenhardt R: Perioperative normothermia to reduce the incidence of surgical-wound infection and shorten hospitalization. *N Engl J Med* 1996, 334:1209–1215.
43. Iserson KV, Huestis DW: Blood warming: current applications and techniques. *Transfusion* 1991, 31:558–571.
44. Ping ST, Stene JK, Grande CM: Anesthesia for Trauma. In *Principles and Practice of Anesthesiology*. Edited by Rogers MC, Tinker JH, Covino BG, Longnecker DE, St. Louis: Mosby-Year Book, Inc.; 1993:2219–2220.

8

Deliberate Hypotension

Edward D. Miller, Jr.

Decrease in arterial blood pressure to hypotensive levels during surgery was first proposed by Cushing in 1917 for intracranial surgery and gained popularity in Great Britain in the late 1940s. In 1950 the introduction of ganglionic blocking agents allowed the blood pressure to be decreased in a more controllable manner and the popularity of this technique soared. Unfortunately, in the United States, there appeared to be an increased instance of mortality associated with the use of this technique and deliberate hypotension or controlled hypotension was not put into use until the 1970s.

Decreasing the blood pressure not only decreased blood loss but also allowed for a better surgical field. As surgical operations became more complex, the need for a drier surgical field became apparent. It was also with the contamination of the blood supply that routine administration of blood transfusions was not accepted by the public. These are the two major reasons (*ie*,a drier field and less use of blood products) why deliberate hypotension was frequently used in the 1980s.

A variety of techniques and drugs exist that can induce deliberate hypotension. Mean arterial blood pressures values of 50 to 65 mm Hg have been chosen because these rates are at the lower limit of autoregulation of the brain. Many agents have their own specific advantages and disadvantages; however, in general, an agent is used that has a relatively rapid onset and that can be quickly terminated when the period of deliberate hypotension is no longer needed. All of the anesthetic techniques have the advantage of decreasing blood flow to skin and muscle and, therefore, are responsible for the dramatic decrease in blood loss seen when this technique is used.

Monitoring for deliberate hypotension must be considered prospectively. In general, if potent vasoactive agents are to be used, the placement of an arterial line for monitoring of blood pressure is necessary. Measurement of central venous pressure, pulmonary wedge pressure, or both are required only in those patients in whom that monitoring would be used because of the type of surgery or the patient's condition. For example, monitoring of central pressures is not required just because deliberate hypotension is being used. Some institutions routinely use neurophysiologic monitoring in cases in which deliberate hypotension is used. However, it is not required and there appear to be no reports documenting the value of this type of monitoring.

Much of the investigation into deliberate hypotension has consisted of examining the effects of hypotension on specific organ function. A variety of methods of examining organ functions have been investigated and in general organ perfusion has been shown to be well-maintained as long as deliberate hypotension is coupled with adequate volume replacement. The introduction of hemodilution used in combination with deliberate hypotension is an area of recent research interest. It appears that patients who undergo hemodilution and then receive deliberate hypotension do not have the same hemodynamic profile they would have if deliberate hypotension alone were used.

Complications from deliberate hypotension appear to be no greater than are those of anesthesia itself. There is a slight suggestion that optic neuropathy may occur in the face of deliberate hypotension coupled with hemodilution. Psychometric testing done in a variety of series has shown no difference between patients who receive deliberate hypotension and those who do not.

Deliberate hypotension has been in clinical use for almost 50 years. From a review of the literature, it appears that there continues to be a growing use of this technique as new drugs are developed. Safety of the technique is well-established. In the early use of this technique problems most often occurred when hypotension was allowed to occur because of hemorrhage. Volume replacement with deliberate hypotension is important to prevent serious complications. Deliberate hypotension, therefore, appears to be a safe and reliable method that results in decreased blood loss.

BLOOD LOSS

REPORTED BLOOD LOSSES FOR TOTAL HIP ARTHROPLASTY

References	Hypotensive Technique	Reported Intraoperative Blood Pressure, *mm Hg*	Blood Loss, mL
Amaranath *et al.* (1975) [1]	Halothane, N_2O	Normotensive	1514 ± 273
	Morphine, N_2O, trimethaphan	< 30% control	884 ± 89
	Morphine, N_2O, SNP	< 30% control	820 ± 96
Thompson *et al.* (1978) [2]	Halothane, N_2O	20% control	1183
	Halothane, N_2O	50 MABP	407 ± 102
	Halothane, N_2O, SNP	50 MABP	326 ± 42
Eerola *et al.* (1979) [3]	Halothane, N_2O	> 80 systolic	2336 ± 212
	Halothane, N_2O, pentolinium	< 80 systolic	730 ± 80
Vazeery and Lunde (1979) [4]	N_2O, fentanyl	94 MABP	1038 (500-1750)
	N_2O, fentanyl, SNP	64 MABP	212 (160-350)
Barbier-Böhm *et al.* (1980) [5]	Halothane, N_2O	Normotensive	900 ± 130
	Halothane, N_2O, SNP	55 MABP	320 ± 35
Qvist *et al.* (1982) [6]	N_2O, fentanyl, droperidol	99 MABP	2093 ± 1332
	Halothane, N_2O	73 MABP	718 ± 482

Figure 8-1. Reported blood losses for total hip arthroplasty. Six comparative studies using a variety of anesthetic techniques to lower mean arterial blood pressure to 50 to 65 mm Hg are shown. Blood loss is decreased by almost 50% in patients undergoing total hip arthroplasty. BP—blood pressure; SNP—sodium nitroprusside; MABP—mean arterial blood pressure; N_2O—nitrous oxide. (From Miller [7].)

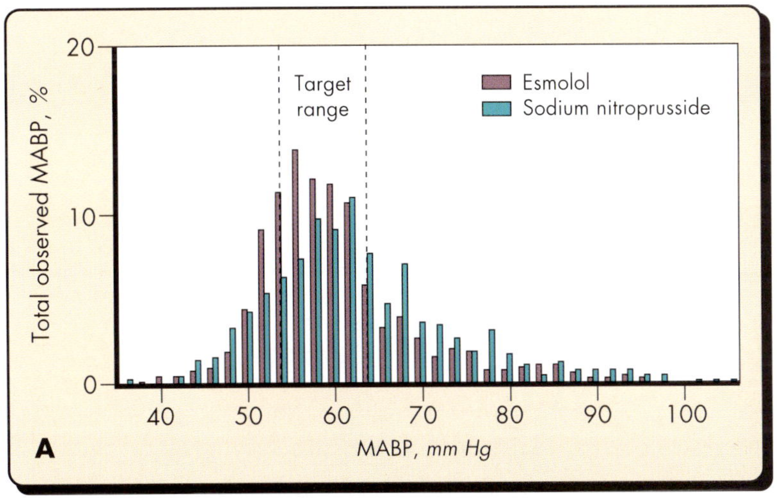

Figure 8-2. Blood loss was decreased by 50% in patients undergoing orthognathic surgery using either sodium nitroprusside (SNP) or esmolol (ESM). ESM was more effective than was SNP because the ability to control blood pressure in the target range (55–65 mm Hg) was more commonly achieved with ESM than with SNP. **A**, Average frequency distributions for mean arterial blood pressure (MABP) in patients receiving ESM or SNP for controlled hypotension. Target range for MABP was 55 to 65 mm Hg. **B**, Duration of surgery, quality of the surgical field, and blood loss in the two study groups. (*From* Blau and coworkers [8]; with permission.)

B. DURATION OF SURGERY, QUALITY OF THE SURGICAL FIELD, AND BLOOD LOSS IN THE TWO STUDY GROUPS*

	Esmolol Group	Sodium Nitroprusside Group	Statistical significance†
Duration of surgery, *min*	214 ± 25	215 ± 15	NS
Duration of hypotension, *min*	95 ± 7	95 ± 9	NS
Surgical field rating‡	1 (1–2.5)	2 (0–4)	$P < 0.05$§
Estimated blood loss, *mL*			
During hypotension	304 ± 48	650 ± 110	$P < 0.01$
Total	436 ± 65	895 ± 101	$P < 0.001$

NS—not significant.
*Results are mean values ± standard error unless otherwise indicated.
†For treatment effect, ESM vs SNP (Student's *t*-test).
‡Median (range); rating scale is 0–5, where 0 is no bleeding, virtually bloodless field, and 5 is massive uncontrollable bleeding.
§Wilcoxon two-sample test.

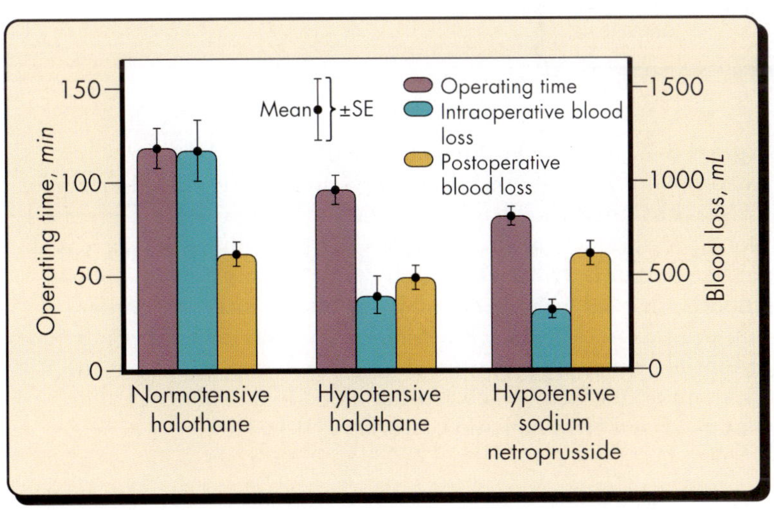

Figure 8-3. The 30 patients undergoing total hip arthroplasty showed a 50% decrease in blood loss intraoperatively when blood pressure was deliberately lowered with sodium nitroprusside or high inspired concentrations of halothane. Not only was blood loss decreased, but operating room time was also significantly decreased. Postoperative blood loss was similar in all three groups. (*From* Thompson and coworkers [2].)

PHYSIOLOGIC TECHNIQUES TO INDUCE DELIBERATE HYPOTENSION

Surgical field at apex
Prevent venous obstruction (no PEEP, no head down position, no spontaneous ventilation)
Adequate anesthesia for this surgical stimulus

Figure 8-4. Physiologic techniques used to induce deliberate hypotension. PEEP—positive end-expiratory pressure.

HEMODYNAMIC REPONSES TO 0.75% BUPIVACAINE IN 29 PATIENTS HAVING TOTAL HIP ARTHROPLASTY*

Variable	Baseline	After Epideural Anesthesia		
		10 min	20 min	30 min
MABP, *mm Hg*	100.3 ± 16.2	65.9 ± 14.5†	57.8 ± 9.8†	56.2 ± 8.9†
HR, *bpm*	69.8 ± 9.8	70.8 ± 11.7	69.0 ± 13.0	67.5 ± 11.7
CVP, *mm Hg*	4.2 ± 2.4	4.8 ± 2.5	4.5 ± 2.5	4.6 ± 2.5
PADP, *mm Hg*	10.2 ± 4.1	11.1 ± 3.8	10.6 ± 3.7	10.3 ± 3.7
SVRI, $dyne \bullet s \bullet cm^{-5} \bullet m^{-2}$	907.2 ± 350.8	581.5 ± 329.9†	448.2 ± 210.3†	454.9 ± 285.3†
CI, $L \bullet min^{-1} \bullet m^{-2}$	2.9 ± 0.5	3.3 ± 0.8‡	3.3 ± 0.8‡	3.3 ± 0.9‡
SVI, $mL \bullet beat^{-1} \bullet m^{-2}$	41.4 ± 8.2	47.2 ± 11.1‡	49.4 ± 12.3†	50.3 ± 13.5†

CI—cardiac index; CVP—central venous pressure; HR—heart rate; MABP—mean arterial blood pressure; PADP—pulmonary artery diastolic pressure; SVI—stroke volume index; SVRI—systemic vascular resistance index.

*Values are mean ± standard deviation.

†$P < 0.0005$ compared with baseline.

‡$P < 0.005$ compared with baseline.

Figure 8-5. Hemodynamic responses to 0.75% bupivacaine, 20 to 25 mL administered through the lumbar epidural route in 29 patients undergoing total hip arthroplasty. Mean arterial blood pressure was maintained at 50 to 60 mm Hg by the infusion of epinephrine through a central venous catheter. It should be noted that cardiac index values ranged from 2.0 to 4.5 L/min/m^2. Despite this large range, the response to the lowering of blood pressure was similar. (*From* Sharrock and coworkers [9]; with permission.)

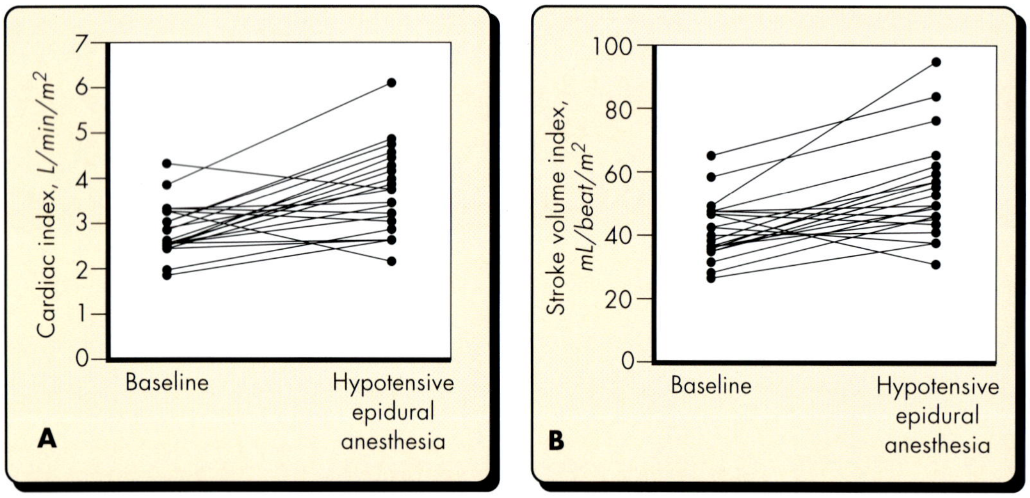

Figure 8-6. Cardiac index (**A**) and stroke volume index (**B**) in patients undergoing total hip arthroplasty under lumbar epidural hypotensive anesthesia (0.75% bupivacaine, 20–25 mL). Despite a twofold difference in baseline cardiac index and stroke volume index, there was significant increase in both these parameters except in two of the 29 patients studied (*From* Sharrock and coworkers [9]; with permission.)

CARDIAC OUTPUT OR BLOOD PRESSURE?

	Trimethaphan	Sodium nitroprusside
Blood pressure	76 → 53	72 → 56
Cardiac output	6.4 → 4.1 (37% decrease)	6.5 → 8.3 (27% increase)
Blood loss	170 ± 102	183 ± 92

Figure 8-7. Twenty healthy patients underwent bilateral osteotomy of the mandible. Blood pressure was decreased to similar levels with either trimethaphan or sodium nitroprusside. Decreased blood pressure with a ganglionic blocker (trimethaphan) decreased cardiac output by 37%. Decreased blood pressure with a vascular smooth muscle dilator (sodium nitroprusside) increased cardiac output by 27%. The decrease in blood loss was similar in both groups, demonstrating that the decrease in blood pressure is the most important factor in decreasing blood loss, and not cardiac output. (*From* Sivarajan and coworkers [10].)

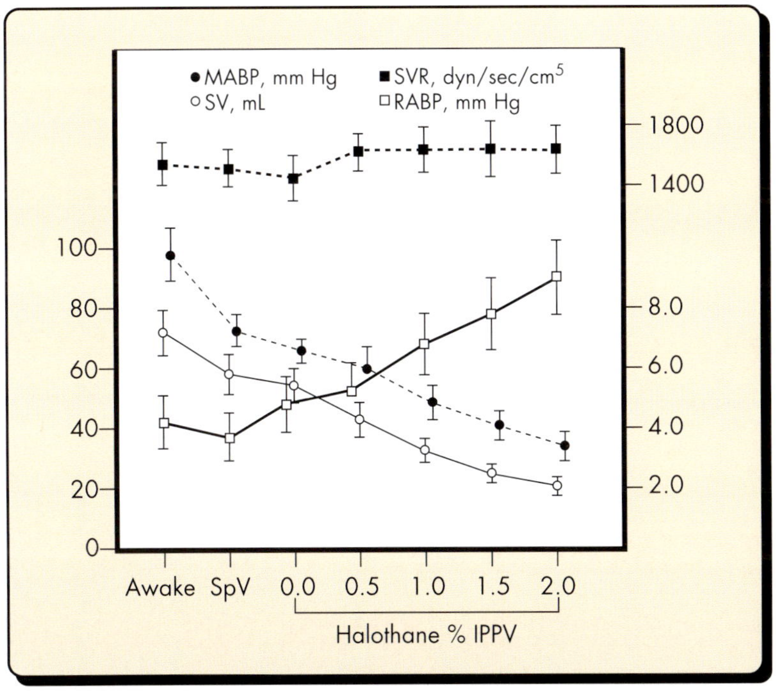

Figure 8-8. The effects of increasing concentrations of halothane in humans. Mean arterial blood pressure (*MABP*) decreases as stroke volume (*SV*) decreases. Intermittent positive pressure ventilation (*IPPV*) and increasing concentrations of halothane increases right atrial blood pressure (*RABP*) suggesting myocardial depression. Systemic vascular resistance (*SVR*) is increased. This early study was one of the first to show that halothane is not a vasodilator, as was commonly thought. It also established that halothane is a myocardial depressant and that the decrease in blood pressure was caused by decreased cardiac output, and not vasodilation. IPPV—intermittent positive pressure ventilation; SpV—spontaneous ventilation. (*From* Prys-Roberts and coworkers [11]; with permission.)

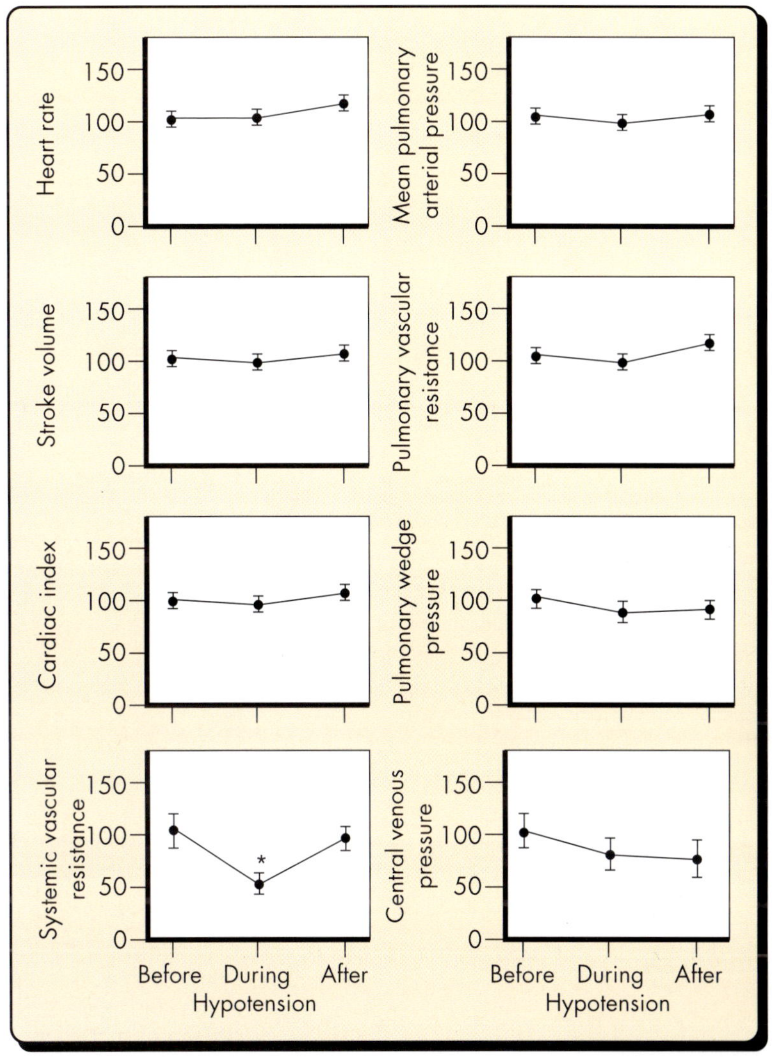

Figure 8-9. Eight cardiovascular parameters in 13 patients undergoing clipping of a cerebral aneurysm. During the prehypotensive period patients received 1% to 2% isoflurane anesthesia. Mean arterial blood pressure was then decreased to 40 mm Hg by increasing the inspired isoflurane concentration to 4%. There is no decrease in cardiac output and only a decrease in systemic vascular resistance. This is in marked contrast to halothane anesthesia. (*From* Lum and Gelb [12]; with permission.)

INTRAVENOUS DRUGS

Sodium nitroprusside
Nitroglycerine
Hydralazine
Trimethaphan
Prostaglandin E
Adenosine and adenosine triphosphate
Labetalol
Calcium channel blockers
Esmolol

Figure 8-10. Intravenous drugs used to induce hypotension.

SODIUM NITROPRUSSIDE

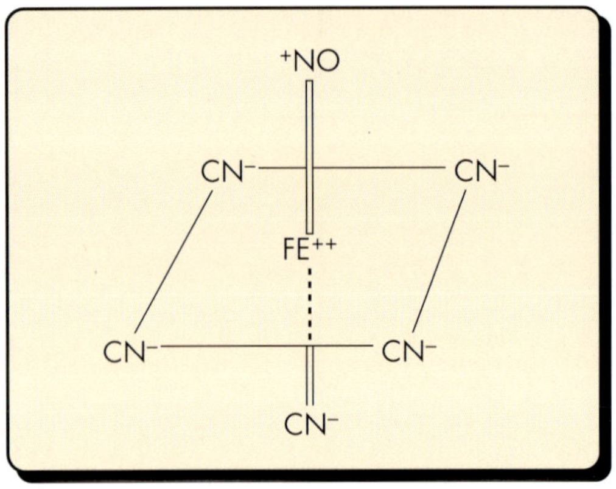

Figure 8-11. Chemical structure of sodium nitroprusside. The five cyanide ions (CN^-) are potential causes of toxicity when excess sodium nitroprusside is given. The nitroso group (*NO*) causes vascular smooth muscle relaxation. Fe^{++}—iron ions.

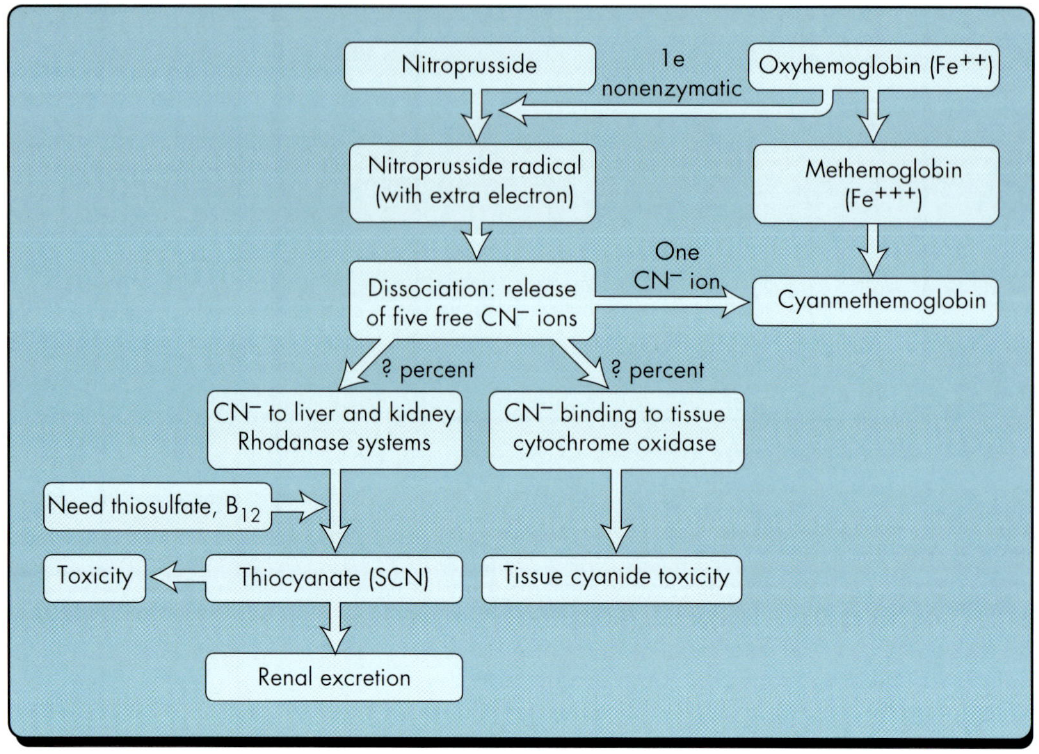

Figure 8-12. The breakdown of sodium nitroprusside leading to the formation of cyanmethemoglobin, thiocyanate, and free cyanide ions (*CN^-*), which bind to the cytochrome oxidase system. It should be noted that treatment of cyanide toxicity is aimed at complexing the cyanide ions with either thiosulfate or forming more methemoglobin through administration of methylene blue.

FACTORS THAT LEAD TO EXCESS SNP ADMINISTRATION

Mechanical hypertension, *eg*, coarctation of the aorta
Renin angiotension system activation
Sympathetic nervous system activation
Contraction of vascular smooth muscle caused by cyanide
Greater amount of SNP required by younger than older patients
Inaccurate blood pressure measurement

Figure 8-13. Factors that lead to excess sodium nitroprusside (*SNP*) administration.

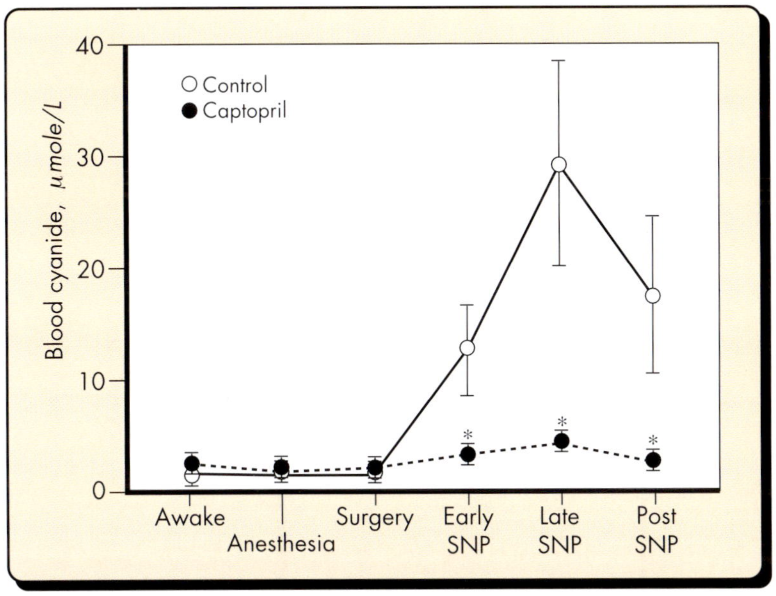

Figure 8-14. Whole blood cyanide measured in two groups of patients during deliberate hypotension with sodium nitroprusside (*SNP*). One group received captopril (converting enzyme inhibitor) before surgery. Blood pressure was decreased to 55 to 60 mm Hg in both groups with SNP. Five times as much SNP was needed in the control group as compared with the group receiving captopril to achieve similar pressure reductions. This explains the elevated cyanide levels in the control group. (*From* Woodside and coworkers [13].)

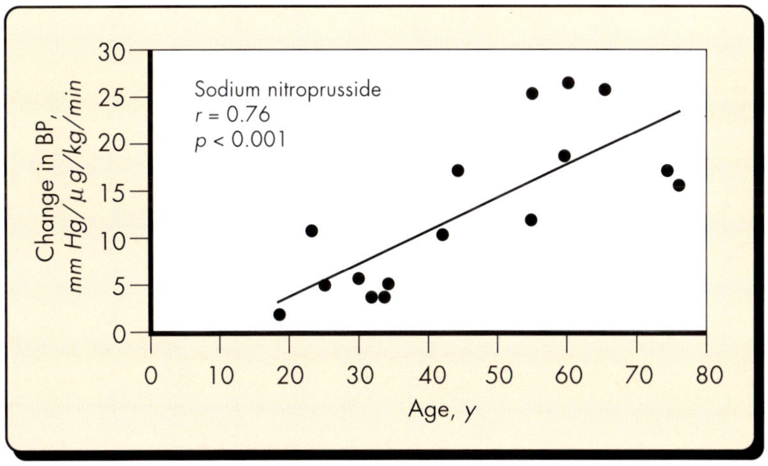

Figure 8-15. The ages of 16 patients plotted against changes in mean arterial blood pressure (BP) per μg/kg/min dose of sodium nitroprusside (SNP). For the same degree of deliberate hypotension, older patients require less SNP than do younger patients. This fact becomes important when the clinician gives SNP to achieve a desired BP without knowledge of the dose of SNP. Early use of SNP resulted in deaths in young patients because the correct dose of SNP was not known and lethal concentrations of the drug were given. (*From* Wood and coworkers [14].)

VASODILATORS AND HEMODYNAMIC RESPONSES

HEMODYNAMIC VALUES BEFORE, DURING, AND AFTER INFUSION OF SNP AND NTG

	SNP			NTG		
	MAP	CI	SVR	MAP	CI	SVR
Baseline	82 ± 5	2.37 ± 0.35	1889 ± 499	86 ± 15	3.23 ± 0.90	1574 ± 450
≤ 10 μg • kg^{-1} • min^{-1}	53 ± 2*	4.44 ± 1.36*	676 ± 295*	67 ± 13*	3.14 ± 0.79	1230 ± 542*
40 μg • kg^{-1} • min^{-1}	—	—	—	68 ± 12*	3.48 ± 0.68	1122 ± 460*
Off drug	96 ± 10*	2.82 ± 1.05	2158 ± 996	84 ± 13	3.30 ± 0.53	1508 ± 389

CI—cardiac index in L • min^{-1} • m^{-2}; MAP—mean arterial pressure in mm Hg; NTG—nitroglycerine; SNP—sodium nitroprusside; SVR—systemic vascular resistance in dyn • s • cm^{-5}.
Values are mean ± standard deviation.
*$P < 0.05$ compared with baseline.

Figure 8-16. Hemodynamic variables in 12 children undergoing deliberate hypotension with either sodium nitroprusside (*SNP*) or nitroglycerine (*NTG*). In all of the six children receiving SNP, blood pressure was decreased to 55 mm Hg with 6 to 8 μg/kg/min. In children receiving NTG, however, blood pressure could not be lowered to a similar degree despite the use of 40 μg/kg/min of NTG. (*From* Yaster and coworkers [15]; with permission.)

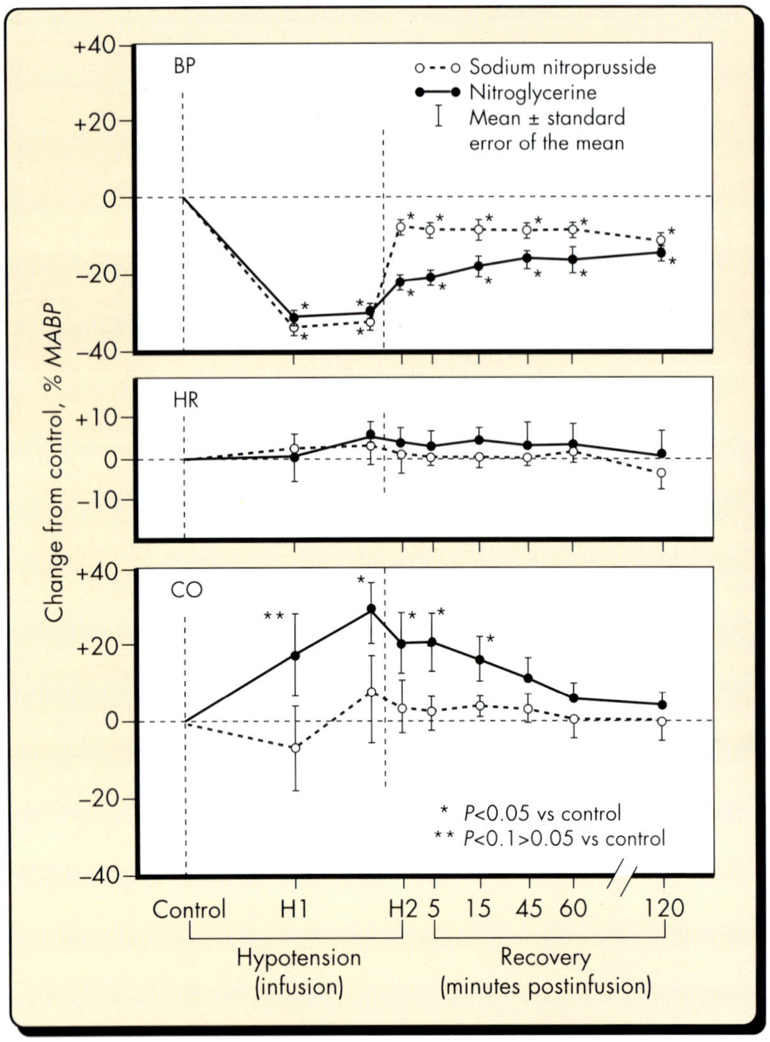

Figure 8-17. Changes in mean arterial blood pressure (*MABP*), heart rate (*HR*), and cardiac output (*CO*) in a group of patients receiving either sodium nitroprusside or nitroglycerine. Note that the changes in blood pressure are the percentage of change from control because deeper levels of hypotension could not be achieved with nitroglycerine. The recovery of blood pressure with nitroglycerine is prolonged compared with nitroprusside. (*From* Todd and coworkers [16]; with permission.)

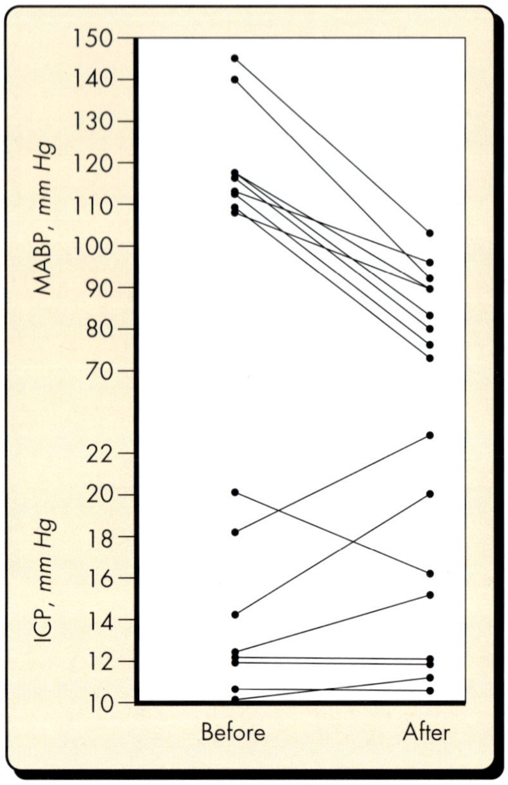

Figure 8-18. The effect of hydralazine on mean arterial blood pressure (*MABP*) and intracranial pressure (*ICP*) in eight patients undergoing intracranial procedures. Blood pressure decreased in all patients; however, ICP increased in four, decreased in one, and remained the same in three. (*From* James and Bedford [17]; with permission.)

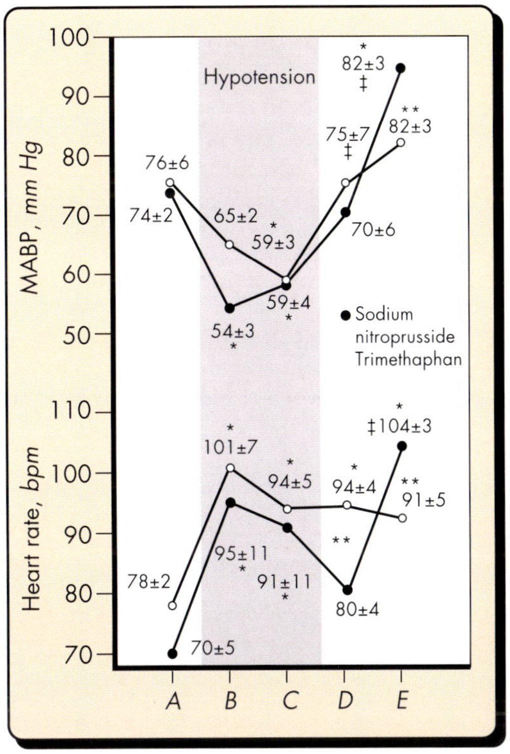

Figure 8-19. Changes in mean arterial blood pressure (*MABP*) and heart rate in patients undergoing deliberate hypotension with either sodium nitroprusside or trimethaphan. *A*, Before surgical incision. *B*, After 60 minutes of deliberate hypotension. *C*, After 120 minutes of deliberate hypotension. *D*, Immediately after termination of hypotension. *E*, 30 to 45 minutes after termination of anesthesia and surgery. *—P < 0.001 for comparison to A; **—P < 0.05 for difference between hypotension groups; ‡—P < 0.05 for difference compared with preceding observation. (*From* Knight and coworkers [18]; with permission.)

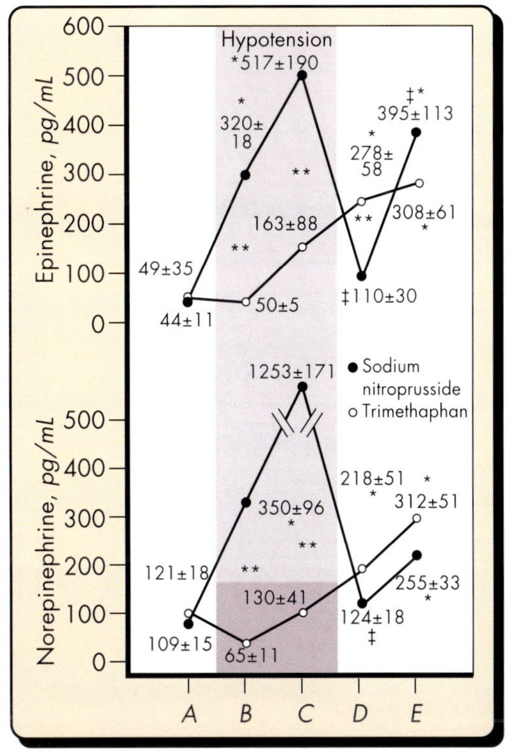

Figure 8-20. Plasma catecholamines in patients before, during, and after deliberate hypotension with either sodium nitroprusside or trimethaphan. Because trimethaphan is a ganglionic blocking agent, no increase in norepinephrine or epinephrine occurs. (See Fig. 8-19 for explanation of A–E.) *—P < 0.001 for comparison to A; **—P < 0.05 for difference between hypotension groups; ‡—P < 0.05 for difference compared with preceding observation. (*From* Knight and coworkers [18]; with permission.)

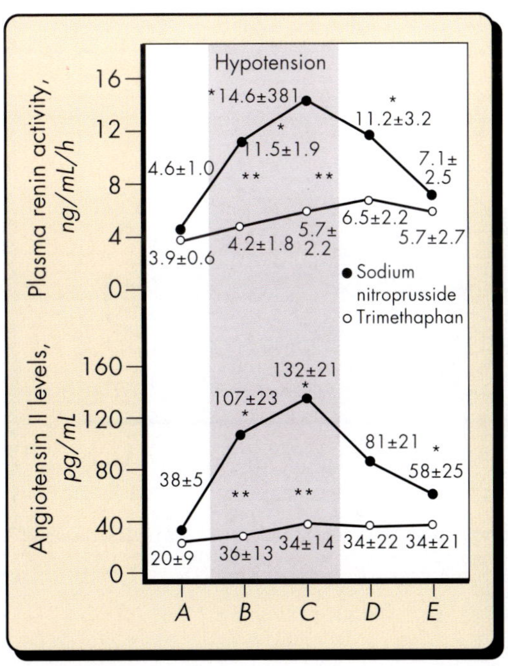

Figure 8-21. Plasma renin activity and angiotensin II concentrations before, during, and after deliberate hypotension with either sodium nitroprusside or trimethaphan. Plasma renin activity and angiotensin II levels do not increase because of the ganglionic blocking properties of trimethaphan. (See Fig. 8-19 for explanation of A–E.) *—P < 0.001 for comparison to A; **—P < 0.05 for difference between hypotension groups; ‡—P < 0.05 for difference compared with preceding observation. (*From* Knight and coworkers [18]; with permission.)

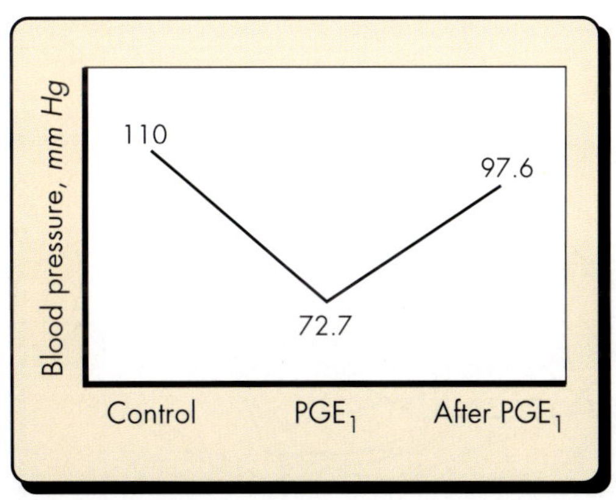

Figure 8-22. Blood pressure response to the infusion of prostaglandin E_1 (PGE_1) in normal subjects. Heart rate was unchanged during this mild deliberate hypotension. Nausea and vomiting are potential problems when this technique is used postoperatively. (*From* Abe and coworkers [19].)

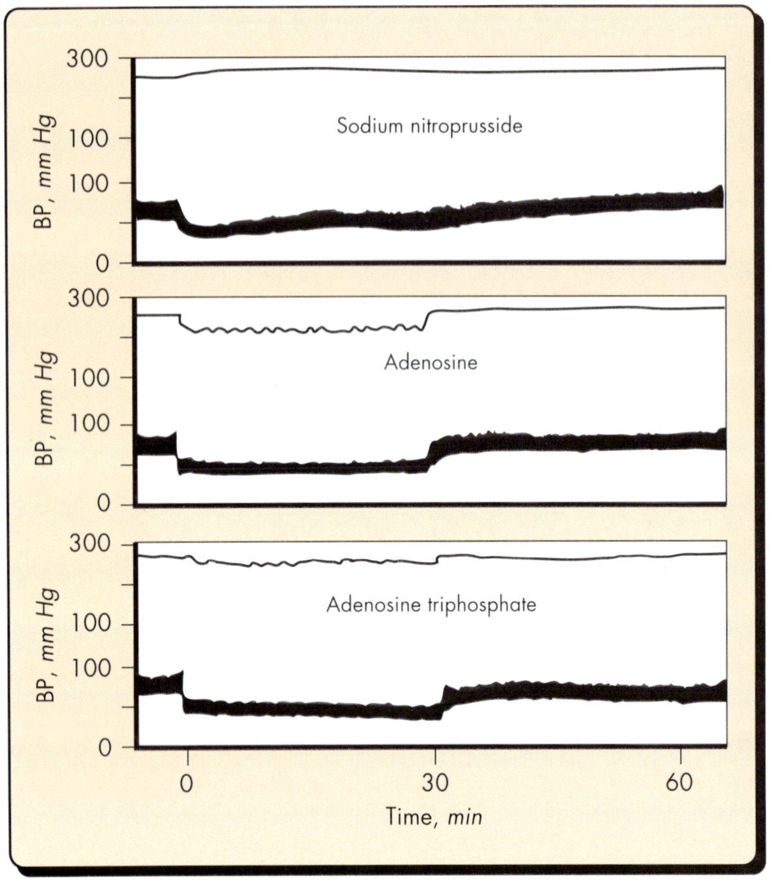

Figure 8-23. Effect of sodium nitroprusside, adenosine, and adenosine triphosphate (ATP) on blood pressure (*BP*) in rabbits. The rapid on–off effect of adenosine and ATP are attractive features. Complete heart block with adenosine, however, has been reported. Clinical trials in the United States have been stopped, and therefore, it is unlikely that this agent will be used in the near future for deliberate hypotension. (*From* Fukunaya and coworkers [20]; with permission.)

HORMONAL RESPONSES TO HYPOTENSION

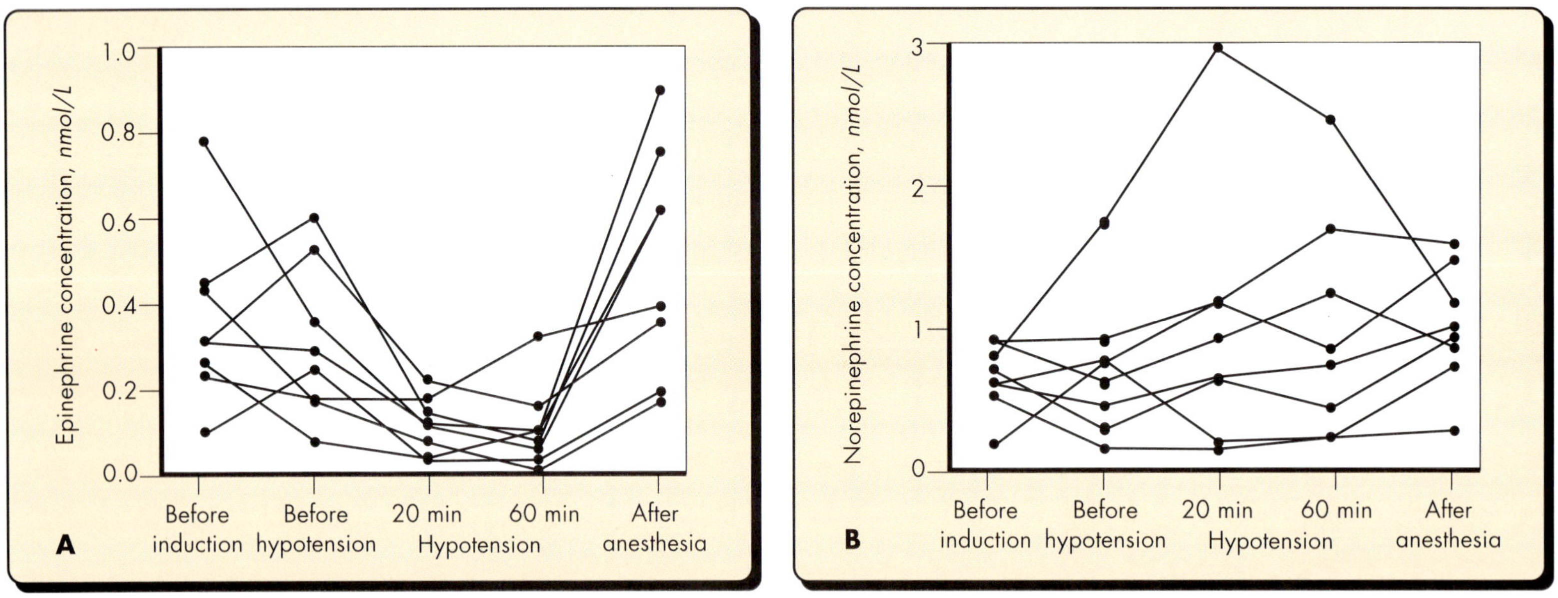

Figure 8-24. Plasma epinephrine (**A**) and norepinephrine (**B**) levels before and during deliberate hypotension induced with labetalol, 0.5 mg/kg, in eight patients. (*From* Toivonen [21]; with permission.)

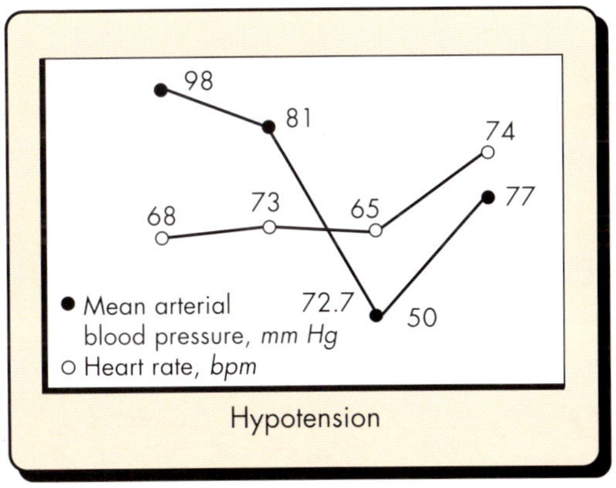

Figure 8-25. Effects of labetalol with isoflurane anesthesia on mean arterial blood pressure and heart rate. Patients received labetalol, 0.5 mg/kg, to induce hypotension. Note that heart rate does not decline further despite increasing amounts of labetalol. Blood pressure, however, shows significant decreases. The five- to sevenfold β blocking to α blocking properties of labetalol do not seem to be as pronounced in this clinical study. (*From* Toivonen [21].)

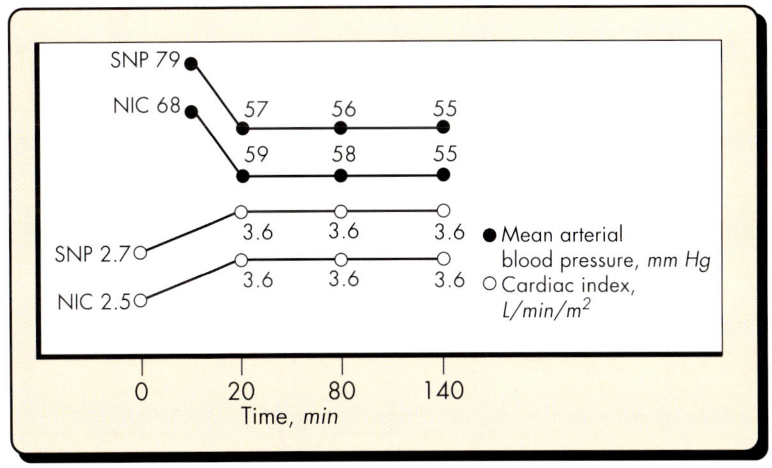

Figure 8-26. Comparison of sodium nitroprusside and nicardipine on blood pressure and cardiac index during deliberate hypotension in 10 patients. Heart rate was similar in both groups. (*From* Bernard and coworkers [22]; with permission.)

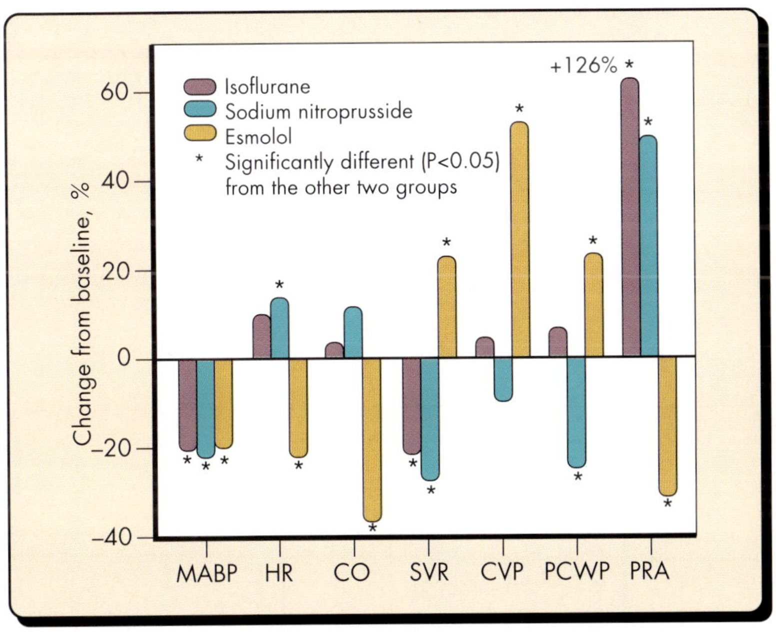

Figure 8-27. Percentage change from baseline for hemodynamic variables and plasma-renin activity (*PRA*) during hypotension induced by esmolol, sodium nitroprusside, or high-dose isoflurane in 30 patients undergoing resection of intracranial arteriovenous malformations. For mean arterial blood pressure (*MABP*) and heart rate (*HR*), $n = 10$ for esmolol and sodium nitroprusside and $n = 9$ for isoflurane. For cardiac output (*CO*), central venous pressure (*CVP*), pulmonary capillary wedge pressure (*PCWP*), and systemic vascular resistance (*SVR*), $n = 9$ for esmolol and isoflurane and $n = 7$ for sodium nitroprusside. For plasma renin activity, $n = 8$ for all groups. (*From* Ornstein and coworkers [23]; with permission.)

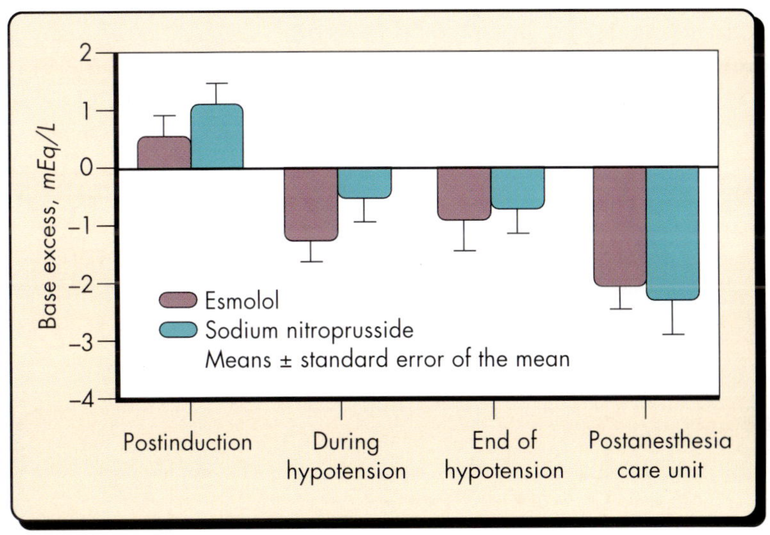

Figure 8-28. Progressive base deficit in two groups of patients receiving either esmolol or sodium nitroprusside for deliberate hypotension. There is no difference between the two groups; however, the change in the deficit over time is significant. (*From* Blau and coworkers [24].)

EFFECT OF HYPOTENSION ON CEREBRAL CIRCULATION

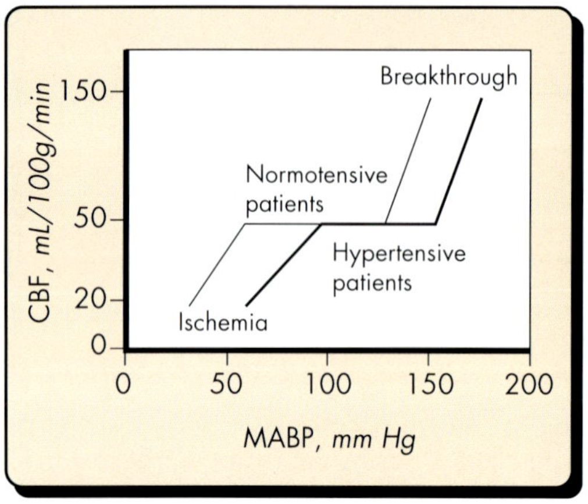

Figure 8-29. Normal autoregulatory curve in humans. Note that in the patient with hypertension, the curve shifts to the right. Deliberate hypotension is adjusted to 50 to 60 mm Hg because blood flow to the brain decreases below that range. CBF—cerebral blood flow; MABP—mean arterial blood pressure.

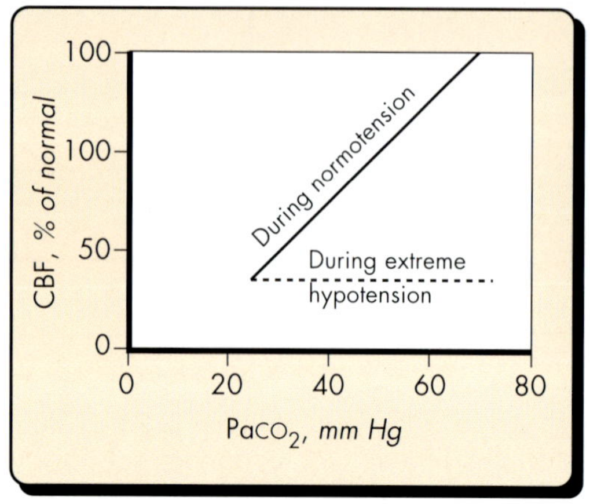

Figure 8-30. Relationship of cerebral blood flow (*CBF*) to carbon dioxide (CO_2) tension during normotension. In extreme deliberate hypotension (mean arterial pressure of 35 mm Hg) there is no change in CBF with changes in CO_2. $PaCO_2$—partial pressure of CO_2 in arterial blood. (*From* Harper and Glaso [25].)

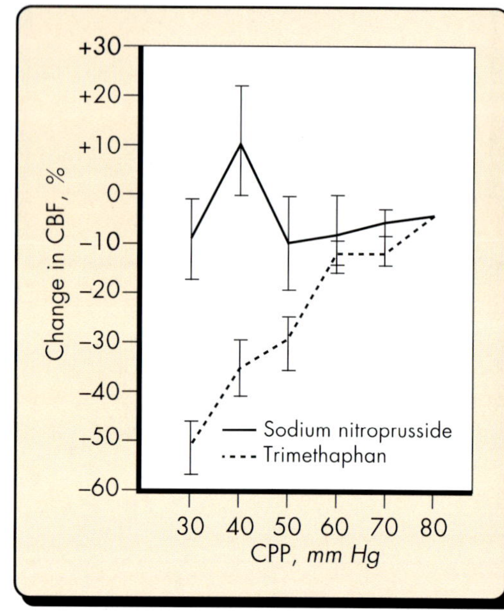

Figure 8-31. Change in cerebral blood flow (*CBF*) in dogs subjected to varying degrees of hypotension induced by trimethaphan or sodium nitroprusside. When cerebral perfusion pressure (*CPP*) was incrementally decreased from 80 to 30 mm Hg, CBF decreased with trimethaphan but not with sodium nitroprusside. (*From* Stoyka and Schutz [26]; with permission.)

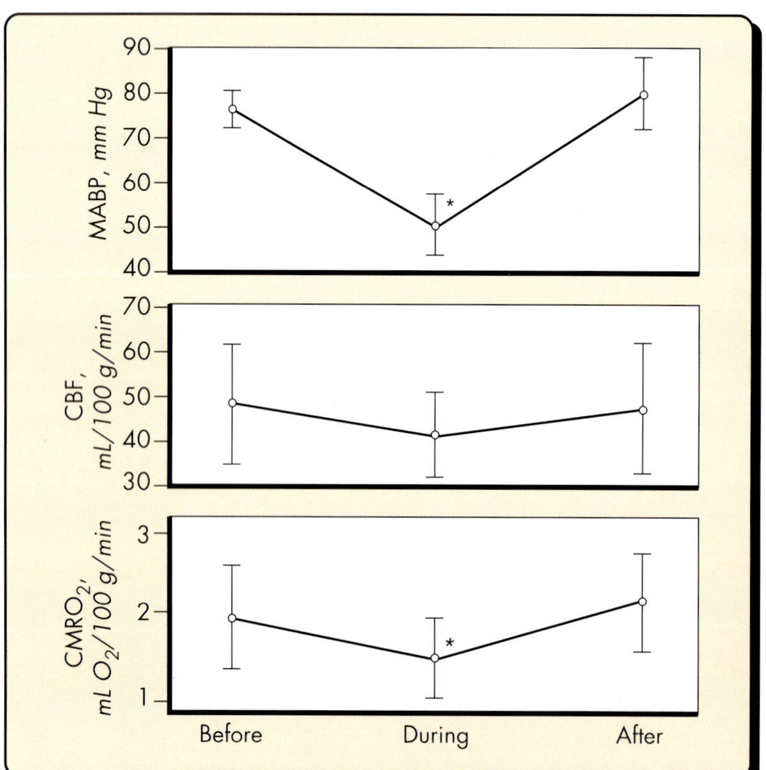

Figure 8-32. Changes in cerebral blood flow (*CBF*) and cerebral rate of oxygen (*CMRO*$_2$) in 12 patients before, during, and after decrease in mean arterial blood pressure (*MABP*) induced by isoflurane. *—P < 0.25 compared wiht prehypotension value. (*From* Neuman and coworkers [27].)

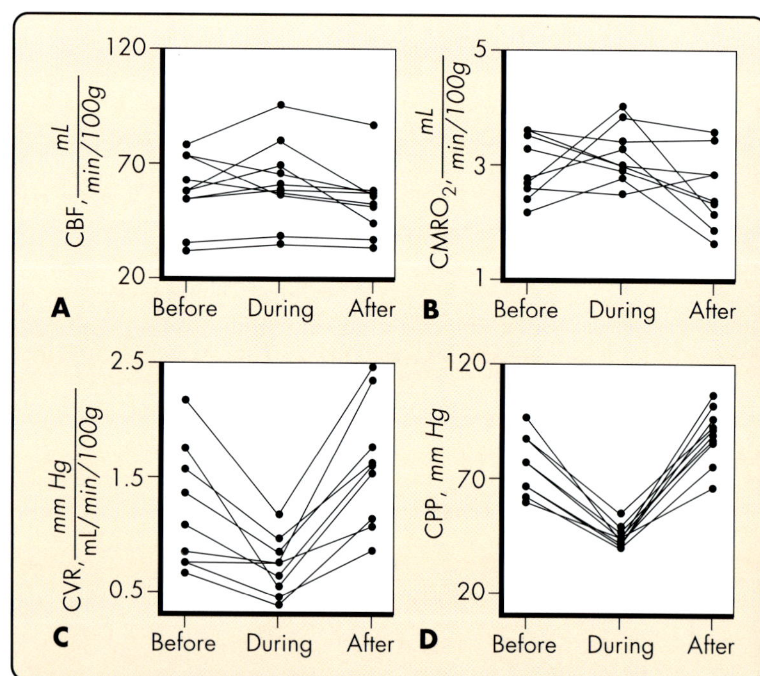

Figure 8-33. Cerebral blood flow (*CBF*) (**A**), cerebral metabolic rate of oxygen (*CMRO*$_2$) (**B**), cerebral vascular resistance (*CVR*) (**C**), and cerebral perfusion pressure (*CPP*) (**D**) in nine patients during deliberate hypotension with sodium nitroprusside. (*From* Larsen and coworkers [28]; with permission.)

COMPARISON OF HEMODYNAMIC CHANGES FROM AWAKE AT 1.4 AND 1.8 (1.7) MAC

Anesthetics	Halothane	Enflurane	Isoflurane	Halothane	Enflurane	Isoflurane
MAC	1.4	1.4	1.4	1.8	1.8	1.7
HR	+3.9 ± 8*	+53 ± 11	+64 ± 12†	+46 ± 11*	55 ± 14	+64 ± 12†
MAP	-29 ± 4‡	-38 ± 3†	-38 ± 4	-36 ± 4‡	-56 ± 3*†	-43 ± 4‡
LAP	+0.6 ± 0.7*	+0.9 ± 1.4	-1.0 ± 0.4†	+1.4 ± 0.5	+2.6 ± 1.3	-0.3 ± 0.8
CO	-9 ± 7	-9 ± 6	-1 ± 6	-13 ± 7‡	-31 ± 5*†	-3 ± 5‡
LV	-54 ± 2‡	-61 ± 2*†	-53 ± 3‡	-65 ± 2‡	-74 ± 2*†	-59 ± 3‡
SV	-34 ± 5	-40 ± 5	-36 ± 6	-40 ± 5‡	-56 ± 4*†	-38 ± 5‡
SVR	-24 ± 5	-34 ± 4	-37 ± 4	-29 ± 6	-40 ± 6	-41 ± 6

CO—cardiac output; HR—heart rate; LAP—left atrial pressure; LV—lung volume in dP/dt_{max}; MABP—mean arterial blood pressure; MAC—monitored anesthesia care; SV—stroke volume; SVR—systemic vascular resistance.
*P < 0.05 vs same MAC isoflurane.
†P < 0.05 vs same MAC halothane.
‡P < 0.05 vs same MAC enflurane.

Figure 8-34. Comparison of hemodynamic changes at various levels of inhalation anesthetic: awake, 1.4, and 1.8 MAC (minimal alveolare concentration) for halothane, enflurane, and isoflurane. Cardiac output was least affected by isoflurane. (*From* Hysing and coworkers [29]; with permission.)

COMPARISON OF REGIONAL BLOOD FLOW CHANGES FROM AWAKE AT 1.4 AND 1.8 (1.7) MAC

Anesthetics	Halothane	Enflurane	Isoflurane	Halothane	Enflurane	Isoflurane
MAC	1.4	1.4	1.4	1.8	1.8	1.7
CoBF	-1 ± 5*	+19 ± 7	+29 ± 7†	+2 ± 6	+8 ± 5	+20 ± 10
ReBF	+16 ± 15	-5 ± 13	-2 ± 16	+19 ± 13*‡	-28 ± 8*†	-7 ± 14†‡
CoVR	-24 ± 6*‡	-46 ± 4†	-50 ± 4†	-32 ± 6‡	-55 ± 3†	-49 ± 5
ReVR	-34 ± 9	-39 ± 9	-31 ± 7	-44 ± 8	-36 ± 8	-33 ± 8

CoBF—coronary blood flow; CoVR—coronary vascular resistance; MAC—monitored anesthesia care; ReBF—renal blood flow; ReVR—renal vascular resistance.
*P < 0.05 vs same MAC isoflurane.
†P < 0.05 vs same MAC halothane.
‡P < 0.05 vs same MAC enflurane.

Figure 8-35. Comparison of regional blood flow changes in the coronary and renal circulation at 1.4 and 1.8 MAC for halothane, enflurane, or isoflurane. Coronary and renal vascular resistance are decreased by all agents from control. (*From* Hysing and coworkers [29]; with permission.)

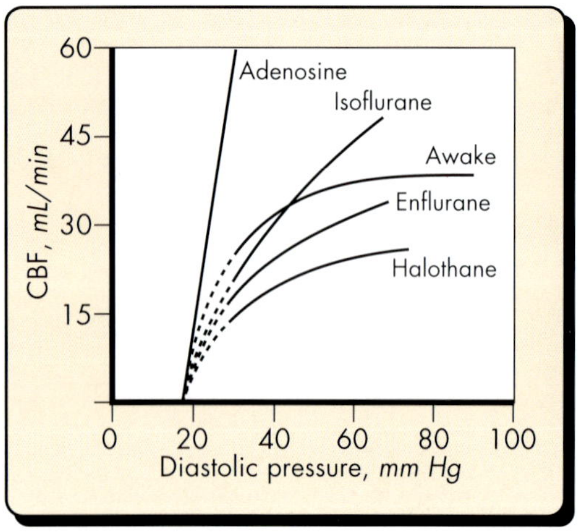

Figure 8-36. Effects of isoflurane, enflurane, and halothane on the autoregulatory curve of the coronary circulation. Coronary blood flow (*CBF*) is most effected by adenosine. Below pressures of 40 mm Hg, there is a sharp decrease in coronary blood flow. (*From* Hickey and coworkers [30]; with permission.)

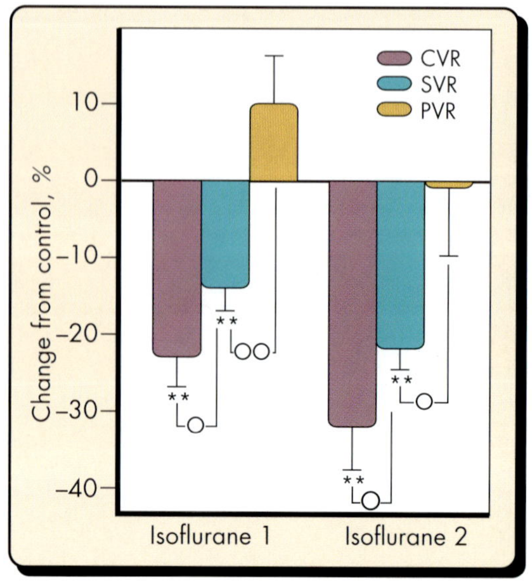

Figure 8-37. Percentage of change in coronary, systemic, and pulmonary vascular resistance (*CVR*, *SVR*, and *PVR*, respectively) from control to either 70 mm Hg (isoflurane 1 equals 1.2%) or 55 mm Hg (isoflurane 2 equals 1.8%.) **—P < 0.01 from control; o,oo—P < 0.05 (o) or < 0.01 (oo) between indicated parameters. (*From* Priebe [31]; with permission.)

EFFECT OF SNP-INDUCED AND NTG-INDUCED HYPOTENSION ON PULMONARY SHUNT, PAO_2, and CO

	Normal Patients		Chronic Obstructive Lung Disease	
	Control	SNP	Control	SNP
Shunt %, *QS/QT*	5.19 ± 0.48	8.81 ± 0.37*	8.14 ± 0.97	8.41 ± 0.82
PaO_2, *mm Hg*	135 ± 10.5	92.3 ± 0.75	110 ± 3.0	105 ± 2.5
CO, *L/min*	4.17 ± 0.26	4.13 ± 0.28	3.75 ± 0.34	3.75 ± 0.75
	Control	NTG	Control	NTG
Shunt %, *QS/QT*	5.13 ± 0.48	6.59 ± 0.56*	8.12 ± 0.97	8.37 ± 0.74
PaO_2, *mm Hg*	146 ± 11.5	105 ± 3.5	105 ± 10.5	119 ± 9.3
CO, *L/min*	4.15 ± 0.26	4.22 ± 0.15	3.78 ± 0.34	3.82 ± 0.27

CO—cardiac output; NTG—nitroglycerin; PaO_2—arterial oxygenation; SNP—sodium nitroprusside.
*P < 0.005 from control.

Figure 8-38. Effect of sodium nitroprusside–induced and nitroglycerine-induced hypotension on pulmonary shunt arterial oxygenation and cardiac output in normal patients and in patients with chronic obstructive lung disease. Shunt fraction increases only in normal patients. Patients with chronic obstructive pulmonary disease, or COPD, do not have further elevation in their already elevated shunt fraction. (*From* Casthely and coworkers [32].)

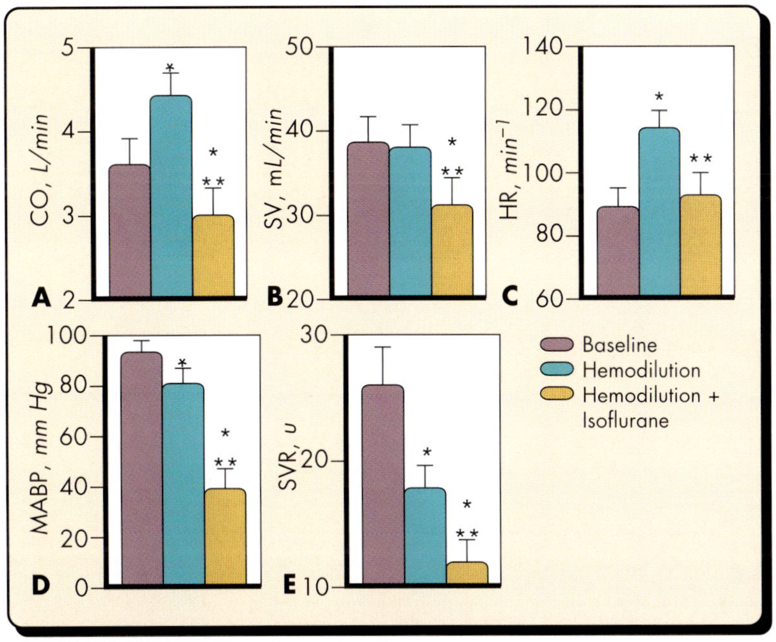

Figure 8-39. The effects of hemodilution (hematocrit, 15%) or hemodilution with isoflurane-induced hypotension on cardiac output (*CO*) (**A**), stroke volume (*SV*) (**B**), heart rate (*HR*) (**C**), mean arterial pressure (*MABP*) (**D**), and systemic vascular resistance (*SVR*) (E). For figures 8-39 and 8-40: *—$P < 0.05$ compared with baseline; **—$P < 0.05$ compared with hemodilution. (*From* Noldge and coworkers [33].) Note that in the presence of hemodilution isoflurane-induced hypotension produces a significant drop in cardiac output due to decreases in both stroke volume and heart rate.

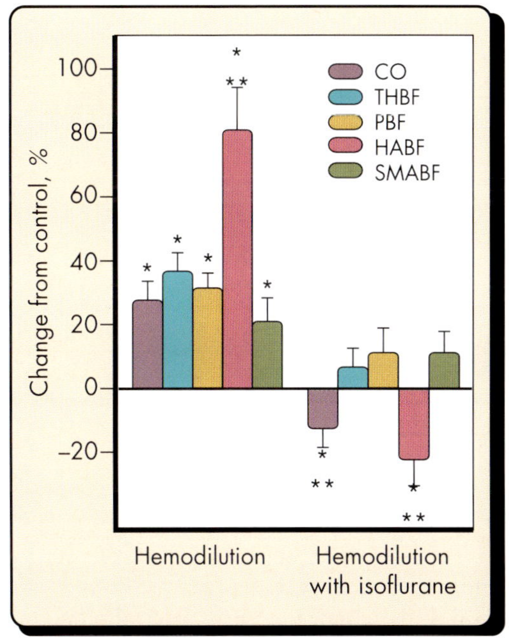

Figure 8-40. Bars represent the percentage of change from control after hemodilution (hematocrit, 15%) or hemodilution and isoflurane-induced hypotension. Cardiac output (*CO*), total hepatic blood flow (*THBF*), portal blood flow (*PBF*), hepatic artery blood flow (*HABF*), and superior mesenteric artery blood flow (*SMABF*) are altered by isoflurane-induced hypotension. (*From* Noldge and coworkers [33].)

EFFECTS OF INDUCED HYPOTENSION ON KIDNEY FUNCTION

	Hypotensive Drug(s)	
Variable	Deep Isoflurane	Labetalol plus Isoflurane
UF, *mL/min*		
Before	0.58 ± 0.12	0.56 ± 0.17
During	0.07 ± 0.02	0.25 ± 0.10
After	1.28 ± 0.17	0.56 ± 0.06
C_{creat}, *mL/min*		
Before	78 ± 14	78 ± 11
During	8 ± 1*	33 ± 8
After	110 ± 17	120 ± 17
U_{osm}, *mOsm/kg/H$_2$O*		
Before	530 ± 27	611 ± 65
During	369 ± 53	568 ± 97
After	470 ± 27	598 ± 43
FE_{Na}, %		
Before	0.28 ± 0.10	0.23 ± 0.05
During	0.16 ± 0.03	0.13 ± 0.04
After	0.58 ± 0.14	0.18 ± 0.04

C_{creat}—creatinine clearance; FE_{Na}—fractional excretion of sodium; U_{osm}—urinary osmolarlity; UF—urinary flow.
*$P < 0.05$ compared with labetalol group.

Figure 8-41. Effects of induced hypotension on kidney function. Mean values for urinary flow, creatinine clearance, urinary osmolarity, and fractional excretion of sodium of labetalol, 0.5 mg/kg, and isoflurane at 1.4%. (*From* Toivonen and coworkers [34]; with permission.)

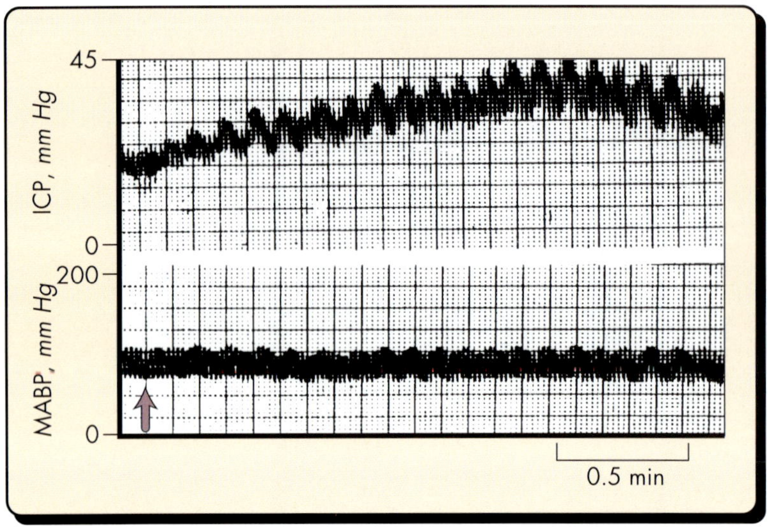

Figure 8-42. Effects of a small dose of sodium nitroprusside on systemic blood pressure and intracranial pressure (*ICP*). *Arrow* indicates the start of the infusion. Little change in mean arterial blood pressure (*MABP*) occurs; however, a considerable increase in ICP is seen in this patient who already has elevated intracranial pressure. (*From* Marsh and coworkers [35]; with permission.)

INDICATIONS AND CONTRAINDICATIONS FOR DELIBERATE HYPOTENSION

Indications
- Intracranial surgery
- Scoliosis surgery
- Total hip arthroplasty
- Large cancer surgery
- Mandible, maxillary osteotomy
- Middle ear surgery
- Patient who is a Jehovah's Witness

Contraindications
- Hypovolemia
- Strokes, transient ischemic attack, carotid bruit
- Major organ dysfunction
- ?? Previous myocardial infarction
- ?? Hypertension

Figure 8-43. Indications and contraindications for deliberate hypotension.

MORTALITY IN DELIBERATE HYPOTENSION

References	Years	Deliberate Hypotension, *N*	Deaths, *N* (%)
Hampton and Little	1950–1953	27,930	96 (0.34)
Enderby	1950–1960	9107	9 (0.10)
Larson	1958–1964	13,264	113 (0.10)
Enderby	1960–1976	9256	2 (0.02)
Pasch and Huk	1977–1984	1802	1 (0.06)
Enderby	1950–1979	20,558	10 (0.04)

Figure 8-44. Mortality in deliberate hypertension.

REFERENCES

1. Amaranath L, Cascorbi HF, Singh-Amaranath AU, *et al.*: Relations of anesthesia to total hip replacement and control of operative blood loss. *Anesth Analg* 1975, 54:641–649.
2. Thompson GE, Miller RD, Stevens WC, Murry WR: Hypotensive anesthesia for total hip arthroplasty: a study of blood loss and organ function (brain, heart, liver and kidney.) 1978, *Anesthesiology* 48:91–99.
3. Eerola R, Eerola M, Kaukinen L, *et al.*: Controlled hypotension and moderate haemodilution in major hip surgery. *Ann Chir Gynaecol* 1979, 69:109–116.
4. Vazeery AK, Lunde O: Controlled hypotension in hip joint surgery. An assessment of surgical haemorrhage during sodium nitroprusside infusion. *Acta Orthop Scand* 1979, 50:433–442.
5. Barbier-Böhm G, Desmonts JM, Conderc E, *et al.*: Comparative effects of induced hypotension and normovolemic hemodilution on blood loss in total hip arthroplasty. *Br J Anaesth* 1980, 52:1039–1046.
6. Qvist TF, Skovsted P, Sørensen MB: Moderate hypotensive anaesthesia for reduction of blood loss during total hip replacement. *Acta Anaesthesiol Scand* 1982, 26:351–358.
7. Von Aken H, Miller ED, Jr: Deliberate Hypotension. In *Anesthesia*, edn. 4. Edited by Miller RD. New York: Churchill-Livingstone; 1994:1481–1504.
8. Blau WS, Kafer E, Anderson J: Esmolol is more effective than sodium nitroprusside in reducing blood loss during orthognathic surgery. *Anesth Analg* 1992, 75:172–178.
9. Sharrock NE, Bading B, Mineo R, Blumenfeld J: Deliberate hypotensive epidural anesthesia for patients with normal and low cardiac output. *Anesth Analg* 1994, 79:899–904.
10. Sivarajan M, Amoy D, Everett G, Buffington C: Blood pressure, not cardiac output, determines blood loss during induced hypotension. *Anesth Analg* 1980, 59:203–207.
11. Prys-Roberts C, Lloyd J, Fisher A, *et al.*: Deliberate profound hypotension induced with halothane: studies of hemodynamics and pulmonary gas exchange. *Br J Anaesth* 1974, 46:105–111.
12. Lum A, Gelb A: Cardiovascular effects of isoflurane-induced hypotension for cerebral aneurysm surgery. *Anal Analg* 1983, 62:742–748.
13. Woodside J. Garner L, Bedford R, *et al.*: Captopril reduces the dose requirement for sodium nitroprusside induced hypotension. *Anesthesiology* 1984, 60:413–418.
14. Wood M, Hyman A, Wood AJ: A clinical study of sensitivity to sodium nitroprusside during controlled hypotensive anesthesia in young and elderly patients. *Anesth Analg* 1987, 66:137–142.

15. Yaster M, Simmons RS, Tolo UT, *et al.*: A comparison of nitroglycerine and nitroprusside for inducing hypotension in children: a double blinded study. *Anesthesiology* 1986, 65:175–180.

16. Todd M, Morris P, Moss J, Philbin D: Hemodynamic consequences of abrupt withdrawal of nitroprusside or nitroglycerine following induced hypotension. *Anesth Analg* 1982, 61:261–266.

17. James D, Bedford R: Hydralazine for controlled hypotension during neurosurgical operations. *Anesth Anag* 1982, 61:1016–1019.

18. Knight PR, Lane G, Hensinger R, *et al.*: Catecholamine and renin-angiotensin response during hypotensive anesthesia induced by sodium nitroprusside or trimethaphan camsylate. *Anesthesiology* 1983, 59:248–253.

19. Abe K, Demizu A, Mima T, *et al.*: Carbon dioxide reactivity during prostaglandin E–induced hypotension for cerebral aneurysm surgery. *Can J Anaesth* 1992, 39:253–259.

20. Fukunaya A, Flache W, Bloor B: Hypotensive effects of adenosine and adenosine triphosphate compared with sodium nitroprusside. *Anesth Analg* 1982, 61:273–278.

21. Toivonen, J: Plasma renin, catecholamines, vasopressin, and aldosterone during hypotension induced by labetalol with isoflurane. *Acta Anaesthesiol Scand* 1991, 35:496–501.

22. Bernard JM, Passute N, Pinaud M: Long-term hypotensive technique with nicardipine and nitroprusside during isoflurane anesthesia for spinal surgery. *Anesth Analg* 1992, 75:179–185.

23. Ornstein E, Young WL, Ostapkovich N, *et al.*: Deliberate hypotension in patients with intracranial or arteriovenous malformations: esmolol compared with isoflurane and sodium nitroprusside. *Anesth Analg* 1991, 72:639–645.

24. Blau WS, Kafer E, Anderson J: Esmolol is more effective than sodium nitroprusside in reducing blood loss during orthognathic surgery. *Anesth Analg* 1992, 75:172–178.

25. Harper AM, Glaso HI: Effects of alterations in arterial carbon dioxide tension on the blood flow through the cerebral cortex at normal and low arterial blood pressures. *J Neurol Neurosurg Psychiatry* 1965, 28:449–456.

26. Stoyka W, Schutz H: The cerebral response to sodium nitroprusside and trimethaphan controlled hypotension. *Can Anaesth Soc J* 1975, 22:275–281.

27. Newman B, Gelb AW, Lam AM: The effect of isoflurane-induced hypotension and cerebral blood flow and cerebral metabolic rate for oxygen in humans. *Anesthesiology* 1986, 64:307–314.

28. Larsen R, Teichmann J, Hilfiker O, *et al.*: Nitroprusside-hypotension: cerebral blood flow and cerebral oxygen consumption in neurosurgical patients. *Acta Anesthesiol Scand* 1982, 26:327–334.

29. Hysing E, Chelly J, Doursont M, Merin R: Comparative effects of halothane, enflurane, and isoflurane at equihypotensive doses of cardiac performance and coronary and renal blood flows in chronically instrumented dogs. *Anesthesiology* 1992, 76:979–984.

30. Hickey R, Sybert P, Verrier E, Cason B: Effects of halothane, enflurane and isoflurane on coronary blood flow autoregulation and coronary vascular reserve in the canine heart. *Anesthesiology* 1988, 68:21–30.

31. Priebe H: Differential effects of isoflurane on regional right and left ventricular performance and on coronary, systemic and pulmonary hemodynamics in the dog. *Anesthesiology* 1987, 66:262–272.

32. Casthely PA, Lear S, Cottrell J, *et al.*: Intrapulmonary shunting during induced hypotension. *Anesth Analg* 1982, 61:231–235.

33. Noldge G, Priebe H, Geigen K: Splanchnic hemodynamics and oxygen supply during acute normovolemic hemodilution alone and with isoflurane induced hypotension in the anesthetized pig. *Anesth Analg* 1992, 75:660–674.

34. Toivonen J, Virtanen H, Kaukinen S: Labetalol attenuates the negative effects of deliberate hypotension induced by isoflurane. *Acta Anaesthesiol Scand* 1992, 36:84–89.

35. Marsh ML, Shapiro H, Smith R, *et al.*: Changes in neurologic status and intracranial pressure associated with sodium nitroprusside administration. *Anesthesiology* 1979, 51:336–339.

9

Malignant Hyperthermia

Steven M. Karan, Edwin W. Lojeski, and Sheila M. Muldoon

Malignant hyperthermia (MH) is a pharmacogenetic disease of skeletal muscle. No pathognomonic physical signs or simple laboratory tests exists to identify susceptible individuals. When exposed to potent inhaled anesthetics or depolarizing muscle relaxants, susceptible individuals can experience fatal skeletal muscle hypermetabolism. However, most susceptible individuals lead normal lives with no limitations on their activities.

Almost 40 years ago MH was originally described as an autosomal dominant syndrome [1]. Since that time, the clinical syndrome has been more accurately defined through the study of MH in humans and the use of an animal model (porcine stress syndrome) [2,3]. By the early 1970s the halothane and caffeine contracture tests were able to identify susceptible people. The North American and European diagnostics centers have developed standard testing protocols to determine the sensitivity and specificity of the tests and to facilitate the interpretation of tests performed at different diagnostic centers. Contracture testing requires that a skeletal muscle biopsy be obtained from the patient. In addition, the patient must travel to a diagnostic center for the biopsy, because contracture testing must be completed within 5 hours of the biopsy excision. Therefore, contracture testing is not practical as a routine screening test for the general population.

In 1979, the Food and Drug Administration approved dantrolene for the treatment of MH. Dantrolene is very effective at reversing MH when it is administered early in the course of the episode [4,5]. It is limited by it poor water solubility (large volumes required for treatment), cost, and availability. Dantrolene continues to be the only commercially available pharmacologic treatment for MH.

The genetic mutation for porcine stress syndrome was identified in 1990. This single mutation has been identified in all breeds of susceptible swine. However, unraveling the genetics of human MH has proven to be more complex. Less than 5% of individuals who are tested have been shown to have the corresponding human mutation. To date, more than 15 genetic defects have been identified in susceptible families; however, no single defect appears to be dominant.

Advances in education, awareness, pharmacology, and technology have helped to decrease MH-related mortality in the United States from 70% to less than 5% over the past three decades. Despite these advances, the cause of human MH remains a mystery. It is generally accepted that elevated intracellular calcium concentrations in skeletal muscle are responsible for the clinical signs of MH. Defects in structural proteins, modulators, and ion channels are currently under investigation as possible causes of human MH. Continued research in these areas may one day lead to a simpler noninvasive test to identify susceptible individuals. Until that time, continued awareness and vigilance are required to minimize the morbidity and mortality of MH.

CLINICAL PRESENTATION

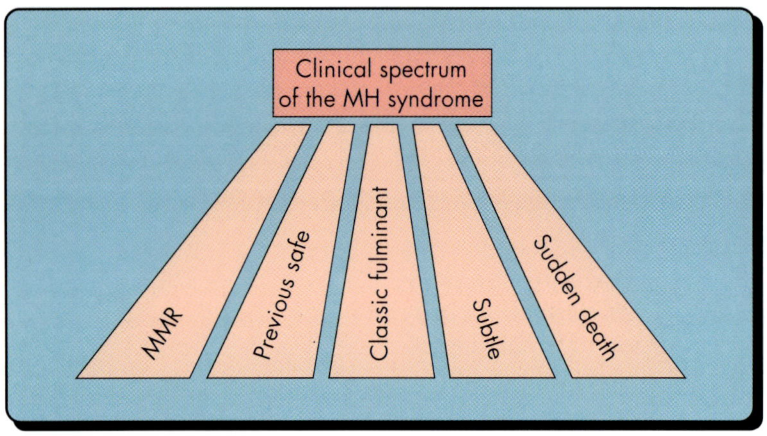

Figure 9-1. Clinical spectrum of the malignant hyperthermia (MH) syndrome. Human MH presents as a broad clinical spectrum. Alone, no clinical sign or laboratory result is pathognomonic for MH. The time of onset can vary from minutes to hours. Possibly owing to environmental and genetic factors, susceptible patients may have had uneventful exposures to triggering agents (succinylcholine and all potent inhaled agents) during previous anesthesia. Sudden or rapid death may be the result of the inability to adequately ventilate the patient (because of muscle rigidity) or the result of fatal arrhythmias. Masseter muscle rigidity (*MMR*) is a contracture of the masseter muscle after succinylcholine administration. The incidence of MMR progressing to a fulminant MH episode is unknown.

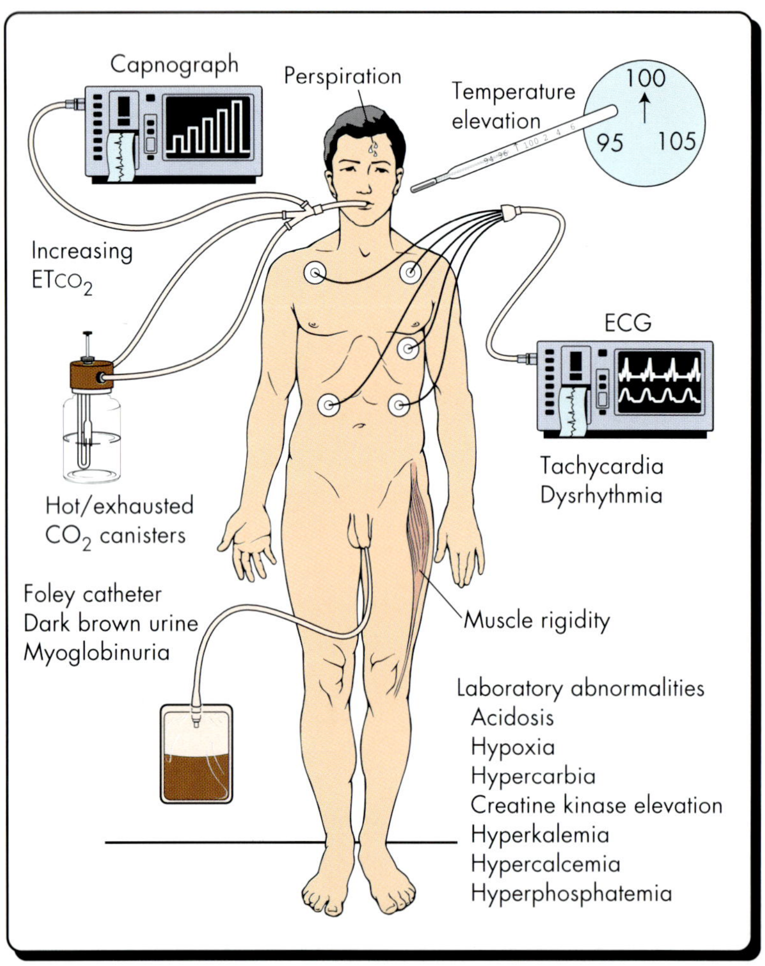

Figure 9-2. Fulminant malignant hyperthermia (MH). An unexplained increase in end-tidal carbon dioxide ($ETCO_2$) provides the earliest, most sensitive, and specific sign of MH. Tachypnea is masked if controlled ventilation and neuromuscular blockade are employed. Without the use of $ETCO_2$ monitoring, an unexpected increase in heart rate may be the most valuable early sign. Tachycardia may be more prominent than are blood pressure elevations early in the course of the episode. Core temperature begins to increase when the body is no longer able to dissipate the heat generated from the increased skeletal muscle metabolism. Rigidity is the most unique sign of MH; however, it is not the most consistent. The progression of body and limb muscle rigidity usually parallels the progression of the clinical syndrome and can interfere with perfusion and ventilation. Alterations in skeletal muscle membrane permeability lead to elevations in serum potassium, sodium, calcium, phosphate, myoglobin, and creatine phosphokinase [6]. Ultimately, the clinical signs are a reflection of the body's inability to respond to an extraordinary increase in metabolic demand. When the metabolic demand can no longer be sustained, the syndrome accelerates and organ system failure occurs. Patients are at risk for recrudescence of the syndrome for up to 24 hours after successful treatment of the initial episode [7]. ECG, electrocardiogram.

DIFFERENTIAL DIAGNOSIS OF INCREASED $ETCO_2$ CONCENTRATION IN MALIGNANT HYPERTHERMIA

I. Equipment
   A. Machine: leak, disconnect, decreased fresh gas flow
   B. Breathing circuit: leak, disconnect, decreased fresh gas flow, obstruction, valve malfunction, depletion or channeling of CO_2 absorbent, improper attachment of circuit to machine
   C. Ventilator: leak, disconnect, improper settings, malfunction, decreased driving pressure
   D. Monitor: leak, disconnect, inaccurate calibration, moisture, baseline drift

II. Metabolic: increased production of CO_2
   A. Fever: iatrogenic, sepsis, thyrotoxicosis, pheochromocytoma, central nervous system injury
   B. Light anesthesia
   C. Malignant hyperthermia

III. Mechanical: decreased elimination of CO_2
   A. Pulmonary: airway obstruction, bronchial intubation, secretions, aspiration, pulmonary edema, asthma, pneumonia, acute respiratory distress syndrome, pneumothorax, hemothorax
   B. Extrathoracic: pressure on chest, retractors, increased abdominal muscle tone, ascites, Trendelenburg position
   C. Central: decreased ventilatory drive in spontaneously ventilating patients (narcotics or inhalational agents)

Figure 9-3. Differential diagnosis of an elevated end-tidal carbon dioxide ($ETCO_2$) concentration. An unexplained increase in $ETCO_2$ provides the earliest, most sensitive, and specific sign of an episode of malignant hyperthermia. Any sustained increase in $ETCO_2$ concentration must be aggressively investigated.

DIFFERENTIAL DIAGNOSIS OF MALIGNANT HYPERTHERMIA

I. Iatrogenic
   Excessive warming measures
   Surgical drapes and coverings

II. Fever
   Infection
   Bacteremia
   Sepsis
   Transfusion reactions (acute hemolytic and nonhemolytic)
   Central nervous system dysfunction
   Allergic reactions

III. Endocrine abnormalities
   Pheochromocytoma
   Thyrotoxicosis (thyroid storm)

IV. Drug induced
   Neuroleptic malignant syndrome
   Cocaine overdose
   Tricyclic antidepressants
   Monoamine oxidase inhibitors (MAOIs)
   Anticholinergics (atropine, glycopyrrolate)
   Amphetamines
   Alcohol withdrawal
   Drug interactions (MAOI and meperidine)

V. Malignant hyperthermia

VI. Autonomic dysfunction
   Riley-Day syndrome

VII. Osteogenesis imperfecta

Figure 9-4. Differential diagnosis of hyperthermia. Temperature elevation in the perioperative period is common and has diverse causes. However, temperature elevation is usually one of the later clinical signs of malignant hyperthermia (MH) and, rarely, is it the only clinical sign. The MH hotline was established in 1982 by the Malignant Hyperthermia Association of the United States (MHAUS) to answer questions about MH and to assist clinicians in the management of ongoing clinical cases. Since 1990, all calls to the MH hotline have been entered into a database for epidemiologic analysis. Approximately 50% of the case consultations calls are considered unlikely to be MH. Most of these calls were initiated on the basis of an isolated peri-operative temperature elevation.

COMPARISON OF THE CLINICAL SIGNS OF MALIGNANT HYPERTHERMIA, THYROTOXICOSIS, AND PHEOCHROMOCYTOMA

	Malignant Hyperthermia	Thyrotoxicosis	Pheochromocytoma
Increased $ETCO_2$	+++	++	++
Tachycardia	+++	+++	+++
Hypertension	+	++	+++
Rigidity	++	+/-	-
Acidosis	+++	-	+
Diagnostic test	Muscle biopsy	Free T4, thyroid-stimulating hormone	Urinary vanillylmandelic acid, plasma catecholamines
Creatine kinase	+++	-	+/-
Myoglobinuria	++	-	-
Response to dantrolene	+++	+/-	-

Figure 9-5. Differential diagnosis of malignant hyperthermia (MH). The differential diagnosis of MH includes sepsis, iatrogenic hyperthermia, hypoventilation, light anesthesia, hyperkalemic cardiac arrest, myotonic reaction, thyrotoxicosis, pheochromocytoma, hypoxia, hypoxic encephalitis, intracranial trauma, neuroleptic malignant syndrome, cocaine toxicity, and drug reactions. Pheochromocytoma [8] and thyrotoxicosis [9] can be difficult to differentiate from MH. Although an elevated end-tidal carbon dioxide ($ETCO_2$) is most frequently associated with MH, it can be seen in all three conditions. Hypertension and tachycardia are the most prominent signs of pheochromocytoma, whereas atrial dysrhythmias and tachycardia are more prominent for thyrotoxicosis. There is no rapid diagnostic test for any of these conditions. However, MH usually responds dramatically to dantrolene therapy, whereas the response to dantrolene in pheochromocytoma and thyrotoxicosis is limited. - —absent; +—mild; ++—moderate; +++—severe. (*Adapted from* Weglinski and Wedel [10].)

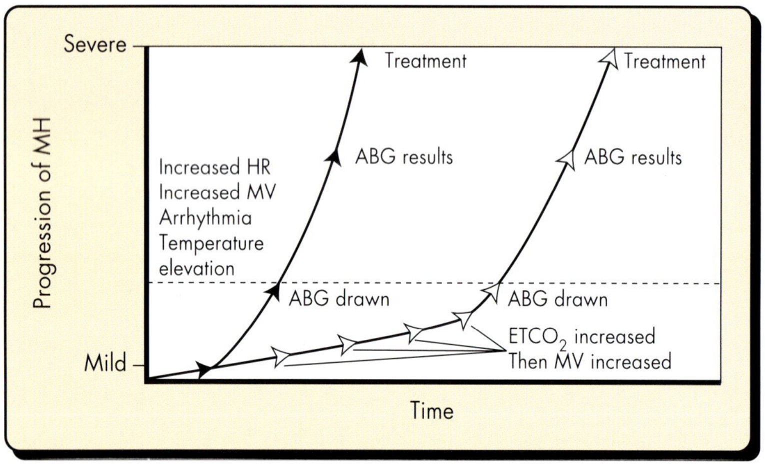

Figure 9-6. Subtle malignant hyperthermia (MH). The influence of capnography on the rate of MH progression. Before capnographic monitoring, routine anesthetic monitoring could not easily detect small or slowly progressive increases in metabolism. Malignant hyperthermia episodes progressed until the metabolic imbalance became pronounced enough to be detected by other signs (increased heart rate (*HR*), increased minute ventilation (*MV*), and arrhythmias), thus delaying the diagnosis and making treatment more difficult (*closed arrows*). Routine capnographic monitoring now allows clinicians to detect increasing CO_2 production by either a rising end-tidal carbon dioxide ($ETCO_2$) or an increasing MV requirement (intermittent increases in MV may be able to maintain the $ETCO_2$ below 40 mm Hg for an extended period of time in some cases). Increasing MV provides early supportive treatment and can mask other diagnostic signs (*open arrows*). In a slowly developing episode, small, intermittent increases in MV may be the only clinical indication of MH [11]. However, increased CO_2 production will eventually outpace efforts to increase MV if MH is not diagnosed and treated. Therefore, $ETCO_2$ and MV must be evaluated together to diagnose slowly progressing MH via increased CO_2 production. ABG, arterial blood gas.

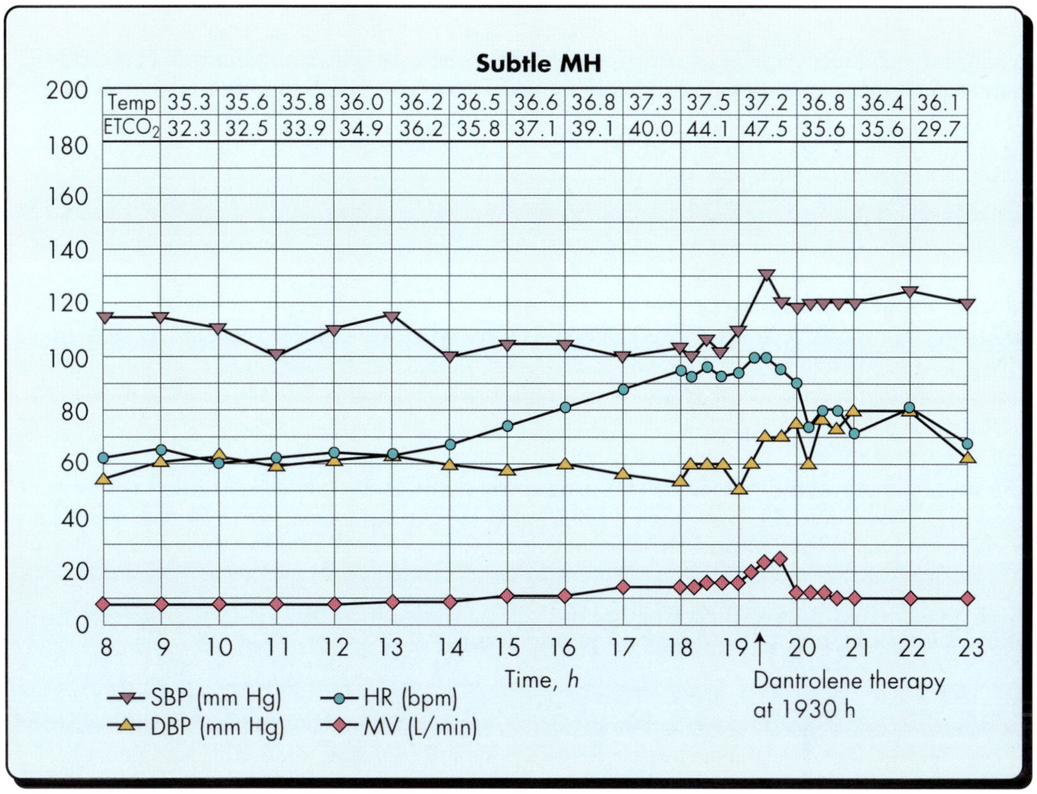

Figure 9-7. Condensed anesthetic record of subtle malignant hyperthermia (MH). An otherwise healthy 26-year-old male with no personal or family history of anesthetic complications, presented for resection of an acoustic neuroma. The patient's anesthetic induction included thiopental, sufentanil, and succinylcholine. His anesthetic was maintained with sufentanil, isoflurane, and vecuronium. The first 6 hours of the case were unremarkable. However, over the next 5 hours the minute ventilation (*MV*) was intermittently increased in an effort to maintain end-tidal carbon dioxide ($ETCO_2$) concentrations below 40 mm Hg. By the 11th hour of the case, the $ETCO_2$ concentration could not be kept below 40 mm Hg despite vigorous hand ventilation. The patient responded dramatically to the discontinuation of isoflurane and the administration of dantrolene. Halothane–caffeine contracture testing was performed approximately 2 months after the event, with seven of seven muscle strips testing positive for MH susceptibility. DBP, diastolic blood pressure; HR, heart rate; SBP, systolic blood pressure.

Estimation of carbon dioxide production

Est CO_2P = [MV(mL/min)] x [$ETCO_2$ (%)] x [1− total functional dead space (%)]

Assumptions: $ETCO_2$ is the alveolar CO_2 concentration; the predicted total functional dead space is 50%; and the predicted MV is 100 mL/kg/min.

A

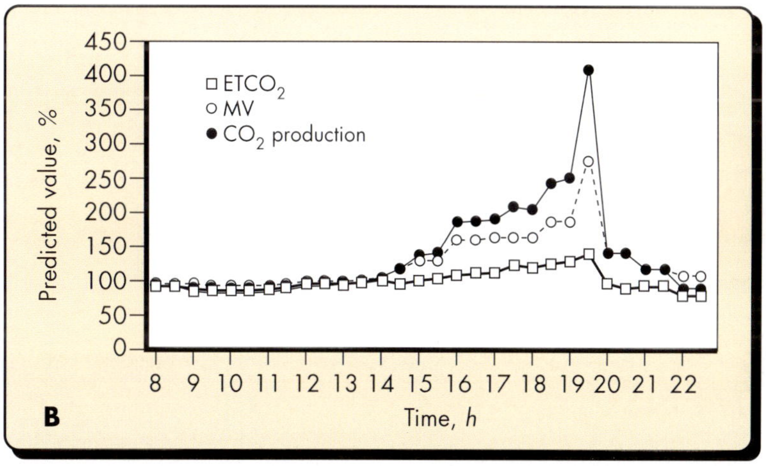

Figure 9-8. Carbon dioxide (CO_2) production. **A**, Precise measurement of CO_2 production during administration of an anesthetic is complicated and currently unavailable in the operating room. However, the equation in this illustration can be used to estimate CO_2 production at intervals during an anesthetic so that the trend can be assessed. By assuming that the total functional dead space is 50% and that end-tidal CO_2 ($ETCO_2$) is equal to alveolar CO_2 concentration, the equation is reduced to two variables: minute ventilation (*MV*) and $ETCO_2$ concentration. **B**, Application of CO_2 production, MV, and $ETCO_2$ concentration trends as a percentage of predicted values for the case of subtle malignant hyperthermia is presented in Fig. 9-7. Est CO_2 P—estimated carbon dioxide production.

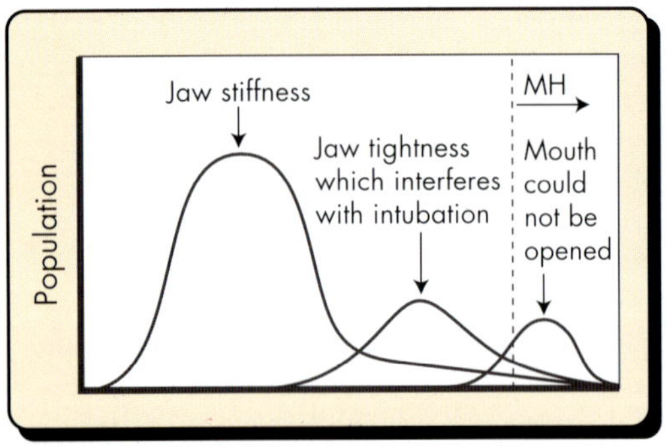

Figure 9-9. Increased jaw tension, masseter muscle rigidity (MMR), and malignant hyperthermia (*MH*). MMR is defined as contracture of the masseter muscle after administration of succinylcholine. It is a transient phenomenon (usually lasting less than 10 minutes) that occurs despite flaccid paralysis of the extremities. Mask ventilation is usually not impaired. Tachycardia, ventricular arrhythmias, and elevations in end-tidal carbon dioxide ($ETCO_2$) are common. Discontinuation of the triggering agents usually result in an uneventful recovery. The incidence of MMR progressing to a fulminant MH episode is unknown. A fulminant episode can begin immediately; however, it is more likely to develop 20 to 30 minutes after the resolution of MMR. Serum creatine phosphokinase levels can be markedly elevated, especially if a second dose of succinylcholine was administered.

When MMR was first described, the mortality of an MH episode was high and no other signs were available to predict the occurrence of an MH episode. Since that time, capnographic monitoring and dantrolene therapy have become available for the early diagnosis and treatment of MH. The lack of a standard widely accepted definition of MMR has also added confusion. In addition, there is a discrepancy between the reported incidence of MMR and the rate of positive contracture test results after MMR. For these reasons, the role of MMR as a predictive sign of MH has recently been questioned. Kaplan [12] proposed a practical guideline for increased jaw tension after succinylcholine administration to help define the types of increased jaw tension [12]. The most common response is "jaw stiffness" that is subclinical and can only be detected using special measuring devices. This is a normal response to succinylcholine and has no prognostic significance for MH. Another response is "jaw tightness which interferes with intubation." This group maybe quite large (1% to 2% in children induced with halothane and succinylcholine) [13]. A small but unknown number of these patients are at risk for MH. The third response is defined as "the mouth could not be opened." This group defines MMR and is predicted to have an increased incidence of MH. (*Adapted from* Kaplan [12]; with permission.)

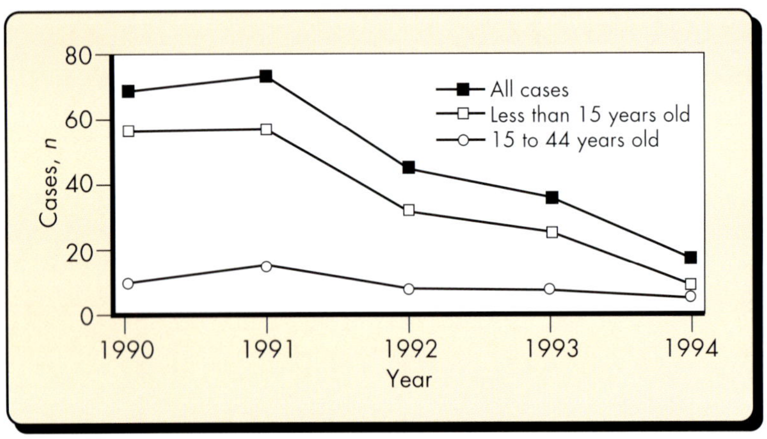

Figure 9-10. Incidence of isolated masseter muscle rigidity (MMR) cases reported to the malignant hypothermia (MH) hotline from 1990 to 1994 [14]. Cases of isolated MMR reported to the MH hotline database have decreased dramatically since 1991. Concurrent with this decline was the recognition of an association in apparently healthy infants and children between succinylcholine administration and hyperkalemic ventricular dysrhythmias leading to cardiac arrest. The debate surrounding these reports and the subsequent Food and Drug Administration warning against the routine use of succinylcholine in pediatric patients may have contributed to this decline. (*From* Karan and coworkers [14]; with permission.)

TREATMENT

MANAGEMENT OF PATIENT WITH A FULMINANT EPISODE OF MALIGNANT HYPERTHERMIA

I. Discontinue all potent inhaled anesthetic agents and hyperventilate with 100% oxygen.

II. Obtain assistance and inform the surgeon to expedite or abort the procedure, if possible.

III. Administer IV dantrolene, 2.5 mg/kg. Be prepared to repeat this dose until the patient responds with a decrease in $ETCO_2$ levels, ventilatory requirement, rigidity, or heart rate.

IV. Monitor acidosis using blood gas analysis to determine if bicarbonate therapy is indicated. Consider central or intraarterial catheter placement for serial measurements.

V. Hyperkalemia is common and is treated with insulin and glucose, 10 units of regular insulin in 1 L $D_{10}W$. Serum potassium and glucose levels must be monitored.

VI. Efforts to cool the patient must correspond with the extent of temperature elevation. Patients can be cooled by decreasing the room temperature, infusion of cold solutions, surface cooling with ice, or using cold solutions for gastric, bladder, and rectal lavage.

Figure 9-11. Treatment of an acute episode of malignant hyperthermia (MH). Early diagnosis and rapid treatment are essential in limiting the morbidity and mortality of MH. Supportive care should be initiated while dantrolene is obtained and prepared for administration. Changing the anesthetic machine or breathing circuit is no longer recommended for the following reasons: 1) hyperventilating with 100% oxygen and discontinuing the potent inhaled anesthetic agent are effective in removing the anesthetic agent from the patient, 2) the risks of inadequate ventilation and airway mismanagement as anesthetic machines or breathing circuits are exchanged are eliminated, and 3) the time required to change the machine or circuit is better spent providing supportive care and dantrolene therapy. The response to dantrolene therapy is usually dramatic. Occasionally, dantrolene doses in excess of 10 mg/kg are required to control an episode. Reassessment of the differential diagnosis is required if the patient's response to large doses of dantrolene is less than expected.

A. CLINICAL APPROACH TO INCREASED JAW TENSION IN MALIGNANT HYPERTHERMIA

	Clinical Signs		Clinical Response		
	Mouth Opening	Intubation	Anesthetic	Surgery	MH Workup
Normal jaw stiffness	Fully opens with firm pressure	No difficulty with laryngoscopy	Continue planned anesthetic	Continue surgery	No
Jaw tightness	Incompletely opens with firm pressure	Laryngoscopy difficult	Switch to nontriggering anesthetic	Continue surgery	Yes
MMR	Cannot be opened	Laryngoscopy impossible	Stop anesthetic	Stop surgery	Yes

B. PATIENT WITH MMR

I. When MMR is diagnosed:
   A. Discontinue the potent inhaled anesthetic agent and continue to ventilate by mask with 100% oxygen.
   B. Do not give a second dose of succinylcholine.
   C. Call for assistance and the MH cart.
   D. Continue to monitor end-tidal carbon dioxide ($ETCO_2$), electrocardiogram, blood pressure, and temperature.
   E. Obtain blood gas analysis if the situation does not rapidly improve.

II. The decision whether to proceed or abort must consider the anesthesiologist's experience, urgency and length of the surgical procedure, human and treatment resources available, monitoring capabilities, and the patient's increased risk to progress to a fulminant MH episode.

III. If the procedure is aborted, it can be rescheduled after the patient's creatine kinase (CK) level has returned to normal.

IV. If the procedure is continued, use a nontriggering anesthetic technique and continue to monitor $ETCO_2$ arterial blood gases, blood pressure, pulse rate, temperature, serum CK level, urine color, and muscle tone for signs of MH.

V. Postoperative management:
   A. Institute intensive care unit–overnight recovery room observation for 24 h to monitor urine output and signs of increased metabolism (increased heart rate, blood pressure, respiration, acidosis, and temperature).
   B. Obtain serial CK measurements every 8 h for 24 h or until the CK level has peaked.
   C. Test urine for the presence of myoglobin:
      If positive, maintain urine output above 1 mL/kg/h until clear.
      If negative, continue to monitor until CK has peaked.

Figure 9-12. Clinical management of patients with increased jaw tension. Controversy exists both in the definition of masseter muscle rigidity (*MMR*) and the management of the patient in whom the response to succinylcholine is abnormal. Suggested strategies range from aborting the procedure and treating with dantrolene to continuing with triggering agents while observing the patient for other signs of malignant hyperthermia (*MH*). Until a consensus on treatment is obtained, the following clinical approach is proposed based on Kaplan's [12] classification discussed in Fig. 9-9. **A**, Clinical signs and response. When the patient's mouth can be opened and intubation is easily accomplished, this is most likely a normal response to succinylcholine. No MH evaluation is necessary and triggering agents can be continued. If the mouth cannot be opened with firm pressure and intubation is difficult, this response is more suspicious for MH. Switching to a nontriggering technique and monitoring closely for other signs of MH are suggested. If the response is that the jaw could not be opened and laryngoscopy is impossible, this is highly suspicious for MH. The surgery and anesthetic should be stopped as soon as possible, and the patient should be observed for further signs of MH. **B**, Management of MMR. Suggested guidelines for the perioperative management of MMR. The patient and family should be informed that they are MH-susceptible and appropriately counseled. Muscle biopsy for contracture testing should be considered as part of the workup. (*From* Karan and coworkers [15].)

ANESTHETIC MANAGEMENT OF THE PATIENT WITH A QUESTIONABLE OR DOCUMENTED HISTORY OF MALIGNANT HYPERTHERMIA

I. Equipment
   A. A "clean" anesthesia machine should be prepared by removing or sealing the vaporizers, replacing the fresh gas hose, and using a new disposable circuit. Next, flush the machine with a fresh gas flow of 10 L/min for 5 min. Prepare the anesthetic machine even if a regional technique or monitored anesthesia care is planned in case of failed technique or emergency.
   B. Capnography with real-time display, electrocardiogram, blood pressure, and electronic temperature monitoring are required.
   C. MH cart must be checked for expired medications.

II. Scheduling
   A. First case of the day.
   B. Observation in the recovery room for 4 to 6 h.
   C. Outpatient surgery is acceptable if the patient can be observed in the recovery room for 4 to 6 h and intensive care support is readily available.

III. Premedication
   A. Dantrolene prophylaxis is at the discretion of the anesthesiologist.
   B. Sedation is at the discretion of the anesthesiologist.

IV. Technique
   A. Monitored anesthesia care.
   B. Regional anesthesia (peripheral or central axis).
   C. Nontriggering agents for general anesthesia.

V. Postoperative care
   A. Monitoring: respiratory rate, blood pressure, heart rate, and temperature.
   B. Laboratory: if the clinical course remains uneventful, tests are not necessary.
   C. Health care providers in the recovery room should be alerted to the patient's MH status.

Figure 9-13. Management of the patient susceptible to malignant hyperthermia (*MH*). Many patients will present for surgery who either have a documented history of MH or a family history suspicious for MH. Often times a workup has not been initiated or is incomplete because of missing records or lack of contracture testing. Although a complete workup is desirable, it is not required. These patients can be safely anesthetized for surgery if the proper precautions are observed. A recommended management plan for these patients is outlined in this illustration. *The essential points are to use a "clean" anesthesia machine, monitor the patient appropriately, avoid triggering agents, and be prepared to treat an acute MH episode should it develop*. It is preferable that these patients be scheduled as the first case of the day to allow time for preparation and to avoid contamination of the room by waste anesthetic gas. Extended observation postoperatively, 4 to 6 hours, is suggested. Routine use of dantrolene prophylaxis is not required, although certain patients may benefit and pretreatment may be appropriate. Pretreatment with dantrolene does not eliminate the need for a non-triggering anesthetic technique.

NECESSARY SUPPLIES FOR THE MH CART

The MH cart must contain the following supplies:

- Dantrolene, 36 vials
- Sterile water for injection, 3 L (for reconstitution of dantrolene, 60 mL per vial)
- 5 to 10 50-mL syringes and 16-gauge needles to mix the dantrolene
- Lidocaine, bolus and continuous infusion
- Procainamide, bolus and continuous infusion
- Sodium bicarbonate, 10 ampules
- Dextrose 50%, 4 ampules
- Furosemide, 200 mg
- 25% Mannitol, 100 g (8 ampules)

Plan for rapid access of the following:

- Refrigerated normal saline solution for infusion and irrigation
- Ice maker or crushed ice
- Central pressure catheters, transducers, and monitors
- Blood collection tubes for laboratory processing of samples: blood gas analysis, electrolytes, and glucose
- Cooling blanket
- Rectal tube and irrigating Foley catheter

Figure 9-14. Necessary supplies for the malignant hyperthermia (MH) cart. Successful treatment of MH relies on prompt recognition of the clinical situation, quick access to supplies, and initiation of appropriate therapeutic measures. The MH cart must be easily identified and stored in an accessible location. The cart also must be routinely checked for outdated supplies. If routine resuscitation drugs are stocked on the regular anesthesia cart, they are not required on the MH cart.

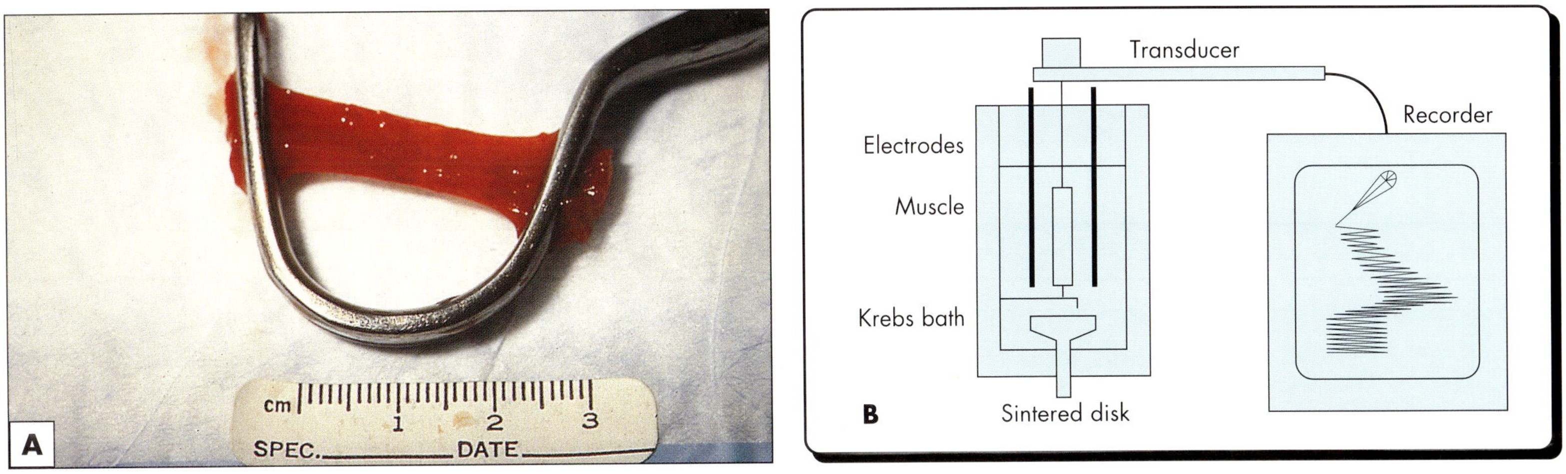

Figure 9-15. Contracture testing. There is no simple screening test or minimally invasive diagnostic test to identify individuals susceptible for malignant hyperthermia (MH). The halothane–caffeine contracture tests are the only tests to accurately identify patients that have had clinical MH episodes [4,16]. In North America, 10 medical centers provide diagnostic contracture testing. Approximately 25 centers are operational in Europe. Current muscle viability standards require that testing be completed within 5 hours, and therefore patients are required to travel to a diagnostic center for testing. Contracture testing cannot be used as a routine screening test because of its invasiveness, complexity, limited access, and cost. A, Muscle biopsy. The skeletal muscle sample is divided into 4 to 6 strips (25–30 mm in length and 2–3 mm in diameter) for diagnostic testing. The sample can only be obtained via open muscle biopsy. **B**, Contracture testing setup. Each end of the muscle strip is tied with a silk thread so that the muscle can be suspended in a tissue bath. One thread is attached to a transducer to measure muscle tension. The bath is filled with Krebs solution and carbogen (95% oxygen and 5% carbon dioxide) is bubbled through the solution via a sintered disk. A water jacket maintains the bath at 37°C. Platinum electrodes are used to stimulate ("twitch") the muscle. After stabilization of the twitch height and baseline tension, either halothane or caffeine is added to the solution.

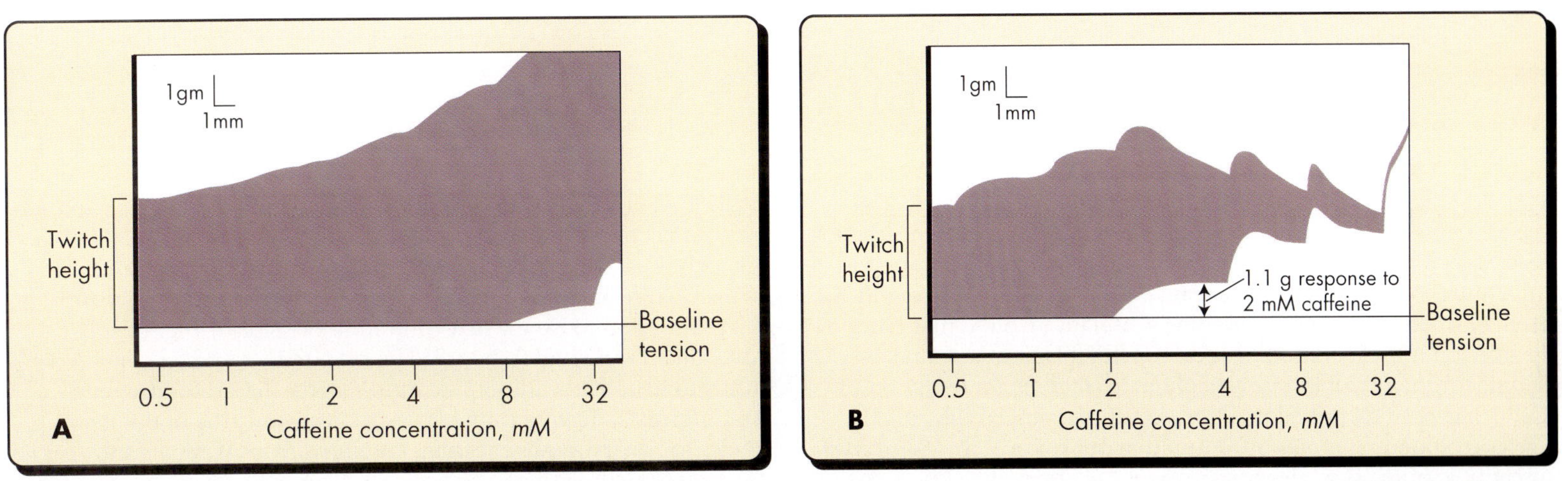

Figure 9-16. Caffeine response (North American protocol). In 1970, Kalow and Britt [4] reported that isolated strips of human muscle demonstrated enhanced contracture response to caffeine when obtained from patients who had muscle rigidity during their episode of malignant hyperthermia (MH). Normal muscle also contracts when exposed to caffeine, but requires higher concentrations. Unlike halothane, caffeine has not been reported to trigger an episode of MH. Standard testing protocols were adopted by European diagnostic centers in 1984 and by North American diagnostic centers in 1987 so that patients and test results from the various diagnostic centers could be pooled for further investigation. The two protocols are slightly different. The North American protocol uses incremental caffeine concentrations of 0.5, 1, 2, 4, 8, and 32 mM, and the European protocol calls for incremental caffeine concentrations of 0.5, 1, 1.5, 2, 3, 4, and 32 mM [17–19]. **A**, Normal caffeine response. Caffeine potentiates twitch height in all muscle strips. However, baseline tension remains unaffected until the bath concentration of caffeine is increased to 8 mM (0.6-g increase in tension). A caffeine contracture test result is considered positive when the muscle strip exhibits an increase in baseline tension of 0.2 g or more in response to a caffeine concentration of 2 mM or less. **B**, Abnormal caffeine response. The muscle strip has a 1.1-g increase in baseline tension in response to a caffeine concentration of 2 mM.

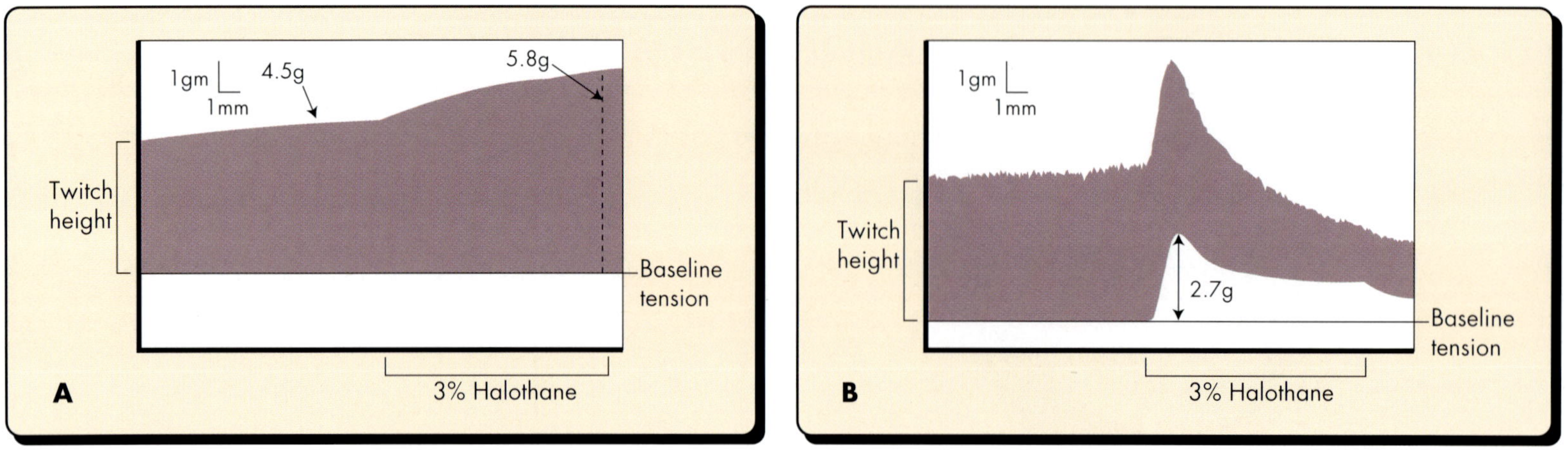

Figure 9-17. Halothane response (North American protocol). In 1971, Ellis *et al.* [16] first reported that muscle strips from patients with MH developed contractures when exposed to halothane *in vitro*. Again, the North American and European protocols are slightly different. The North American protocol uses a single dose of halothane, 3%, and the European protocol uses incremental doses of halothane (0.5%, 1%, 2%, and 3%) [17–19]. Interpretation of the results also differs between protocols. The European protocol requires a positive response from both halothane and caffeine. If the patient's muscle responds to only one drug, the result is labeled as MH equivocal by the European protocol. A patient is reported as being MH susceptible by the North American protocol if any muscle strip exhibits a positive response to either halothane or caffeine. The North American MH Registry database of over 2500 contracture test results has been used to determine the sensitivity and specificity of the North American protocol at 97% and 78%, respectively. **A**, Normal halothane response. Halothane potentiates twitch height in all muscle strips similar to caffeine. The twitch height in this strip increases from 4.5 to 5.8 g of tension. However, there is no change in baseline tension in response to 3% halothane. A positive response to 3% halothane is an increase in baseline tension of 0.7 or more g of tension. **B**, Abnormal halothane response. The muscle strip has a 2.7-g increase in baseline tension in response to 3% halothane.

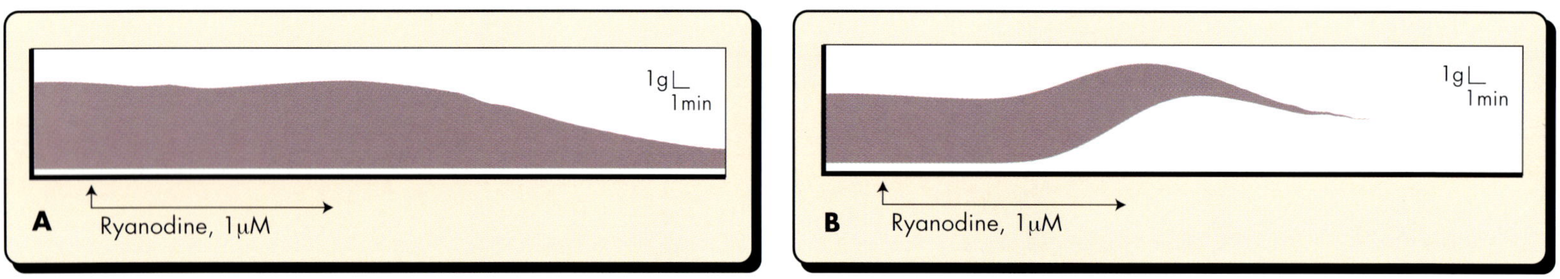

Figure 9-18. Ryanodine response (European Protocol): Many pharmacologic agents have been shown to induce contracture in muscle from MHS patients, but only halothane and caffeine have been accepted as reliable testing agents internationally. Ryanodine and chlorocresol are currently being evaluated as adjunct agents for MH contracture testing. Ryanodine is a plant alkaloid that binds to the skeletal muscle ryanodine receptor (RYR1), a calcium release channel of the sarcoplasmic reticulum. A single point mutation of RYR1 has been identified in all breeds of pigs susceptible to MH. The corresponding mutation is found in approximately 5% of MH susceptible humans. Chlorocresol exerts a caffeine-like effect on skeletal muscle but at a much lower concentration (micro- vs millimolar). **A**, Normal ryanodine response. The muscle strip is exposed to a 1 μM concentration of ryanodine once a 10 minute stable baseline period is achieved. Three times are recorded for each muscle strip: 1) start of contracture, 2) time when contracture reaches 0.2 grams, and 3) time when contracture reaches 1.0 grams. **B**, Abnormal ryanodine response. The ryanodine response times from susceptible patients are significantly shorter than response times from normals. Testing is underway to determine the optimal cut points for the ryanodine testing. (*Adapted from* Wappler and coworkers [20]; with permission.)

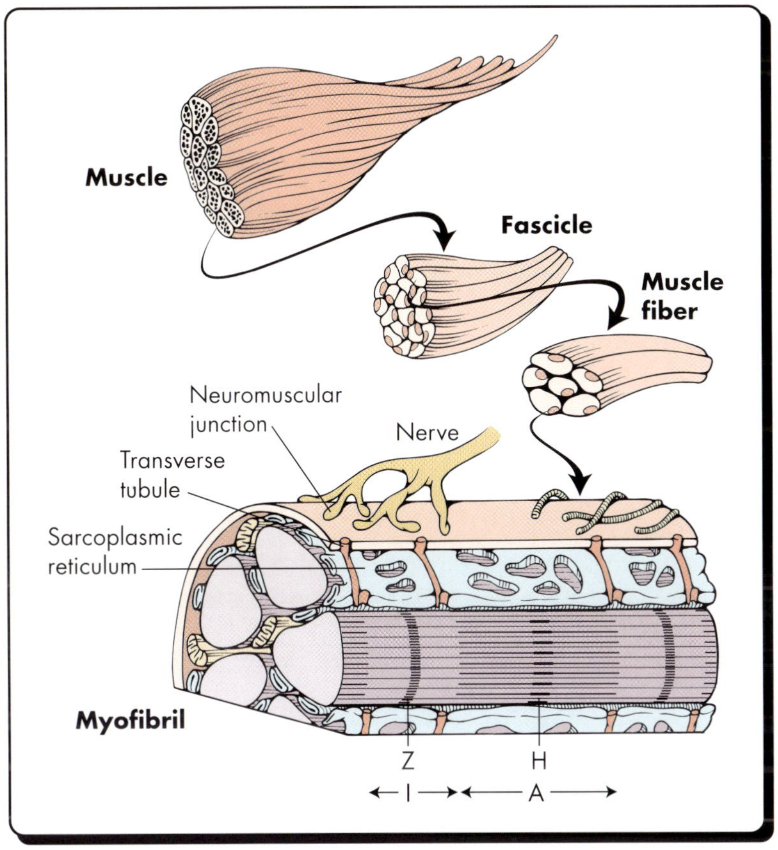

Figure 9-19. Skeletal muscle. Using an isolated perfused porcine hind limb preparation, Gronert and coworkers [21] demonstrated that the malignant hyperthermia (MH) defect resides in skeletal muscle. The isolated limb responded to triggering anesthetic agents in a manner similar to that of intact MH-susceptible pigs. Possible sources of skeletal muscle abnormalities include neuromuscular transmission, excitation-contraction coupling, structural proteins, contractile proteins, and the regulation of any of these systems. Although the exact site of the defect in MH is not completely understood, intracellular calcium is increased during episodes. Abnormalities in the regulation of intracellular calcium or possibly EC coupling are more likely to be the source of the defect in MH because neuromuscular transmission, structural proteins, and contractile proteins are normal in MH susceptible individuals.

Muscle fibers are comprised of myofibrils, which contain the contractual proteins actin and myosin. The myofibrils are densely packed in the cell, accounting for three fourths of the volume. The myofibrils have a characteristic regularly repeating transverse band pattern. Each unit is called a sarcomere. The sarcoplasmic reticulum is the major organelle for the storage and release of calcium. The cell wall of a skeletal muscle cell is called the sarcolemma. Invaginations of the sarcolemma are called transverse tubules and occur at regular intervals. The transverse tubules rapidly spread action potentials from the sarcolemma to the interior of the muscle. They also contain calcium channels that communicate with the sarcoplasmic reticulum to initiate calcium release and result in mechanical contraction. This conversion of sarcolemma depolarization into mechanical activity is called excitation-contraction coupling. M, mitochondria; N, nerve; SC, sarcolemma; SR, sarcoplasmic reticulum; T, T tubule. (*Adapted from* Fischbeth [22]; with permission.)

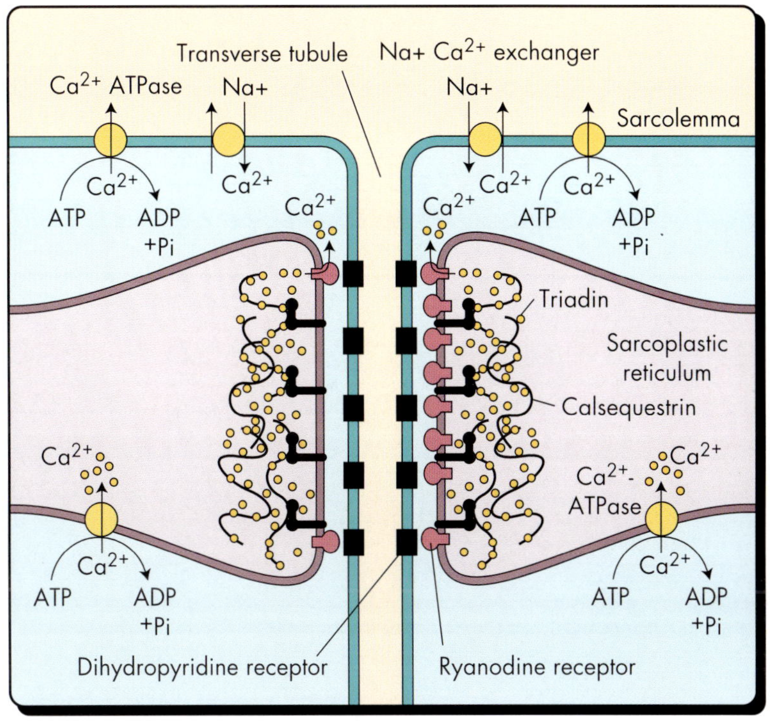

Figure 9-20. Calcium regulation in skeletal muscle. A closer look is given at the proteins involved in calcium regulation and excitation-contraction coupling. The dihydropyridine receptor is the voltage-regulated calcium channel that spans the transverse tubule. Depolarization of the sarcolemma and transverse tubule result in opening of this channel and a net influx of calcium. The ryanodine receptor, a calcium channel that spans the sarcoplasmic reticulum, is adjacent to the dihydropyridine receptor. Calcium is released from the sarcoplasmic reticulum (SR) through the ryanodine receptor. Uptake of calcium into the SR occurs away from the transverse tubule via adenosine triphosphate (*ATP*)–dependent calcium pumps. How the dihydropyridine receptor interacts with the ryanodine receptor to release calcium from the SR has yet to be discovered. Several proteins have been recently discovered in this area and are under investigation as to any role they may have in modulating calcium release. These proteins include triadin, calsequestrin and FK binding protein. The FK binding protein binds to the ryanodine receptor and is proposed to modulate its gating. ADP, adenosine diphosphate; ATPase, adenosine triphosphatase; Ca^{++}, calcium ions; Na^{+}, sodium ions; P_i, free phosphate. (*From* Mickelson and Louis [23]; with permission.)

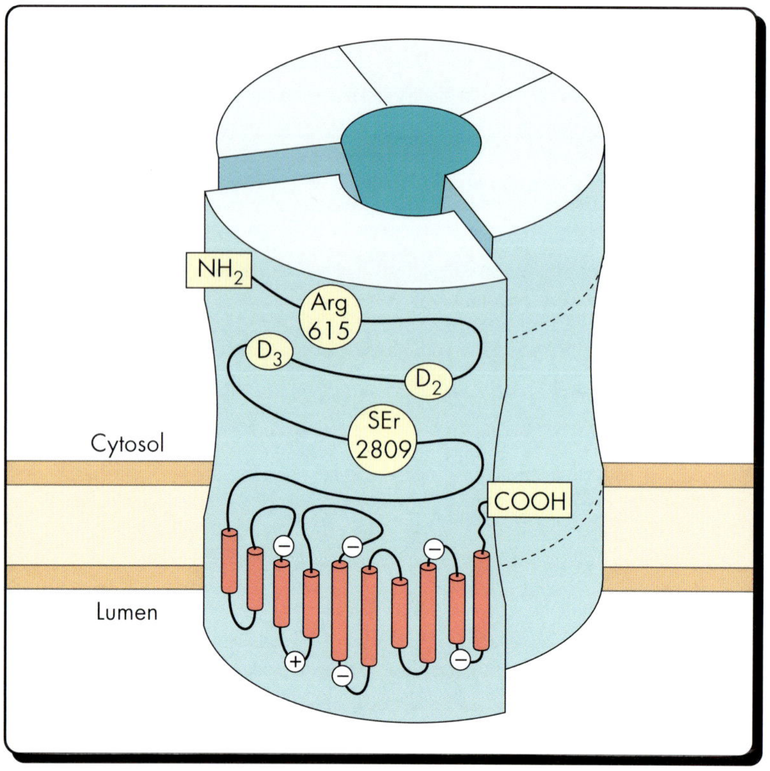

Figure 9-21. The ryanodine receptor. Each ryanodine receptor is composed of four identical monomers of approximately 5000 amino acids. At least three distinct genes encode for isoforms of the ryanodine receptor. The RYR-1 isoform is expressed in skeletal muscle. The proposed membrane organization places the transmembrane sequences in the COOH terminal of each subunit. The remainder of the subunit (approximately 80%) is cytosolic, with binding sites for adenosine triphosphate, calcium, magnesium, and a variety of drugs including volatile anesthetics. The functional significance of the NH_2 terminal domains that contain the Arg615Cys mutation (the pig mutation) and many of the proposed human MH mutations (15 to date) is not understood. The Arg615Cys mutation does not affect conductance or ion selective properties of the ryanodine channel; however this region may be important in the transmission of signals from the transverse tubule and dihydropyridine receptor, determining whether the ryanodine channel is in the open or closed state. (*From* Sorrentino and Volpe [24]; with permission.)

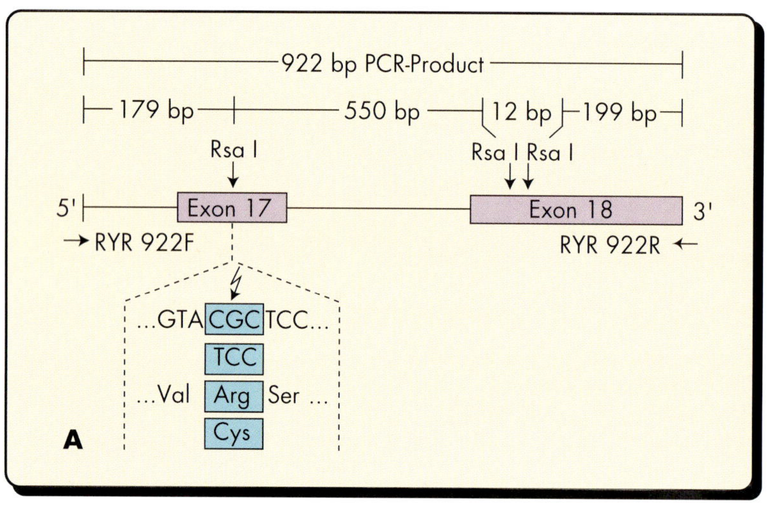

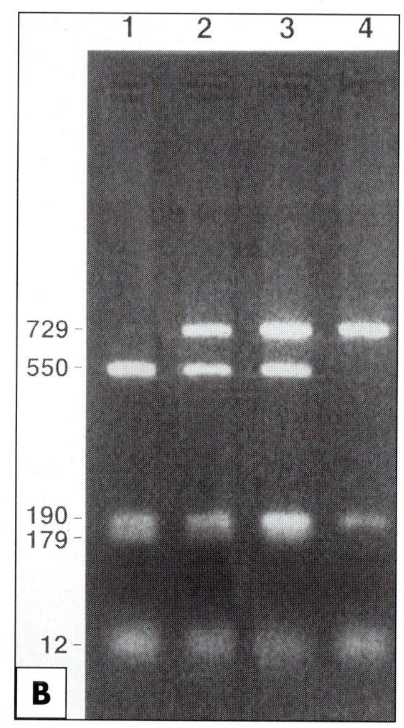

Figure 9-22. Identification of human genetic defects in malignant hyperthermia (MH). Genomic DNA is isolated from the leukocytes of a peripheral blood sample. Once isolated, specific base pair (*bp*) fragments are amplified for further analysis. Defects can then be identified by sequencing of the fragment, which is expensive and time-consuming, or by using restriction enzymes. Restriction enzymes cut DNA at specific sequence sites. They are valuable in detecting defects when the defect either eliminates or creates a cut in the bp fragment. **A**, An example is the human equivalent of the MH swine defect, an arginine (*arg*) to cysteine (*cys*) substitution at amino acid position 614 of the ryanodine receptor [25]. This substitution is the result of a C1840T mutation located in the 922 bp fragment. When the *Rsa I* restriction enzyme is added to a 922 bp fragment that does not contain the substitution, the fragment is cut in three places creating fragments of 12, 179, 199, and 550 bp. However when the substitution is present, one of the sites is eliminated, creating only 3 fragments of 12, 199, and 729 bp. **B**, These fragments can be separated on an agarose gel, identifying individuals as normal, homozygous, or heterozygous for the defect. In normal individuals (*lane 1*) the 729 fragment is not present because it has been cut into the 179 and 550 fragments. In homozygous individuals (*lane 4*) the reverse occurs, the 729 fragment is present and the 179 and 550 fragments are absent. In heterozygous individuals (*lanes 2 and 3*) all three bands appear because one strand is affected and the other is normal. A—adenine; C—cytosine; G—guanine; ser—serine; T—thymine; val—valine.

GENETIC MUTATIONS OF THE HUMAN RYANODINE RECEPTOR GENE	
Mutation	**Association**
Glycine 248 to arginine	MH
Glycine 341 to arginine	MH
Arginine 614 to cysteine	MH
Glycine 2433 to arginine	MH
Arginine 163 to cysteine	MH/CCD
Isoleucine 403 to methionine	MH/CCD
Tyrosine 522 to serine	MH/CCD
Arginine 2434 to histidine	MH/CCD

Figure 9-23. Genetic mutations of the human ryanodine receptor gene. The mutations detected to date on chromosome 19 of the human ryanodine receptor gene and disease associations. MH, malignant hyperthermia; CCD, central core disease. (*Adapted from* MacLennan [26].)

REFERENCES

1. Denborough MA, Lovell RH: Anesthesia deaths in a family. *Lancet* 1960, 2:45.
2. Britt BA: The Clinical Aspects of Hyperthermia. In *Malignant Hyperthermia Current Concepts*. Edited by Felipe MA, Gottmann S, Khambatta HJ. Darmstadt: Normed Verlag; 1989:28:91–107.
3. Berman MÇ: Changes underlining halothane induced malignant hyperpyrexia in landrace pigs. *Nature* 1970, 225:653–655.
4. Kalow W, Britt BA, Terreau ME, *et al.*: Metabolic error of muscle metabolism after recovery from malignant hyperthermia. *Lancet* 1970, 2:895–898.
5. Rosenberg H, Seitman D: Pharmacogenetics. *Clin Anesth* 1989, 17:459–472.
6. Harrison GG: Porcine malignant hyperthermia. *Int Anesth Clin* 1978, 17:25–61.
7. Mathieu A, Bogosian AJ, Ryan JF: Recrudescence after survival of an initial episode of malignant hyperthermia. *Anesthesiology* 1979, 51:454–455.
8. Allen GC, Rosenberg H: Phaeochromocytoma presenting as acute malignant hyperthermia: a diagnostic challenge. *Can J Anaesth* 1990, 37:593–595.
9. Stevens JJ: A case of thyrotoxic crisis that mimicked malignant hyperthermia. *Anesthesiology* 1983, 59:263.
10. Weglinski MR, Wedel DJ: Differential diagnosis of hyperthermia during anesthesia and clinical import. *Anesth Clin North Am* 1994, 12:475–489.
11. Karan SM, Crowl F, Muldoon SM: Malignant hyperthermia masked by capnographic monitoring. *Anesth Analg* 1994, 78:590–592.
12. Kaplan RF: Clinical controversies in malignant hyperthermia susceptibility. *Anesth Clin North Am* 1994, 12:537–551.
13. Littleford JA, Patel LR, Bose D: Masseter muscle spasm in children: implications of continuing the triggering anesthetic. *Anesth Analg* 1991, 72:151–160.
14. Karan SM, Greenberg CP, Hall SL, *et al.*: The MH hotline is a useful epidemiological tool in determining recent trends in MH. *Anesthesiology* 1996, 85:A978.
15. Karan SM, Lojeski EW, Muldoon SM: Hyperthermia and Hypothermia. In *Principles and Practice of Anesthesiology*, edn 2. Edited by Longnecker DE, Tinker JH, Morgan GE. St Louis: Mosby, 1993:2499–2520.
16. Ellis FR, Harriman DGF, Keaney NP, *et al.*: Halothane-induced muscle contracture as a cause of hyperpyrexia. *Br J Anaesth* 1971, 43:721–722.
17. Larach MG, for the North American Malignant Hyperthermia Group: Standardization of the caffeine halothane muscle contracture test. *Anesth Analg* 1989, 69:511–515.
18. European Malignant Hyperpyrexia Group: A protocol for the investigation of malignant hyperpyrexia (MH) susceptibility. *Br J Anaesth* 1984, 56:1267–1269.
19. European Malignant Hyperpyrexia Group: Laboratory diagnosis of malignant hyperpyrexia susceptibility (MHS). *Br J Anaesth* 1985, 57:1038.
20. Wappler F, Roewer N, Kochling A, *et al.*: *In vitro* diagnosis of malignant hyperthermia susceptibility with ryanodine-induced contractures in human skeletal muscles MH diagnosis by ryanodine contracture. *Anesth Analg* 1996, 82:1230–1236.
21. Gronert GA, Milde JH, Theye RA: Role of sympathetic activity in porcine malignant hyperthermia. *Anesthesiology* 1977, 47:411–415.
22. Fischbeck KH: Structure and function of striated muscle. *Clin Neurobiol* 1986, 15:185–97.
23. Michelson JR, Louis CF: Malignant hyperthermia: excitation-contraction coupling, Ca^{2+} release channel, and cell Ca^{2+} regulation defects. *Pharmacol Rev* 1996, 76:537–591.
24. Sorrentino V, Volpe P: Ryanodine receptors: How many, where and why? *TiPS* 1993, 14:98–103.
25. Gillard EF, Otsu K, Fujii J, *et al.*: Polymorphisms and deduced amino acid substitutions in the coding sequence of the ryanodine (RYR1) gene in individuals with malignant hyperthermia. *Genomics* 1992, 13:1247–1254.
26. MacLennan DH: Discordance between phenotype and genotype in malignant hyperthermia. *Curr Opin Neurol* 1995, 8:397–401.

10

Airway Emergencies

Joseph W. Szokol and Jeffery S. Vender

The anesthesiologist may be confronted with several airway emergencies that demand immediate attention. One such emergency is barotrauma. Barotrauma, or ventilator-associated extra-alveolar air, is a potentially life-threatening event that occurs among 4% to 15% of patients receiving mechanical ventilation [1]. This percentage is even higher in those patients with underlying pulmonary pathology such as adult respiratory distress syndrome, chronic obstructive pulmonary disease, or asthma. Some of the associated risk factors for barotrauma or volutrauma include high peak airway pressures, high levels of positive end-expiratory pressure, and large tidal volumes. The most commonly found barotrauma-associated events are mediastinal and subcutaneous emphysema, and pneumothorax. The ability to recognize and treat the cardiovascular and respiratory changes caused by barotrauma can be life-saving. But it must be appreciated that the capability to recognize barotrauma may be hampered by the sometimes poor sensitivity of radiographs and the occasionally late clinical signs.

Another airway crisis is aspiration. The prevention and management of aspiration is one of the hallmarks of anesthetic practice, and its avoidance can prevent serious injury to the patient. Since Mendelson [2] first described the syndrome that is now called aspiration pneumonia, countless articles and texts have been written about it. It is one of the most feared complications of airway management. The incidence is estimated at between 3.1 to 4.7 per 10,000 patients receiving anesthesia, with certain subgroups at a greater risk, such as those with a higher American Society of Anesthesiologists classification or with intestinal obstruction. The risk of aspiration is also increased in patients with underlying neurologic disorders, decreased gastric motility with a concomitant larger gastric fluid volume, and those with reduced gastric pH [3].

An anterior mediastinal mass is a potential airway crisis that most often occurs with lymphomas, teratomas, and thymomas. The possibility of complete airway obstruction brought on by positive airway pressure must be anticipated by the anesthesiologist. If a biopsy of an anterior mediastinal mass is needed, it is often best undertaken under local anesthesia. If this is not feasible and the diagnosis would be interfered with by either the administration of steroids or radiation to shrink the size of the tumor, the anesthesiologist should attempt to preserve spontaneous ventilation. Rigid bronchoscopy must be readily available should the need arise.

Epiglottitis usually has been an airway emergency of childhood. It is usually an acute bacterial illness involving the upper airway that is potentially fatal if airway obstruction is allowed to progress. The disease has changed over the past decade with the introduction of the *Haemophilus influenzae* b vaccine in children. The previous predominance of children versus adults in the incidence of the disease has dramatically changed, with more adults being affected than children. This is also important because the management in adults is quite different. Whereas placement of an artificial airway in children is the general rule, it is the exception in the adult because of the adult's larger diameter airway. In adults, too, the supraglottic structures may be visualized by laryngoscopy without the need for intubation. In the pediatric age group, this maneuver may result in complete airway obstruction. Whereas the placement of an artificial airway in the past often meant tracheostomy, oral intubation is safely accomplished with little or no morbidity in skilled hands. The key to this disease is its rapid diagnosis and appreciation of its capacity for life-threatening airway obstruction.

PNEUMOTHORAX AND BAROTRAUMA

TYPES OF PNEUMOTHORAX

Primary spontaneous (simple) pneumothorax
Secondary spontaneous (complicated) pneumothorax
Catamenial pneumothorax
Pneumothorax associated with drug abuse
Iatrogenic pneumothorax
Pneumothorax associated with mechanical ventilation
Traumatic pneumothorax
Tension pneumothorax

Figure 10-1. Types of pneumothorax. Primary spontaneous pneumothorax occurs in patients without underlying lung disease. It usually occurs in young, tall, slender male patients. Secondary pneumothoraces occur in those patients with underlying lung disease. Pneumothorax has also been associated with drug abuse and is believed to be related to the inhalational route of drug abuse, in which the abuser performs a Valsalva maneuver with generation of pressures greater than 200 cm H_2O. Iatrogenic pneumothorax occurs most commonly during attempted central line placement, with the risk between 3% and 6% for subclavian placement and about 1% to 2% with internal jugular catheterization. Traumatic pneumothorax may be caused by blunt or penetrating trauma and may have associated hemopneumothorax and other vascular injuries.

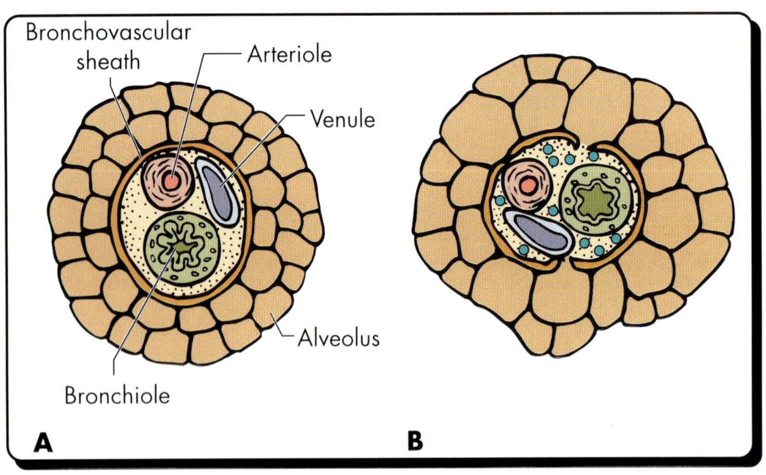

Figure 10-2. Alveoli and bronchioles. **A**, Normal structure. Extra-alveolar air occurs when there is a tear in the base of the perivascular alveoli in the presence of a pressure gradient between the alveoli and vascular sheath. Thus, conditions that cause intra-alveolar pressure to increase or perivascular interstitial pressure to decrease may lead to the occurrence of air outside of the alveolar sac (*arrows* in B). This air in the vascular sheath is called pulmonary interstitial emphysema and develops before evidence of barotrauma is apparent. This gas then decompresses through other fascial planes to eventually produce clinical signs of barotrauma, such as mediastinal emphysema and pneumothorax [4]. (*Adapted from* Maunder and coworkers [5].)

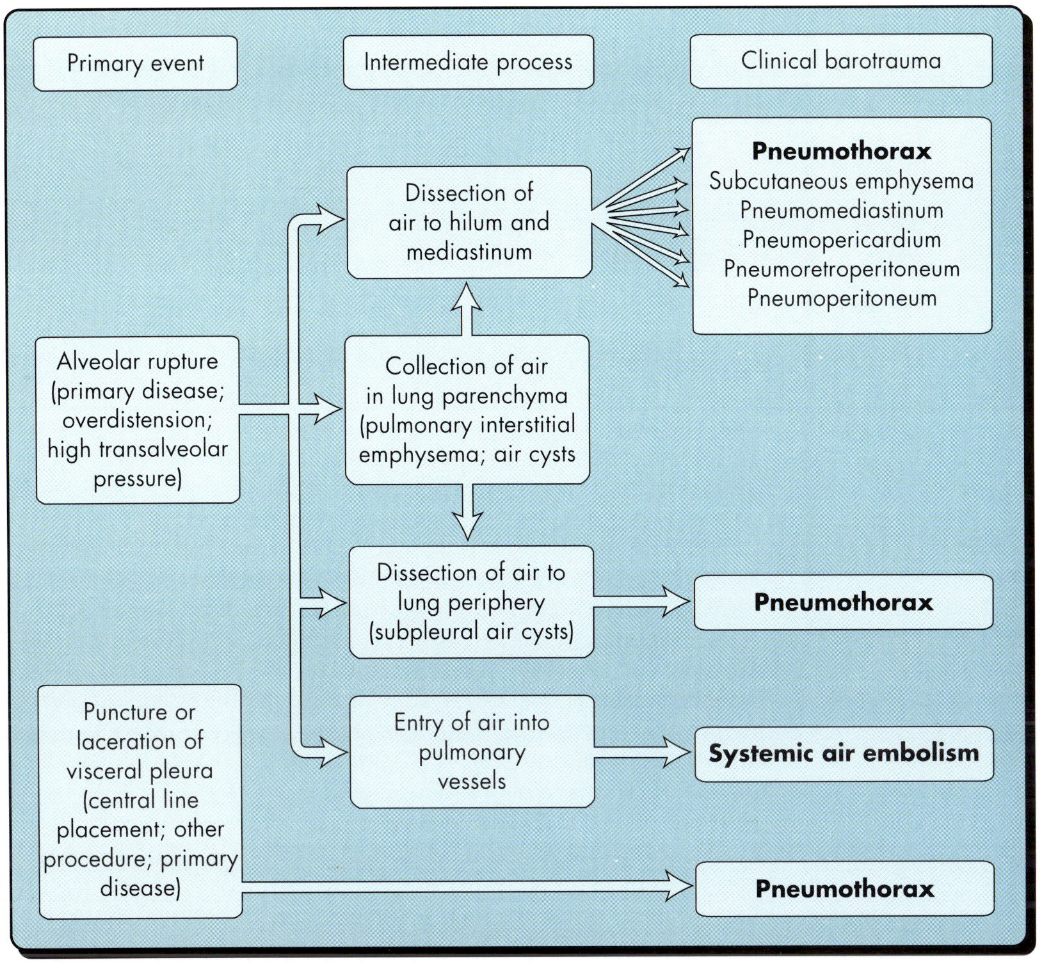

Figure 10-3. Results of alveolar rupture. There are three ways in which extra-alveolar air may occur. The first involves a pressure gradient between the alveoli and their surrounding space, as may occur during high peak inspiratory pressures and positive end-expiratory pressure. The second involves a traumatic injury to the alveoli, such as during attempted central line placement. The third and rarest form involves gas-forming organisms. Once there is disruption of the alveoli, the air dissects along bronchoalveolar sheaths to the lung hilum and mediastinum. From there the air can enter subcutaneous tissues, forming subcutaneous emphysema; the pericardium, forming a pneumopericardium; or enter the retroperitoneum or peritoneum. The air can also break through the mediastinal parietal pleura, resulting in a pneumothorax. Rarely, the air can be embolized into the systemic circulation, causing death [6]. (*Adapted from* Pierson [4].)

RISK FACTORS FOR BAROTRAUMA

	No Barotrauma	Mediastinal emphysema	Pneumothorax
Patients, *n*	105	29	20
Age, *y*	57±17	50±19*	55±22
PIP, *cm*	44±12	55±14*	55±12*
PEEP, *cm* H_2O	3.3±3.6	8.0±7.3*	7.7±8.3*
Rate	20±9	27±8*	27±6*
TV, *mL/kg*	12.1±2.7	12.6±3.1	13.0±3.9
VE, *L/min*	15.4±5.0	20.8±6.1*	21.4±5.6*

*Significant difference.

Figure 10-4. Risk factors for barotrauma. Peak inspiratory pressure, the level of positive end-expiratory pressure (PEEP), rate of ventilation, and minute ventilation are all risk factors for barotrauma and the subsequent development of mediastinal air and pneumothorax. The elevated peak inspiratory pressures (PIP) and PEEP may not be the cause of barotrauma but rather reflect the underlying disease pathology that necessitates the higher levels of airway pressure. Increased PIP is generally recognized as a risk factor for barotrauma, whereas increased levels of PEEP have not always been implicated in the creation of barotrauma [7]. Evidence suggests that it is the transalveolar pressure and alveolar distention, rather than the airway pressure itself, that causes ventilator-associated lung injury. In animal studies, the deleterious effect of high-pressure ventilation can be minimized if alveolar distention is prevented by chest binding [8]. Also, PIP does not always reflect alveolar pressure. PIP is affected by the airflow rate into the lungs, the resistance of the endotracheal tube, secretions, and bronchoconstriction. (*From* Gammon and coworkers [7]; with permission.)

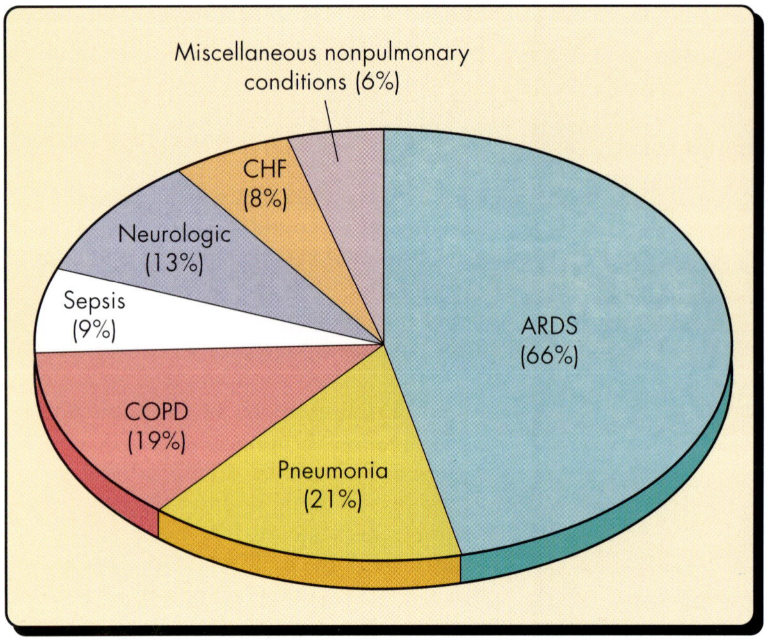

Figure 10-5. Incidence of barotrauma by admitting diagnosis. When barotrauma occurs in the patient on a ventilator it is assumed that mechanical ventilation alone is to blame, and that high peak airway pressures and positive end-expiratory pressure (PEEP) contribute to lung injury. However, barotrauma should be viewed not as a cause of mechanical ventilation but rather as a factor associated with mechanical ventilation, and that the underlying disease process, such as adult respiratory distress syndrome (ARDS) or chronic obstructive pulmonary disease (COPD), may play the more important role in predisposing a patient to barotrauma. Indeed, it is unusual for barotrauma to occur in someone with normal lungs, such as postoperative ventilated coronary artery bypass graft patients, or patients ventilated for a high cervical lesion. Rather, patients with underlying lung pathology who require mechanical ventilation are the ones most apt to need higher peak inspiratory airway pressures and PEEP and thus are more liable to have evidence of barotrauma [7]. CHF—chronic heart failure. (*Adapted from* Gammon and coworkers [7].)

CLINICAL FACTORS THAT INDICATE A HIGH INDEX OF SUSPICION FOR PNEUMOTHORAX
Peak airway pressures > 50 cm H_2O
PEEP > 15 cm H_2O
ARDS, COPD, or asthma
Use of tidal volumes > 12 mL/kg

Figure 10-6. Clinical factors that should create a high index of suspicion for pneumothorax. Physical signs of pneumothorax, such as diminished breath sounds and increased percussion resonance, are not readily apparent unless there is a tension pneumothorax. Other signs that may be present are worsening oxygenation or an increase in peak inspiratory pressure. In the mechanically ventilated patient, a pneumothorax most commonly is discovered on routine chest radiograph. Chest radiograph is best done with the patient in either the lateral decubitus position or upright with the film taken during exhalation. These positions may not be easily accomplished in the critically ill ventilated patient. Chest computed tomography (CT) is a more useful tool but not available at bedside. A study of CT scans of the chest found that in 30% of cases studied, a pneumothorax was not detected initially by the clinician or with plain radiographs of the chest. One half of these progressed to tension pneumothorax [9]. Finally, a pneumothorax may present with an a agitated patient, hypotension, or cardiovascular collapse as occurs in tension pneumothorax. Thus, a high index of suspicion is necessary in those patients who have underlying lung pathology or require high airway pressure or positive end-expiratory pressure (PEEP). ARDS—adult respiratory distress syndrome; COPD—chronic obstructive pulmonary disease.

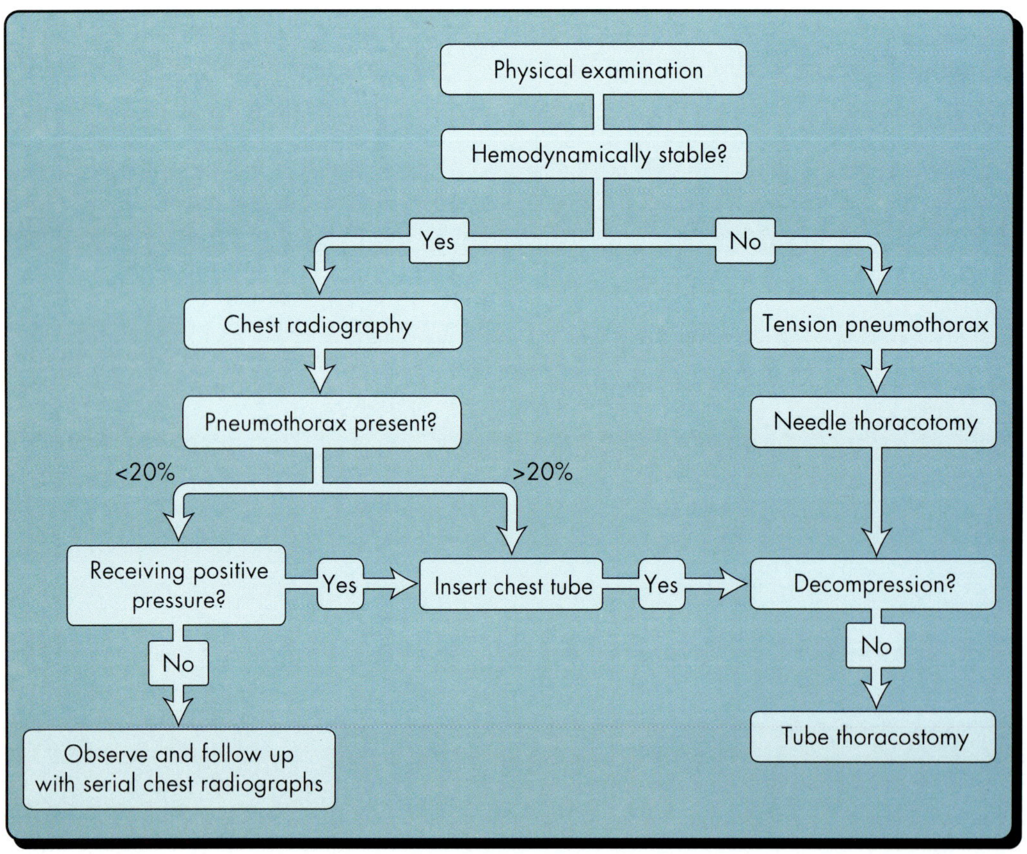

Figure 10-7. Treatment of pneumothorax. The patient who is receiving mechanical ventilation and presents with confirmation of a pneumothorax must receive a chest tube to decompress the pneumothorax and to prevent its enlargement. The individual who presents with a pneumothorax that is estimated to occupy less than 20% of the lung's volume and who is hemodynamically stable with good oxygenation may be followed up by serial radiography and close observation. (*Adapted from* Chomka Leya and Bandala [10].)

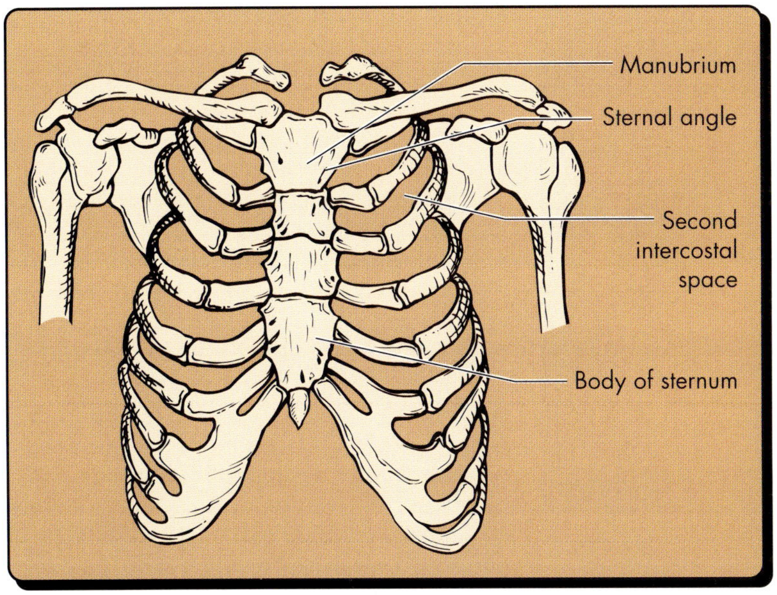

Figure 10-8. Needle thoracostomy. The occurrence of a pneumothorax in the patient receiving positive pressure ventilation necessitates the placement of a chest tube. If the patient has evidence of a tension pneumothorax and exhibits hemodynamic or respiratory instability, a needle thoracostomy should be undertaken immediately. The procedure involves using a 14-gauge angiocatheter and inserting it into the second intercostal space in the midclavicular line of the side of the pneumothorax. The needle is "walked off" the superior portion of the third rib into the second intercostal space. This is done to prevent laceration of the intercostal vessels. If the tension is not released then a tube thoracostomy should be done in the same location. Once a tension pneumothorax is decompressed, a chest tube must be inserted to prevent reaccumulation of air. The angiocatheter, once it has released the tension in the chest, should not be removed until a chest tube is in place.

ASPIRATION

AIRWAY REFLEXES
Pharyngeal (gag and swallow)
Laryngeal
Tracheal (cough)
Carinal

Figure 10-9. Airway reflexes. Competent airway reflexes are an important mechanism in the body's defense against aspiration. Those patients with decreased function of these reflexes may be at greater risk of aspiration. Those with neurologic disorders such as cerebrovascular accidents, connective tissue diseases, and neuromuscular disorders such as myasthenia gravis may lack the normal protective reflexes. Whereas some disease states may attenuate certain airway reflexes, 10% to 15% of healthy patients may have a diminished or absent gag and swallow reflex. As sedation is employed and increased, the pharyngeal and laryngeal reflexes are diminished before the tracheal and carinal reflexes, which are somewhat more resistant to anesthetic agents.

RISK FACTORS FOR ASPIRATION	
Altered Neurologic States	Gastrointestinal Disorders
Cerebrovascular accident	Intestinal obstruction
Drug overdose	Obesity
Acute alcohol ingestion	Intra-abdominal masses
Postictal states	Decreased gastric emptying
Sedative administration	Hiatal hernia
General anesthesia	Achalasia
Cardiopulmonary resuscitation	Esophageal stricture or spasm
Central nervous system disorders	Iatrogenic
	Nasogastric tubes

Figure 10-10. Risk factors for aspiration. Patients with either increased gastric volumes or increased gastric acidity are at greater risk of aspiration. Pregnancy is one condition that may combine both of these factors. Alcohol stimulates gastric secretion and may place a patient at increased risk. The lower esophageal sphincter (LES) may have its intrinsic resting tone altered by either food, drugs, tobacco, or disease states predisposing to an increased risk of aspiration. The LES may also remain open with the presence of a nasogastric tube. The obese patient is believed to be at a high risk of aspiration because of both increased gastric volume and reduced stomach pH. Diabetic patients also are at an increased risk because of autonomic dysfunction and delayed gastric emptying.

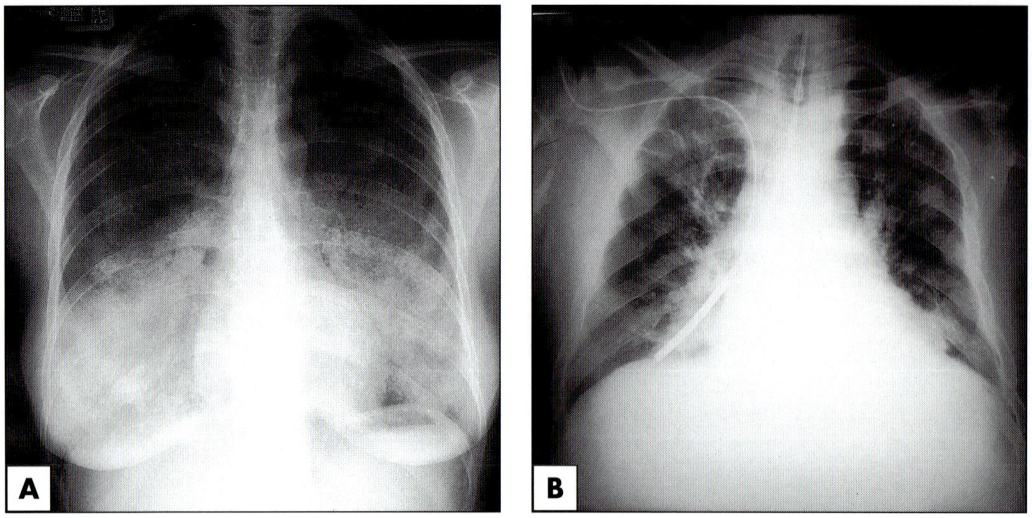

Figure 10-11. Chest radiographs of an aspiration and a nasogastric tube in the lung. **A**, Bilateral pneumonia from a pulmonary aspiration. The right lower lobe is the most often affected segment of the lung in cases of aspiration in patients in the supine position. The left upper lobe is the least often involved lobe. **B**, A feeding tube may be inadvertently placed into the right main stem bronchus. If this is not recognized and hyperalimentation or other substances are infused through the tube, disastrous consequences may result. The practice of injecting air into a nasogastric tube and auscultating over the stomach is not foolproof. Placement of a nasogastric or other type of feeding tube with radiographic confirmation of correct positioning is mandatory in the ventilated and sedated patient. (Courtesy of Joel R. Bernstein, Evanston Hospital, Evanston, IL.)

CLASSIFICATION OF ASPIRATIONS

Toxic	Nontoxic
Acids	Water
Alcohol	Saline
Volatile hydrocarbons	Milk
Oils	Blood
Fats	Barium
	Gastric fluid with pH > 7.3
	Bacterial

Figure 10-12. Classification of aspiration. Aspirations can be divided into three main categories: toxic, nontoxic, and bacterial. Acid aspiration is the classic toxic aspiration. Damage to the tracheal-bronchial tree can be immediate or delayed for several hours. Gross changes include edema, necrosis, atelectasis with disruption of bronchial epithelium, and infiltration of polymorphonuclear cells. In acid aspiration, the severity of damage is related to both the pH of the fluid and volume; the pH is a more important factor, with the severity of damage increasing with decreasing pH. Fluids with a pH greater than 2.5 pose less of a hazard than those with a pH less than 2.5. The volume of aspirated material is also important; 0.4 mL/kg or higher may be needed to produce serious side effects [11]. The aspiration of nontoxic liquids is usually reversible and nonspecific, but a significant fall in PaO_2 can occur from reflex bronchospasm and destruction of surfactant, which can lead to atelectasis.

Near-drowning is a prototypical nontoxic aspiration. Eighty-five percent of near-drowning patients have large amounts of aspirated water (15% develop severe laryngospasm and do not aspirate much fluid). The damage is determined by the volume and tonicity of the fluid aspirated: saltwater drowning has a high incidence of hypovolemic shock and hemoconcentration, whereas freshwater drowning is usually accompanied by hypervolemia, hemodilution, and occasional hemolysis. Near-drowning victims may also have ingested drugs or alcohol and have diminished protective airway reflexes, and the occurrence of toxic gastric aspiration must be considered [12]. Bacterial aspiration, caused by lack of protective airway reflexes, is most often due to the patient's own oropharyngeal secretions, the severity strongly influenced by the patient's own underlying sinusitis or gingivodental disease. The resulting pneumonia, lung abscess, or empyema may present hours to weeks later.

CLINICAL PRESENTATION OF ASPIRATION

Dyspnea
Wheezing
Rales
Ronchi
Cough
Fever
Tachycardia
Hypotension
Cyanosis

Figure 10-13. Clinical presentation of aspiration. The aspiration of small food particles produces a foreign body–type reaction in the airway, which involves mononuclear cell inflammation. The aspiration of acidic gastric material leads to a neutrophilic response that begins immediately and progresses over many hours. This leads to edema, inflammation, and damage to type I epithelial cells. Surfactant production is diminished and alveolar collapse occurs. Capillaries become leaky and fibrin and plasma leak into the pulmonary interstitium, with resultant loss of intravascular volume and hypotension. Aspiration may also lead to mechanical obstruction of a bronchial tree or distal obstruction. Airway resistance is increased by the aspirated material and by desquamation of the lining of the lung with subsequent reflex bronchospasm and airway edema. Hypoxemia occurs because of obstruction, edema, bronchospasm, and alveolar collapse [13].

RISK OF PULMONARY ASPIRATION IN ELECTIVE AND EMERGENCY GENERAL ANESTHESIA BY ASA PHYSICAL STATUS CLASSIFICATION			
ASA Physical Status	**Elective**	**Emergency**	***P* value**
I	4 of 36,916 (1:9299)	1 of 2949 (1:2949)	0.319
II	11 of 82,435 (1:7494)	3 of 5036 (1:1679)	0.043
III	31 of 74,301 (1:2397)	8 of 4413 (1:552)	< 0.001
IV and V	6 of 8409 (1:1401)	3 of 1029 (1:343)	0.066
Total	52 of 202,061 (1:3886)	15 of 13,427 (1:895)	< 0.001

Figure 10-14. Pulmonary aspiration by American Society of Anesthesiologists (ASA) status. In a retrospective review of 172,334 consecutive adult patients performed at the Mayo Clinic over a period of 6 years, it was found that as a patient's ASA physical status went up, so did his or her risk of pulmonary aspiration. This risk of pulmonary aspiration also increased if the patient underwent emergency rather than elective surgery. The patient's age, gender, food intake fewer than 3 hours prior to surgery, presence of obesity, and the nature of the surgical procedure were not independent predictors of pulmonary aspiration. In the patients undergoing emergency surgery, the most common predisposing condition for aspiration was bowel obstruction. (*Adapted from* Warner and coworkers [14].)

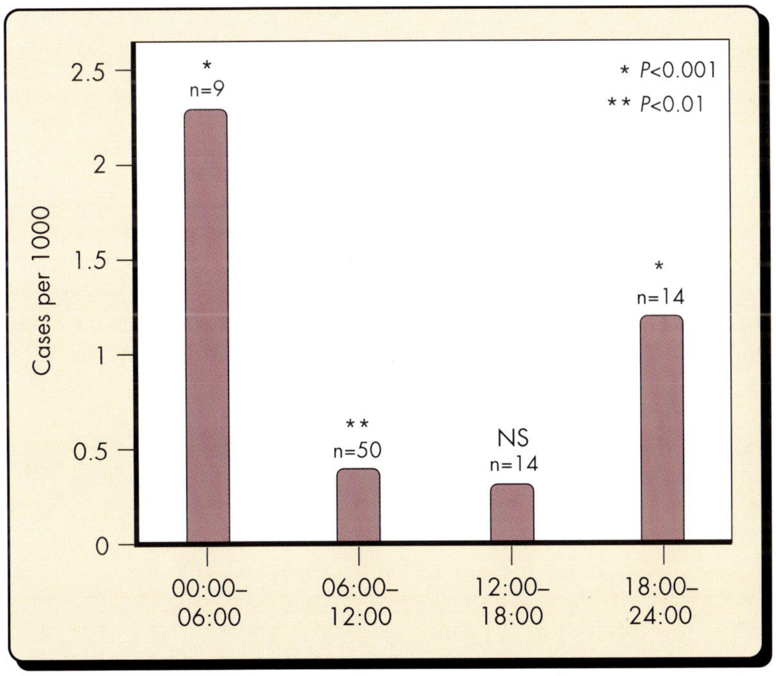

Figure 10-15. Higher incidence of aspiration at night. The incidence of aspiration is higher during the night because less experienced or junior anesthesiologists are more often on night call than senior or more experienced physicians. The incidence of aspiration among patients presenting at night is approximately six times higher than those presenting during the day. Many of these emergency cases involve bowel obstruction, a particularly high-risk condition. The pediatric population is also at a higher risk of aspiration [13]. NS–not significant. (*Adapted from* Olsson [15].)

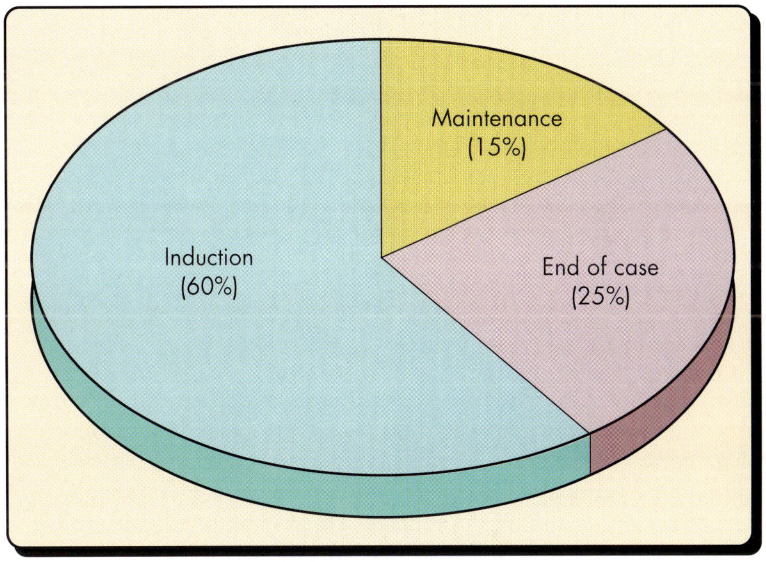

Figure 10-16. Point occurrence of aspiration. Although much of the anesthesiologist's clinical focus is to prevent aspiration at induction of anesthesia with the use of short-acting antacids and cricoid pressure, not all cases of aspiration occur during induction and direct laryngoscopy. About 15% of all aspiration cases occur during the maintenance of the anesthetic, and 20% to 36% of all aspiration causes occur at extubation. The most important clinical event that occurs with postextubation aspiration occurs in the patient who gags and subsequently vomits. The prudent anesthesiologist should bear in mind that the conclusion of a case presents a risk of aspiration almost as great as during induction, and any methods used to reduce gastric pH and volume should continue throughout the conduct of the anesthetic. (*Adapted from* Olsson and coworkers [15].)

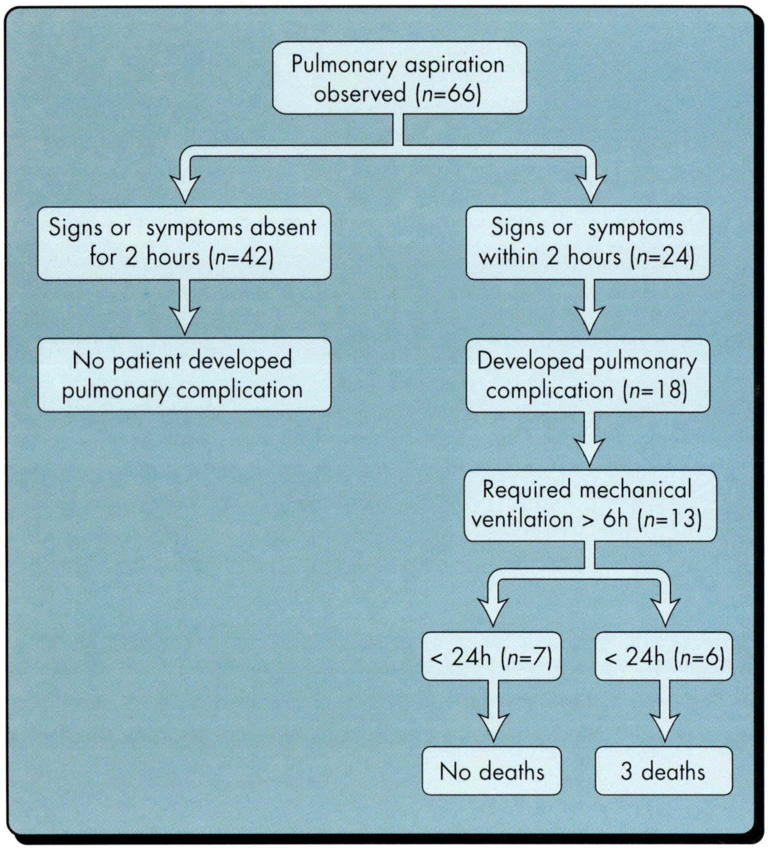

Figure 10-17. Relationship of symptoms or signs of aspiration to outcome. In the patient who does aspirate, the outcome is directly related to whether or not signs and symptoms of pulmonary aspiration are present within 2 hours of either the occurrence of the aspiration or completion of the surgical procedure. If the patient does not develop a new cough or wheeze, a drop in oxygen saturation while breathing room air of greater than 10% from the preoperative value, an alveolar-arterial oxygen gradient equal to or greater than 300, or radiologic evidence of an aspiration, then the patient is unlikely to develop serious pulmonary sequelae. This asymptomatic group of patients need not be sent to an intensive care unit and may be safely observed in a regular ward. The majority of patients who do present with signs of pulmonary aspiration will develop pulmonary complications and will most likely require mechanical ventilation (*Adapted from* Warner and coworkers [14].)

MANAGEMENT OF PULMONARY ASPIRATION

Prevention
- Position
- Antacids
- H_2-receptor antagonists
- Metoclopramide

Airway Management
- Suctioning of oropharynx
- Intubation of airway protection
- Bronchoscopy if particulate aspiration is suspected

Oxygen Therapy

PEEP/CPAP

Lavage

Bronchodilators

Fluid Therapy

Ineffective Therapy

- Corticosteroids
- Antibiotics

Figure 10-18. Management of aspiration. Because aspiration has very serious sequelae, prevention and attenuation of the consequences of aspiration is an important part of anesthetic practice. The duration of fasting (npo) status of the patient, especially in those with risk factors of increased gastric volume or reduced gastric pH, must be enforced. The use of nonparticulate antacids to reduce gastric acidity is important but may not be protective at the end of the case. H_2-receptor antagonists alone may be as effective as a combination of antacids, receptor blockade, and gastric motility agents [16]. Possibly 67% of aspirations may occur after difficulties in airway management or intubation; thus alternative methods of securing the airway must be kept in mind [17]. The use of prophylactic nasogastric tubes to decompress the stomach is uncomfortable to the patient and may not completely empty the gastric pouch, especially of particulate matter [18]. If a rapid sequence technique is to be used, cricoid pressure must be applied. If aspiration does occur, the oropharynx should be suctioned as should the endotracheal tube before the application of positive pressure ventilation. If particulate aspiration is suspected, bronchoscopy should be used to remove the foreign body, which would otherwise lead to intense inflammation and eventual granuloma formation. If oxygenation becomes difficult, mechanical ventilation with the use of positive end-expiratory pressure should be employed. Lavage of the bronchial tree is not recommended as it may worsen pneumonitis. Corticosteroids do not have a beneficial role in aspiration pneumonitis and should not be used. Prophylactic antibiotics are also avoided because the low pH of gastric fluid is usually sterile, unless there is aspiration of feculent material (and thus risk secondary infection) [19]. Finally, aspiration may lead to leakage of large amounts of fluids from capillary beds, and aggressive fluid resuscitation may be required. CPAP—continuous positive airway pressure.

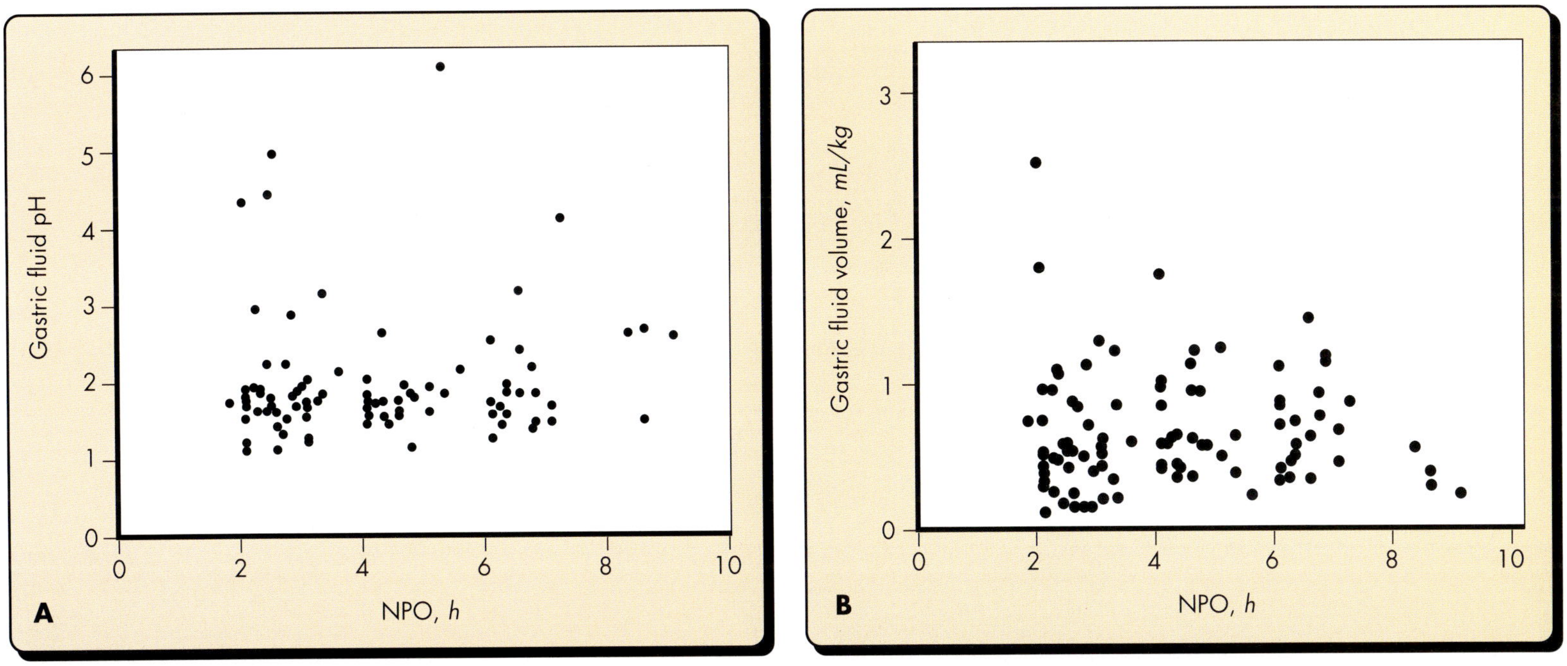

Figure 10-19. Effect of duration of fasting (NPO) status on gastric volume and pH. The general recommendations for NPO status for healthy adult patients has been no solids or clear liquids for up to 8 hours prior to surgery. Most pediatric anesthesiologists in the past would also have recommended a 6- to 8-hour fast for children. But many well-designed studies now support the notion that the time of last clear-fluid intake bears little if no relationship to the pH (**A**) or volume (**B**) of gastric contents [20]. One study in adults found that the ingestion of 240 mL of either water, coffee, or pulp-free orange juice led to a lower gastric volume than at baseline [21]. In healthy patients, with no known risk factors for aspiration, it may be acceptable to allow clear liquids until 2 hours before surgery. (*Adapted from* Crawford and coworkers [20].)

ANTERIOR MEDIASTINAL MASSES

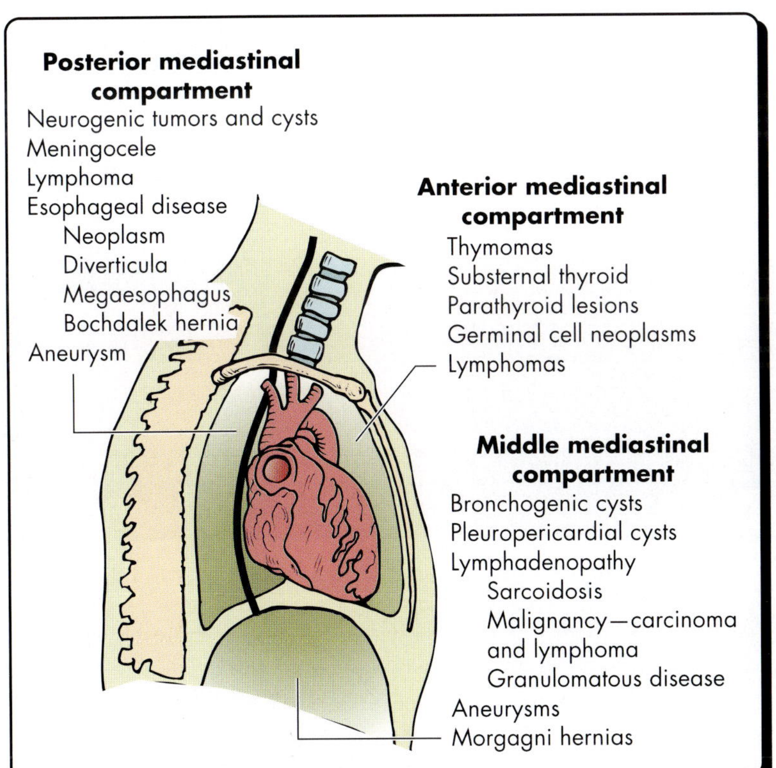

Figure 10-20. The mediastinum. The anterior mediastinal compartment is bounded anteriorly by the sternum and posteriorly by the pericardium, thoracic aorta, and the brachiocephalic vessels. The anterior mediastinum comprises the thymus gland or its remnants, branches of the internal thoracic artery and vein, variable amounts of adipose tissue, and mediastinal lymph nodes. (*Adapted from* Andreoli [22].)

ANTERIOR MEDIASTINAL MASSES	
Lymphoma	Hemangioma
Thymoma	Lipoma
Teratoma	Fibroma
Retrosternal goiter	Fibrosarcoma
Germ-cell neoplasms	Parathyroid adenoma

Figure 10-21. Anterior mediastinal masses. Primary tumors and cysts of the anterior mediastinum affect patients of all age groups but are more common in young and middle-aged adults. Most of these lesions are asymptomatic and are discovered on routine chest radiography. Benign lesions of the mediastinum are usually asymptomatic, whereas malignant lesions tend to produce clinical findings. The most common lesions occurring in the anterior mediastinum are thymomas, lymphomas, and germ-cell tumors [23]. Some lesions may appear in the guise of a tumor but may actually be aberrant parathyroid thyroid tissue, cystic hygroma, or a substernal goiter. In children, approximately two thirds of mediastinal tumors produce symptoms, whereas in adults only about one third do so [24].

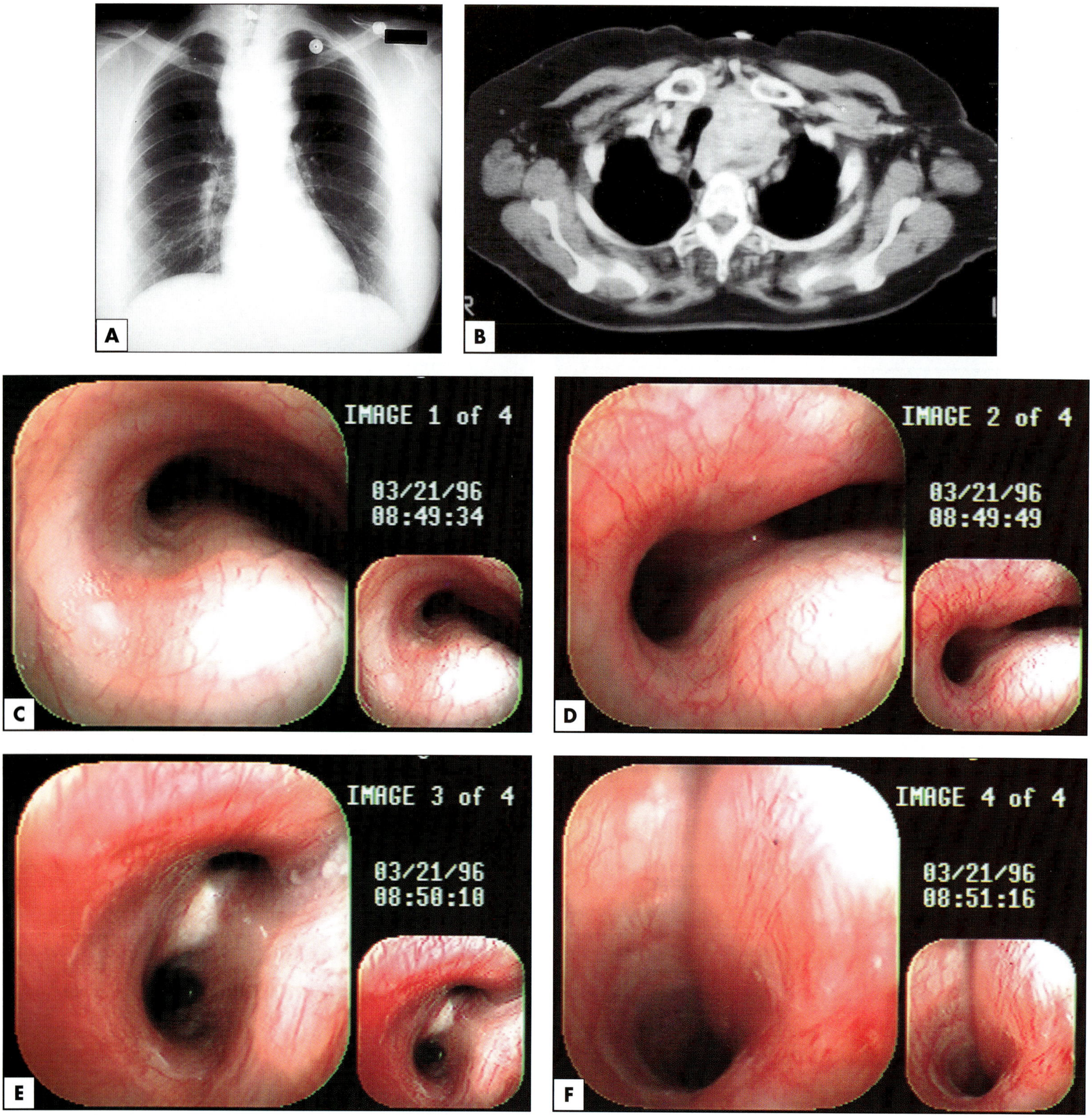

Figure 10-22. Plain radiograph, computed tomographic (CT) scan, and flexible bronchoscopy of an anterior mediastinal mass. **A**, This plain radiograph of the chest demonstrates a patient who presented with a widened mediastinum on routine radiography. This patient was asymptomatic. **B**, CT scan of the chest from a patient with a malignancy in the anterior mediastinum. The scan shows lateral and forward displacement of the trachea owing to the size of the tumor. **C** and **D**, Flexible bronchoscopy of a patient with a mediastinal mass showing partial compression of the right main stem bronchus by an anterior mediastinal mass. However, there is no obstruction of the trachea (**E** and **F**).

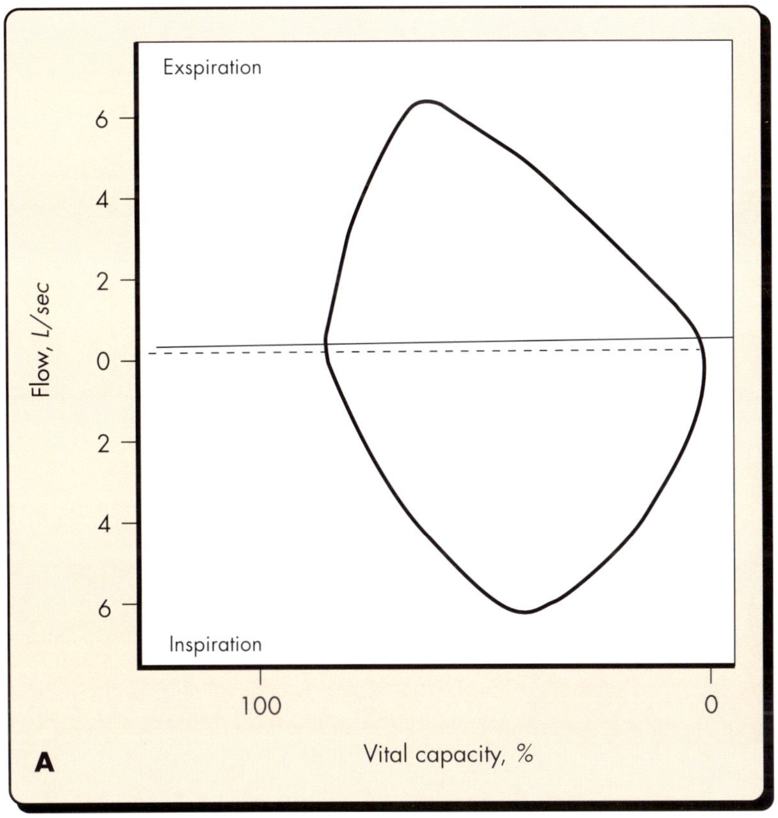

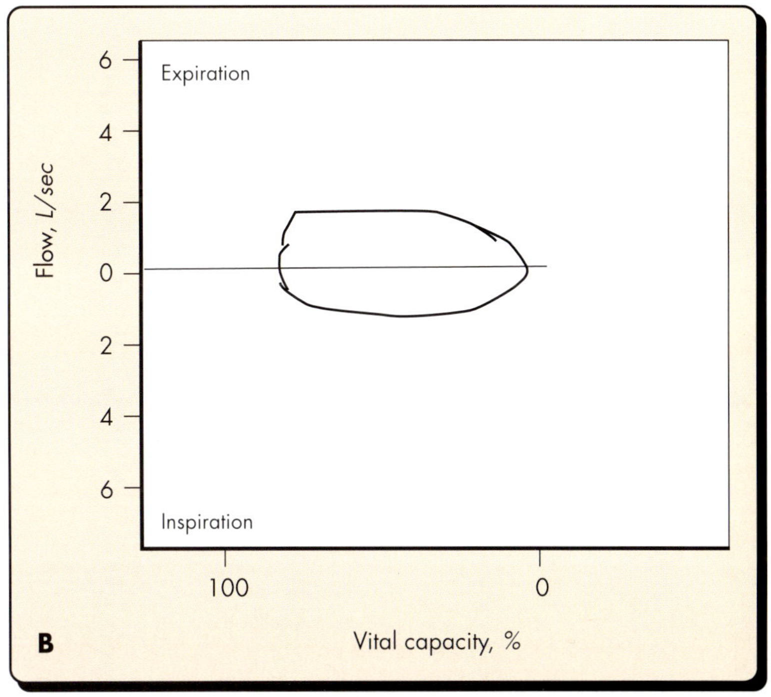

Figure 10-23. Flow-volume loop in anterior mediastinal mass. Flow-volume loops are helpful in determining if upper airway obstruction exists, but also may help the clinician determine the location of the obstruction. **A**, Normal flow-volume loop. In a patient with an anterior mediastinal mass it is important to obtain a flow-volume loop in both the upright and supine positions; although the patient may be asymptomatic sitting or standing, life-threatening airway obstruction may reveal itself in the supine position. In a patient with an anterior mediastinal mass with significant involvement of the airway, the flow-volume loop would be similar to breathing through a fixed external resistance (**B**). There would be little if no change in the caliber of the airway with either inspiration or expiration. Thus, on expiration the flow would show a plateau that has a constant flow over the effort-dependent portion of vital capacity.

SYMPTOMS OF SUPERIOR VENA CAVA SYNDROME

Edema and cyanosis of face, neck, and chest
Conjunctival edema
Dilation of collateral veins in neck and chest
Evidence of increased intracranial pressure

Figure 10-24. Symptoms of superior vena cava syndrome. Enlargement of a mass in the anterior mediastinum may lead to compression of vessels draining blood from the head and upper extremities, leading to dyspnea and swelling of the face, neck, arms, and upper chest. The eyes are usually affected first. Headache, dizziness, tinnitus, and a bursting sensation in the head on bending forward may be present. Elevation of venous pressure may lead to jugular venous and cerebral vascular thrombosis [25]. The patient also may have hoarseness owing to edema of the vocal cords. Increased intracranial pressure may present as nausea, seizures, and obtunded mental state. If the patient with an anterior mediastinal mass does have evidence of superior vena cava syndrome, intravenous access should be obtained below the site of obstruction, and the high likelihood of complete obstruction of the airway on induction of anesthesia should be strongly suspected.

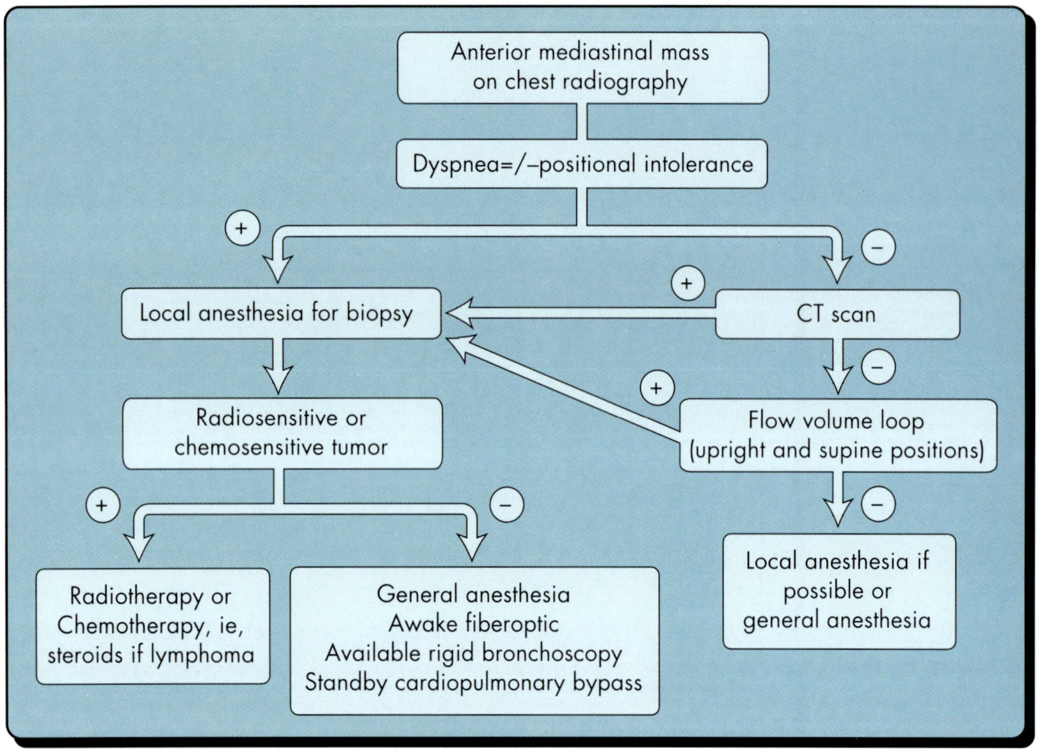

Figure 10-25. Anesthesia for anterior mediastinal masses. More than one half of all anterior mediastinal masses are asymptomatic, discovered as an incidental finding on chest radiography. But children younger than 2 years of age are more likely to be symptomatic because of the smaller diameter of the airway, and also because the trachea is more compressible than in the adult. Computed tomography (CT) scans are extremely helpful in defining the extent of the lesion. In those lesions in which the tracheal narrowing is greater than 50%, a strong likelihood exists of airway problems during anesthesia [26]. Flow-volume loops in both the erect and supine position are helpful to determine the dynamic nature of airway compression. If signs of superior vena cava obstruction are present, a transthoracic echocardiogram may also be employed preoperatively to ascertain the involvement of the great vessels. If the patient is symptomatic or the lesion is compressing, the airway consideration should be given to either irradiation or steroids to shrink the lesion. If irradiation and steroids are not an option, then a biopsy should be performed under local anesthesia if at all possible. If a general anesthetic is required, the ability to maintain the patient's own spontaneous ventilation may be lifesaving. A physician skilled with a rigid bronchoscope should be standing by if airway obstruction results and it is necessary to bypass the mass. Also, the mass may act as a ball-value type mechanism whereby air can be forced passed the obstruction but not exhaled. A chest tube would be indicated in this situation. A cardiopulmonary bypass setup may be placed at the ready, but the ability to rapidly initiate bypass rapidly once complete obstruction occurs might be too time consuming in the face of complete airway loss. If dynamic airway obstruction does occur, the ability to change the patient from the supine position to prone might relieve the obstruction.

ACUTE EPIGLOTTITIS

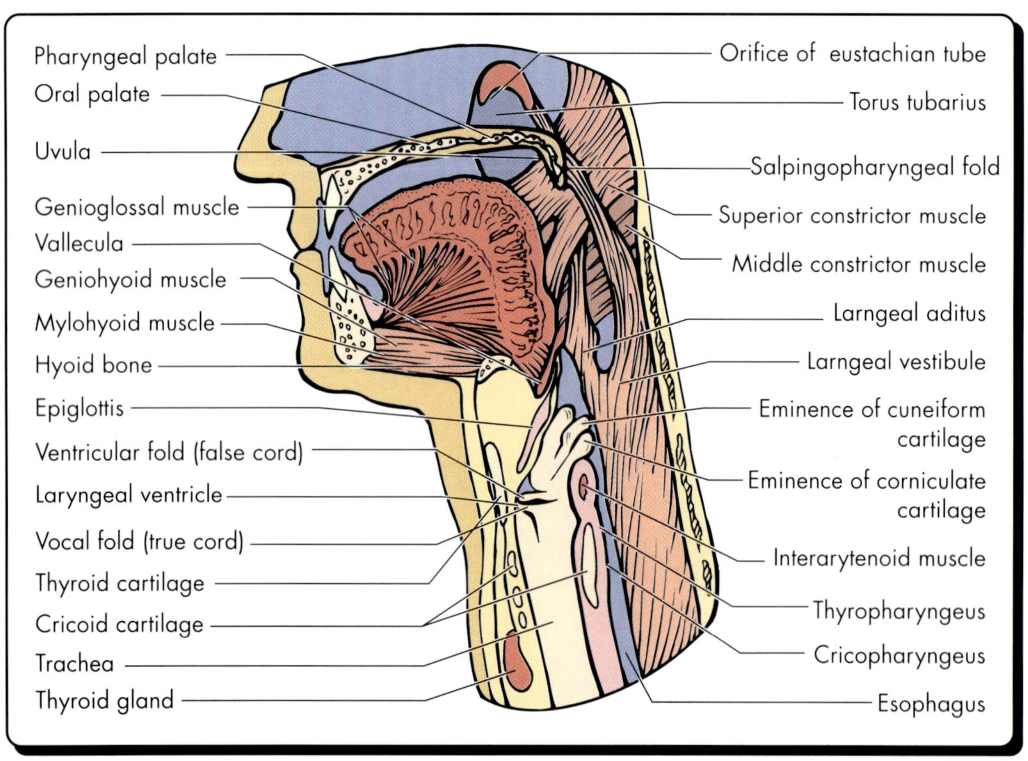

Figure 10-26. Anatomy of the neck and larynx. This figure illustrates the supraglottic and subglottic structures in the neck, including the epiglottis. (*Adapted from* Woodson [27].)

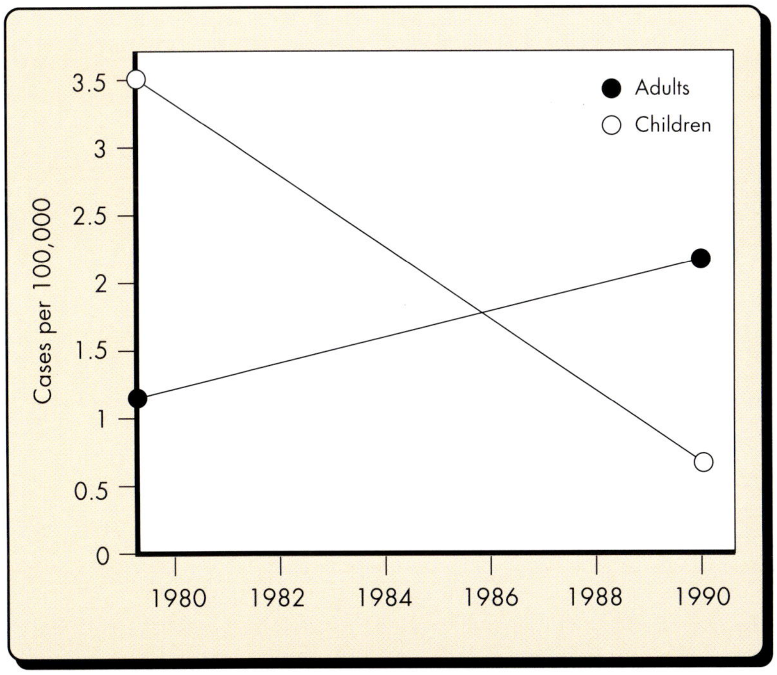

Figure 10-27. Changing pattern of epiglottitis incidence. The introduction of *Haemophilus influenzae* type b vaccine (Hib) in 1985 has changed the child to adult predominance of epiglottitis. Whereas the pediatric incidence of epiglottitis has decreased dramatically, the adult incidence has remained stable or increased (owing in part to a greater appreciation of the disease). In a recent study from Rhode Island, the adult occurrence increased substantially [28]. In this study, children most often presented with shortness of breath, stridor, and an elevated temperature. Adults usually had a sore throat, odynaphagia, and neck pain. Sixty-eight percent of the pediatric patients required an artificial airway, whereas only 21% of adults needed one. With the introduction of the Hib vaccine, epiglottitis is on the decline and epiglottitis may become a disease almost exclusively involving adults (*Adapted from* Frantz and Rasgon [29].)

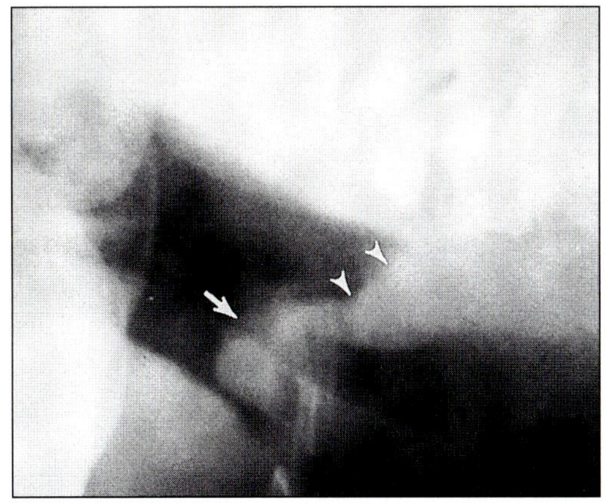

Figure 10-28. Lateral radiograph of neck. The lateral neck radiograph shows a patient with supraglottic inflammation. The *arrow* points to a markedly thickened epiglottis with thickening also affecting the aryepiglottic folds (*arrowheads*). Epiglottitis is more appropriately termed *supraglottic inflammation* because the inflammatory process involves not only the epiglottis but also the aryepiglottic folds, often extending to the vallecula, and may even reach the posterior pharyngeal wall. Up to 25% of children may have evidence of subglottic narrowing. Also, edema of the epiglottis may occur with foreign bodies, tumors, burns, granulomatous diseases, and angioneurotic edema. (*Adapted from* Wippold and coworkers [30]; with permission.)

CLINICAL DISTINCTION BETWEEN EPIGLOTTITIS AND CROUP

Epiglottitis	Croup
2 to 6 years of age	< 2 years of age
5% of children with stridor	80% of children with stridor
Bacterial (*Haemophilus influenzae)*	Viral
Rapid onset	Onset over 24 to 72 hours
Toxic appearance	Nontoxic appearing
Inspiratory stridor	Inspiratory stridor
Pharyngitis	Croupy cough
Fever (often > 39°C)	Rhinnorhea
Lethargic or restless	Fever (rarely > 39°C)
Tachypnea	Lymphocytosis
Cyanosis	Subglottic area narrowing on radiography
Neutrophilia	
Swollen epiglottis on radiography	

Figure 10-29. Clinical distinction between epiglottitis and croup. Epiglottitis may be better termed *supraglottitis* because it usually is a bacterial infection not only involving the epiglottis but also supraglottic structures, such as the arytenoids and uvula. The swelling can be so severe that the vallecula forces the epiglottis to obstruct the tracheal inlet on inspiration, causing obstruction. The cause is usually owing to *Haemophilus influenzae* infection, but can also include *Staphylococcus aureus*, β-hemolytic *Streptococcus*, and *Diplococcus*. The incidence in the past has been many times higher in children than adults. As opposed to croup or laryngotracheobronchitis, epiglottitis is usually a bacterial infection of acute onset and is life-threatening. The patient with epiglottitis is febrile, drooling because of the inability to swallow oropharyngeal secretions, and has inspiratory stridor. (*Adapted from* Stoelting and Dierdorf [31].)

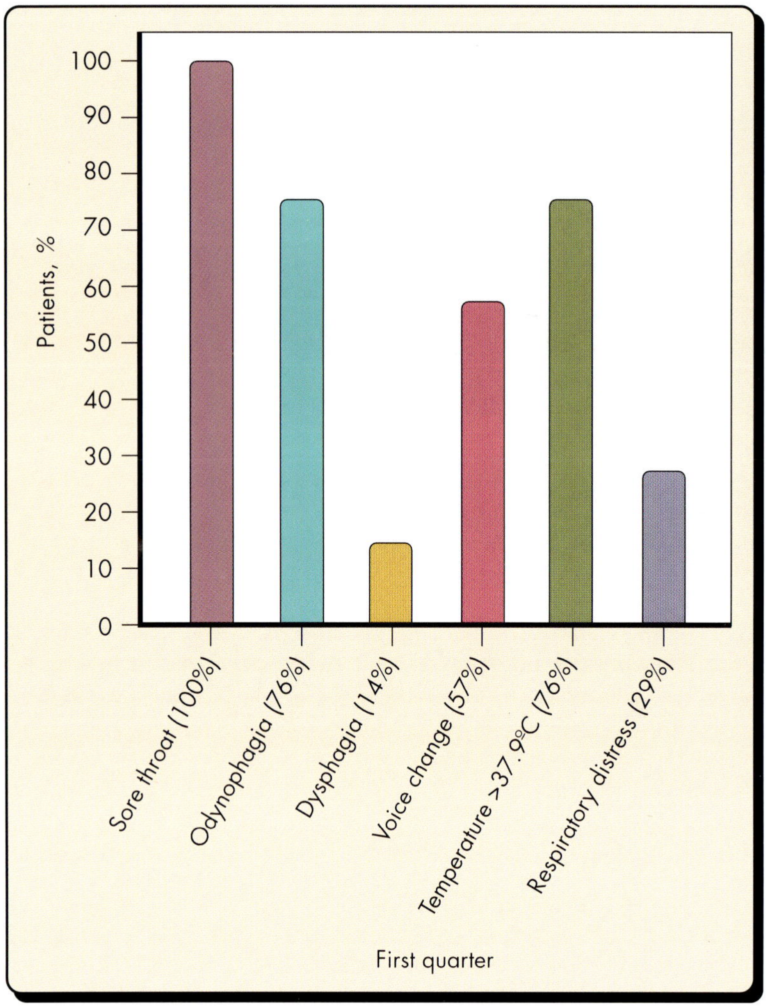

Figure 10-30. Presenting symptoms of epiglottitis in adults. There has been controversy regarding whether to intubate or perform a tracheostomy on all patients that present with inflammation of the supraglottic structures, analogous to the situation in children. But many have recently argued that intubation in the adult is not mandatory, and the adult patient can safely be observed in an intensive-care setting. Those patients presenting with severe respiratory distress should have an airway immediately established. Those without airway compromise can be safely observed until the supraglottic inflammation subsides [32,33]. (*Adapted from* Crosby and Reid [32].)

MANAGEMENT OF EPIGLOTTITIS

Lateral neck radiography if time permits
Avoid supine position or positioning for films
Tracheostomy equipment set up in the operating room
Intravenous access obtained as soon as tolerated
Preoperative vagolytics
Preoxygenation
Inhalation induction with halothane, with or without N_2O
Intubate with endotracheal tube 0.05- to 1-mm smaller than normal
Change to nasal tube once the airway is secured
Transport to the intensive care unit when patient is ventilated and sedated
Intravenous antibiotics

Figure 10-31. Management of epiglottitis. In a case of suspected acute epiglottitis, a lateral radiograph of the neck should be omitted if the patient requires immediate airway management. If time does permit a radiograph, a physician trained in airway management must accompany the patient at all times. Once the operating room is set up and a tracheostomy and rigid bronchoscopy equipment are available, the patient is transported to the operating room. The patient should be allowed to sit up if he or she finds this better tolerated. Induction may be done with the patient initially upright and is usually accomplished with an inhalation technique. Some use nitrous oxide to speed induction of anesthesia, but many prefer 100% oxygenation. Once the patient is anesthetized, upper-airway obstruction may result. Gentle application of positive pressure will usually correct this. The patient is then intubated with an endotracheal tube 0.05- to 1-mm in diameter smaller than normal. Once the airway is secured, the endotracheal tube may be changed to a nasal one, which may be better tolerated when the patient awakens. The patient is then transferred to the intensive care unit, sedated and ventilated, and antibiotics are continued. The patient is extubated 24 to 48 hours later if the clinical picture dictates. In the past, epiglottitis was managed with tracheostomy, but current literature favors endotracheal intubation as the preferred method of airway management [34]. The patient is extubated when there has been a defervescence in temperature, a demonstrated ability to breath around the endotracheal tube with the cuff deflated, and if visual examination finds diminished edema and inflammation.

REFERENCES

1. Marcy TW: Barotrauma: detection, recognition, and management. *Chest* 1993, 104:578–584.
2. Mendelson CL: The aspiration of stomach contents into the lungs during obstetric anesthesia. *Am J Obstet Gynecol* 1946, 52:191–205.
3. Tasch MD, Stoelting RK: Aspiration prevention, prophylaxis, and treatment. In *Airway Management: Principles and Practice*. Edited by Benumof J. St. Louis: Mosby; 1996:183–201.
4. Pierson DJ: Barotrauma and bronchopleural fistula. In *Principles and Practice of Mechanical Ventilation*. Edited by Tobin MJ. New York: McGraw Hill; 1994: 813–836.
5. Maunder RJ, Pierson DJ, Hudson LD: Subcutaneous and mediastinal emphysema: pathophysiology, diagnosis, and management. *Arch Intern Med* 1984, 144:1447–1453.
6. Jantz MA, Pierson DJ: Pneumothorax and barotrauma. *Clin Chest Med* 1994, 15:75–91.
7. Gammon RB, Shin MS, Buchalter SE: Pulmonary barotrauma in mechanical ventilation: patterns and risk factors. *Chest* 1992, 102:568–572.
8. Caldwell EJ, Powell RD, Mullooly JP: Interstitial emphysema: a study of physiologic factors involved in experimental induction of the lesion. *Am Rev Respir Dis* 1970, 102:516–525.
9. Tocino IM, Miller MH, Fairfax WR: Distribution of pneumothorax in the supine and semierect critically ill adult. *AJR Am J Roentgenol* 1985, 144:901–905.
10. Chomka Leya C, Bandala LC: Respiratory complications. In *Post Anesthesia Care*. Edited by Vender JS, Spiess BD. Philadelphia: WB Saunders; 1992:76–93.
11. Broe PJ, Toung TJK, Cameron JL: Aspiration pneumonia. *Surg Clin North Am* 1990:60.

12. Vender JS: Pulmonary aspiration. In *Case Studies in Critical Care Medicine*. Edited by Cane RD, Shapiro BA, Davison R. Chicago: Year Book Medical Publishers, Inc.; 1990:251–265.

13. Benumof J: *Airway Management: Principle and Practice*. St Louis: Mosby; 1996:183–201.

14. Warner MA, Warner ME, Weber JG: Clinical significance of pulmonary aspiration during the perioperative period. *Anesthesiology* 1993, 78:56–62.

15. Olsson GL, Hallen B, Hambraeus-Jonzon K: Aspiration during anaesthesia: a computer-aided study of 185,358 anaesthetics. *Acta Anaesthesiol Scand* 1986, 30:84–92.

16. Maltby JR, Elliott RH, Warnell I, *et al.*: Gastric fluid volume and pH in elective surgical patients: triple prophylaxis is not superior to ranitidine alone. *Can J Anaesth* 1990, 37:650–655.

17. Kallar SK, Everett LL: Potential risks and preventive measures for pulmonary aspiration: new concepts in perioperative fasting guidelines. *Anesth Analg* 1993, 77:171–182.

18. Taylor WJ, Champion MC, Barry AW, *et al.*: Measuring gastric contents during general anaesthesia: evaluation of blind gastric aspiration. *Can J Anaesthesia* 1989, 36:51–54.

19. Dal Santo G: Acid aspiration: pathophysiological aspects, prevention and therapy. *Int Anesthesiol Clin* 1986, 24:31–52.

20. Crawford M, Lerman J, Christensen S, *et al.*: Effects of duration of tasting on gastric fluid pH and volume in healthy children. *Anesth Analg* 1990, 71:400–403.

21. Shevde K, Trivedi N: Effects of clear liquids on gastric volume and pH in healthy volunteers. *Anesth Analg* 1991, 72:528–531.

22. Andreoli TE, ed.: *Cecil: Essentials of Medicine*. Philadelphia: WB Saunders; 1986:470–471.

23. Weisbrod GL, Herman SJ: Imaging. In *Thoracic Surgery*. Edited by Pierson FG, Deslauriers J, Ginsberg RL. New York: Churchill Livingstone; 1995:1333–1359.

24. Shields TW: Primary lesions of the mediastinum and their investigation and treatment. In *General Thoracic Surgery*. Edited by Shields TW. Baltimore: Williams and Wilkins; 1994:1724–1769.

25. McFadden PM, Jamplis RW: Superior vena cava syndrome. In *General Thoracic Surgery*. Edited by Shields TW. Baltimore: Williams and Wilkins; 1994:1716–1723.

26. Shamberger RC, Holzman RS, Griscom NT, *et al.*: CT quantification of tracheal cross-sectional area as a guide to the surgical and anesthetic management of children with anterior mediastinal masses. *J Pediatr Surg* 1991, 26:138–142.

27. Woodson GE: Anatomy of the neck and larynx. In *Otolaryngology: Head and Neck Surgery*. Edited by Meyerhoff WL, Rice DH. Philadelphia: WB Saunders; 1992:668–682.

28. Mayo-Smith MF, Spinale JW, Donskey CJ, *et al.*: Acute epiglottitis: an 18-year experience in Rhode Island. *Chest* 1995, 108:1640–1647.

29. Frantz TP, Rasgon BM: Acute epiglottitis: changing epidemiologic patterns. *Otolaryngol Head Neck Surg* 1993, 109:457–460

30. Wippold FJ II, Glazer HS, Siegel M: Diagnostic imaging of the larynx. In *Otolaryngology: Head and Neck Surgery*. Edited by Cummings CW, Fredrickson JM, Harker LA, *et al.* St. Louis: Mosby-Year Book; 1993:1785–1805.

31. Stoelting RK, Dierdorf SF: *Anesthesia and Co-Existing Disease*. New York; Churchill Livingstone; 1993:607–609.

32. Crosby E, Reid D: Acute epiglottitis in the adult: is intubation mandatory? *Can J Anaesth* 1991, 38:914–918.

33. Frantz TD, Rasgon BM, Quesenberry CP: Acute epiglottitis in adults: analysis of 129 cases. *JAMA* 1994, 272:1358–1360.

34. Schloss MD, Gold JA, Rosales JK, *et al.*: Acute epiglottitis: current management. *Laryngoscope* 1983, 93:489–493.

11

Hemodynamic Emergencies

Brian Woodcock

Hemodynamic emergencies during anesthesia may occur with any type of surgery. The diagnosis of the cause of cardiovascular collapse may not be immediately apparent. However, prompt diagnosis of the cause and management to correct the problem are required to prevent ischemic injury. When the cause of hypotension is not immediately apparent, temporizing measures such as intravenous fluids and vasopressors may be necessary to attempt to elevate the blood pressure and maintain perfusion while the underlying cause of the problem is being investigated.

Cardiovascular collapse during anesthesia most frequently initially presents as hypotension. Low blood pressure may be due to a decrease in cardiac output with a normal or high systemic vascular resistance (*eg*, in hypovolemia or cardiogenic shock) or may be caused by vasodilatation with a normal or increased cardiac output (*eg*, in anaphylaxis or sepsis). Shock is a state of reduced perfusion to the tissues. Hypotension may be the presenting feature in a shocked state; however, blood pressure can be maintained in low cardiac output by intense vasoconstriction. Although blood pressure is easy to measure and monitor, restoration of blood pressure by the administration of vasoconstrictors may not correct the shocked condition. The primary objective should be to restore perfusion (cardiac output) and then normalize blood pressure.

The cause of hypotension may be expected, such as hypovolemia owing to surgical bleeding, or may be from an unexpected emergency such as tension pneumothorax, cardiac tamponade, pulmonary embolism, arrhythmias, or anaphylaxis.

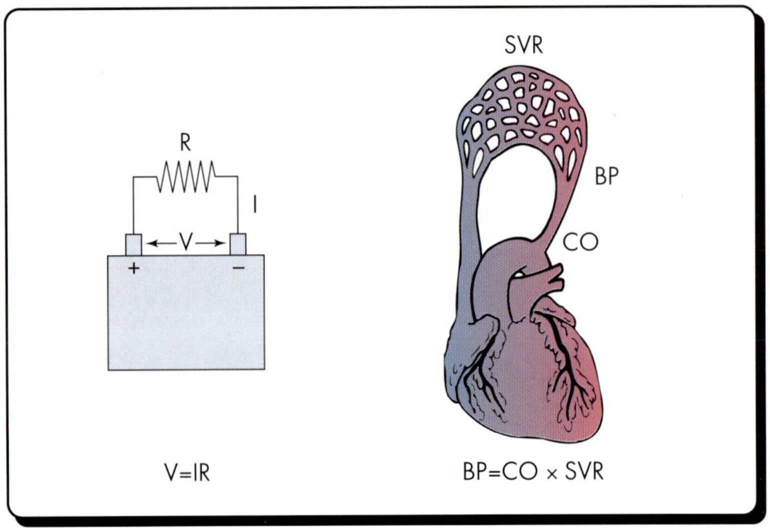

Figure 11-1. In the physics of electricity, Ohm's law states that the potential difference across a circuit (V) is directly proportional to the current (I) and the resistance (R). In a directly analogous way this can be applied to the human body: The potential difference across the circulation is the blood pressure (BP), the current of flow through the body is the cardiac output (CO), and the resistance is the systemic vascular resistance (SVR). It can be seen that a decrease in blood pressure can be caused by a decrease in cardiac output (*eg*, hypovolemia or cardiogenic shock) or a decrease in SVR (*eg*, anaphylaxis or sepsis).

CAUSES OF SHOCK WITH HIGH SVR

- Hypovolemia
  - Preoperative fasting
  - Unrecognized bleeding
  - Gastrointestinal fluid loss
- Cardiogenic shock
  - Myocardial ischemia
  - Myocardial contusion
  - Myocardial depression from anesthetic agents
  - Arrhythmias
- Tension pneumothorax
- Pulmonary embolus
- Cardiac tamponade

Figure 11-2. Shock with a high systemic vascular resistance (*SVR*) value is primarily from a decrease in cardiac output. The decrease in cardiac output may be caused by a decrease in preload to the heart (*hypovolemia*) or a decrease in the inotropic state of the heart (cardiogenic shock from myocardial ischemia or myocardial contusion after trauma). The preload seen by the left ventricle may also be compromised by external factors affecting blood flow through the right ventricle and pulmonary vasculature (tension pneumothorax, pulmonary embolus, and cardiac tamponade).

CAUSES OF SHOCK WITH LOW SVR

- Abnormal vasodilators
  - Sepsis
  - Anaphylactic or anaphylactoid shock
  - Overdose of vasodilators
  - Endocrine vasodilatation
  - Anesthetic agents
  - Carcinoid tumor (histamine)
  - Thyrotoxicosis
  - Liver failure
  - Toxic shock syndrome
- Failure of normal vascular tone
  - Neurogenic shock
  - Spinal shock
  - Epidural and subarachnoid anesthesia
  - Periphral shunts
  - Severe thiamine deficiency
  - Adrenal insufficiency

Figure 11-3. Shock with a low systemic vascular resistance (SVR) value is owing to the presence of abnormal vasodilators or the failure of normal vascular tone. In sepsis and toxic shock syndrome, bacterial products and mediators of the body's inflammatory response cause loss of vascular tone. Histamine causes vasodilatation during anaphylactic reactions and during the flushing attacks of carcinoid syndrome. Thyroxine can vasodilate in thyroid storm. Intravenous and inhaled anesthetic agents can cause vasodilatation in excess. In liver failure, metabolic products ("middle molecules") accumulate. In the presence of a peripheral shunt (such as a vascular shunt for dialysis) or a large arteriovenous malformation, vasoconstriction in other beds is unable to increase the overall SVR. In neurogenic shock there is loss of the normal sympathetic control of vascular tone. This can be caused by sympathetic block during spinal and epidural anesthesia. In wet beriberi due to thiamine deficiencies a high cardiac output heart failure occurs with vasodilatation. In adrenal failure vascular tone may fail.

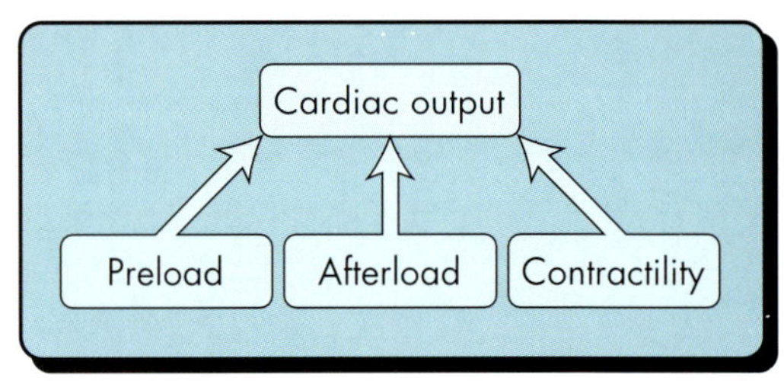

Figure 11-4. Cardiac output is dependent on preload, afterload, and contractility [1]. In the face of shock syndrome these factors can be manipulated pharmacologically to increase cardiac output. Preload should be optimized before changes in the afterload or contractility are made. Vasodilators should only be given when the heart is adequately filled because, as Ohm's law shows, a decrease in systemic vascular resistance that cannot be compensated for by an increase in cardiac output will cause a decrease in blood pressure. Inotropes should also only be administered when the preload has been optimized. There is nothing to be gained from flogging with inotropes an empty heart that merely needs some volume.

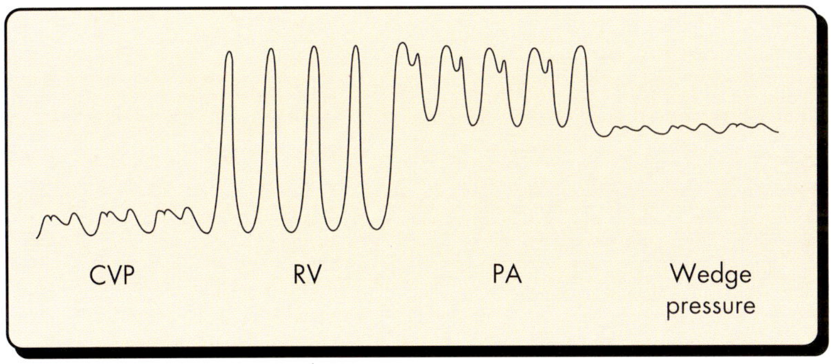

Figure 11-5. Tracing of the waveforms during flotation of a pulmonary artery (*PA*) catheter through the right heart into the pulmonary artery and into the wedge position. The preload of a patient should be evaluated as close as possible to the left ventricle. The central venous pressure (*CVP*) may reflect preload in the normal heart; however, in the presence of tricuspid valve abnormalities, right ventricular failure or ischemia, cor pulmonale, or other causes of increased pulmonary vascular resistance (PVR) there may be no relationship between the CVP and left ventricular filling. The pulmonary artery wedge pressure (PAWP) is the closest estimate of left ventricular filling pressure in the absence of left heart catheterization. The pulmonary artery diastolic pressure is close to or slightly above the PAWP if the heart rate is less than 90 bpm [2] and the PVR is not excessively high. RV—right ventricle.

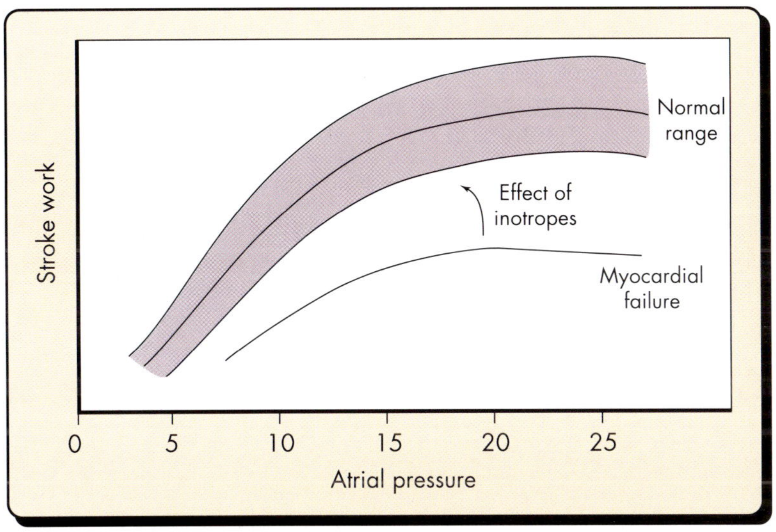

Figure 11-6. The Frank-Starling curve of the heart demonstrates the effect of increasing preload on the contractility or stroke work of the left ventricle [1]. An inadequate preload can cause a decrease in cardiac output and hypotension. This decrease frequently causes hemodynamic instability during anesthesia; although surgical blood loss may not be immediately apparent, it should always be considered and corrected as soon as possible. Through the normal range of preload any increase in the initial stretch of the muscle fibers results in an increase in the force of contraction. However, an excessive initial stretch, (*eg*, an atrial pressure greater than 25 mm Hg), may result in decompensation and a decrease in cardiac output. Initial maneuvers in the management depend on increasing preload to move to a point higher up the Frank-Starling curve. Poor myocardial function may require the use of inotropes to move up to a higher curve, to a point at which adequate stroke work and cardiac output are produced.

TENSION PNEUMOTHORAX

CAUSES OF PNEUMOTHORAX DURING ANESTHESIA

- Iatrogenic
  - Barotrauma
    - Mechanical ventilation
    - Hyperbaric oxygen
  - Procedures
    - Central cannulation
    - Intercostal blocks
    - Stellate ganglion and brachial plexus blocks
    - Back, neck, kidney, or upper abdominal surgery
    - Thoracotomy or thoracocentesis
    - Laparoscopy
    - Biopsy of lung or pleura
    - Cardiopulmonary resuscitation
    - Insertion of nasogastric feeding tube
- Trauma
  - Open chest wound
  - Esophageal or tracheobronchial rupture
  - Rib fracture
- Spontaneous pneumothorax
  - Primary
  - Secondary
    - Infection
    - Tumors
    - Asthma
    - Chronic obstructive pulmonary disease

Figure 11-7. Pneumothorax during anesthesia is most commonly from iatrogenic causes. Central venous catheter placement or nerve blocks in the neck can cause a pneumothorax that may not be perceived immediately. The results of an initial chest radiograph may be negative but then a pneumothorax may develop after positive-pressure ventilation [3].

Breach of the pleura during surgery in adjacent areas may not be recognized until the pneumothorax causes hemodynamic compromise. Pneumothorax may occur as a result of barotrauma during positive-pressure ventilation, particularly if high inspiratory pressures or positive end-expiratory pressure (PEEP) are required. Mechanical ventilation, in patients with a pneumothorax from any cause, is likely to increase the size of the pneumothorax and increase the risk of a tension pneumothorax occurring. Patients with significant chest trauma may benefit from insertion of bilateral chest tubes before intubation and ventilation, even in the absence of evidence of pneumothorax. Nitrous oxide diffuses readily into air-filled spaces and should be avoided in the presence of a pneumothorax. Spontaneous primary pneumothorax characteristically occurs in young men of tall build. These patients, particularly those with a prior occurrence, may be more prone to pneumothorax during positive-pressure ventilation. Spontaneous secondary pneumothorax can result from infection, tumors, asthma and chronic obstructive pulmonary disease.

CLINICAL SIGNS OF PNEUMOTHORAX

Dyspnea
Cough
Pleuritic chest pain
Increased pressures on mechanical ventilation
Decreased chest wall movement
Hyperresonance to percussion
Diminished breath sounds
Decreased vocal resonance
Tachypnea
Cyanosis
Tachycardia
Hypotension
Tracheal and mediastinal shift
Subcutaneous emphysema

Figure 11-8. Clinical symptoms of dyspnea, cough, and chest pain may be volunteered by patients who are awake. Diagnosis may be masked and delayed in patients who are anesthetized because they cannot complain of early symptoms. Pneumothorax may only be suspected when respiratory or hemodynamic compromise has occurred. In patients who are ventilated there may be other signs of barotrauma such as subcutaneous emphysema, pulmonary interstitial emphysema on chest radiography, or pneumopericardium that can cause a crunching murmur on auscultation. In a tension pneumothorax, valve action allows air to enter the thoracic cavity but not leave it. Pressure increases with every breath, causing distortion of the great vessels and cardiac compression. Tension pneumothorax may cause severe hypotension and tachycardia, together with hypoxemia, and may be lethal. Tension pneumothorax is more likely to occur during mechanical ventilation. Suspicion of tension pneumothorax, with tracheal and mediastinal shift, may require active measures to relieve the intrathoracic pressure before a chest radiograph can be obtained (*see* Figs. 11-10 and 11-11).

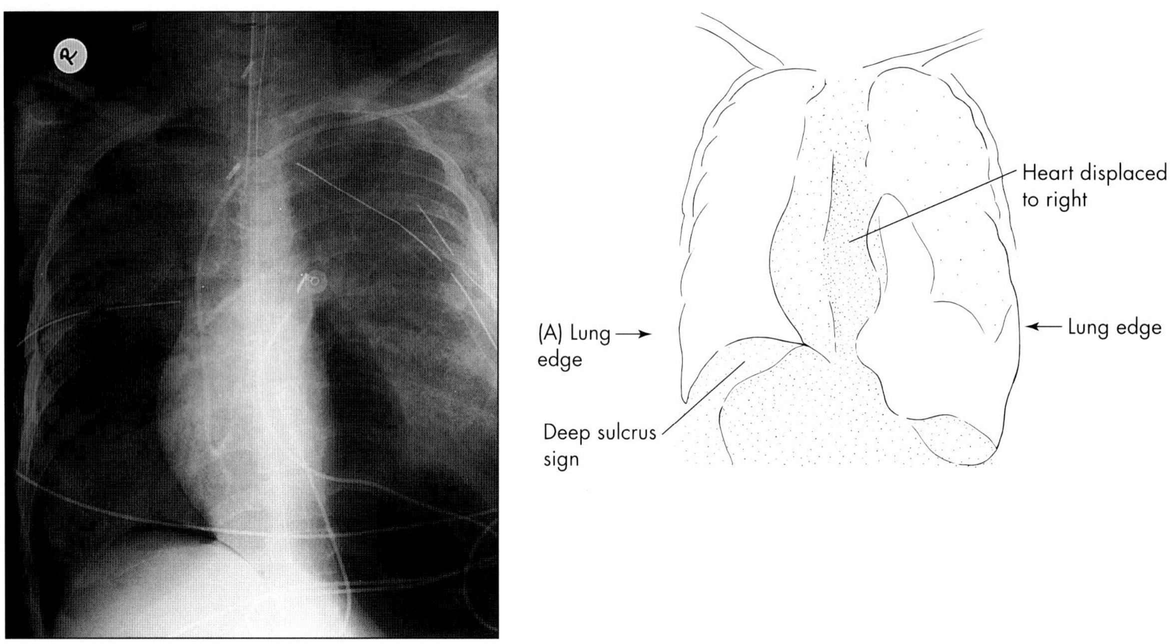

Figure 11-9. In this chest radiograph bilateral pneumothoraxes can be seen. At the right base a thin white line is seen, which marks the lung edge, and there is an absence of lung markings peripheral to the line. On the left side, a large medial and basal tension pneumothorax is seen. The heart is displaced into the right hemithorax, and the left diaphragm is depressed by the tension pneumothorax. Subcutaneous emphysema can be seen in the left axilla and delineating the right pectoral muscles. In some patients a skin fold between the back and the radiographic plate may cause a white line mimicking a pneumothorax. In patients who are in a supine position, air may not rise to the apex of the thoracic cavity. The pneumothorax may be seen as a "deep sulcus" sign in which air in the lower thorax widens the costophrenic angle and may be seen superimposed on the hemidiaphragm. This is visible on both sides in this chest radiograph. Although estimation of the size of the pneumothorax from the chest radiograph may be inaccurate [4], an average interpleural distance of 2 to 2.5 cm roughly corresponds to a 25% pneumothorax. In the absence of tension effects and in a spontaneously breathing patient, a pneumothorax of less than 20% may be observed, 20% to 50% of patients may respond to simple aspiration, and more than 50% of patients require chest tube placement. Pneumothoraxes in patients who are ventilated are more likely to progress, requiring thoracostomy tube placement.

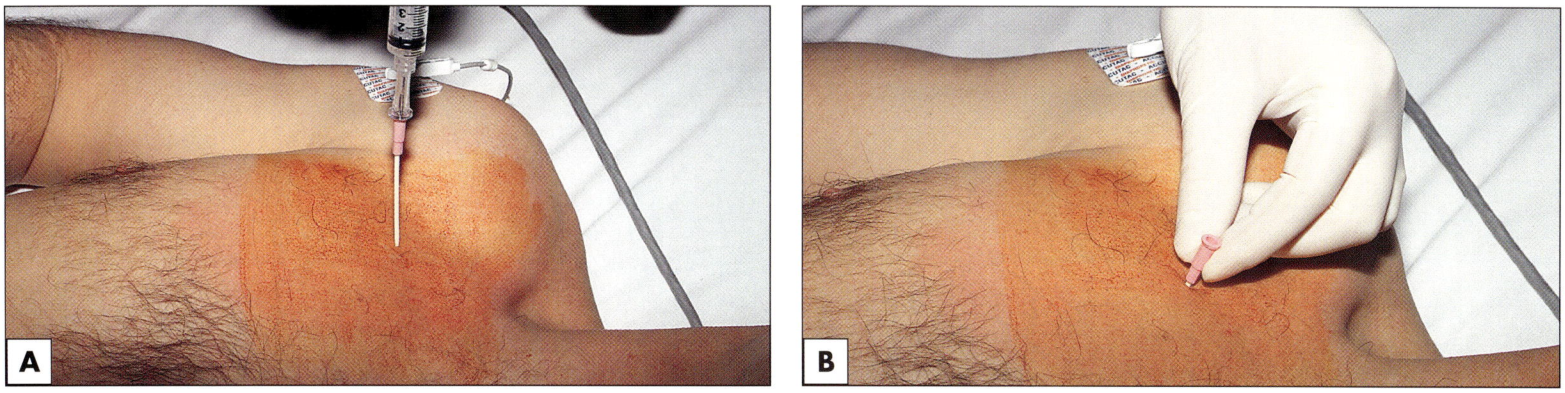

Figure 11-10. "Needling" the chest for tension pneumothorax. This procedure is performed with readily available equipment and can be accomplished rapidly before a chest tube is obtained and inserted. **A**, A 12- or 14-gauge intravenous cannula is inserted in the second intercostal space in the midclavicular line. The cannula is inserted on the side of the pneumothorax, if known, or it can be inserted bilaterally, if the side is not evident clinically or if bilateral pneumothoraxes are suspected. **B**, Entry into a tension pneumothorax is confirmed by air rushing rapidly through the needle. There is risk of causing pulmonary damage with needle insertion if a pneumothorax is not present, and this technique should be reserved for the patient who is rapidly deteriorating and cannot tolerate any delay for chest radiography.

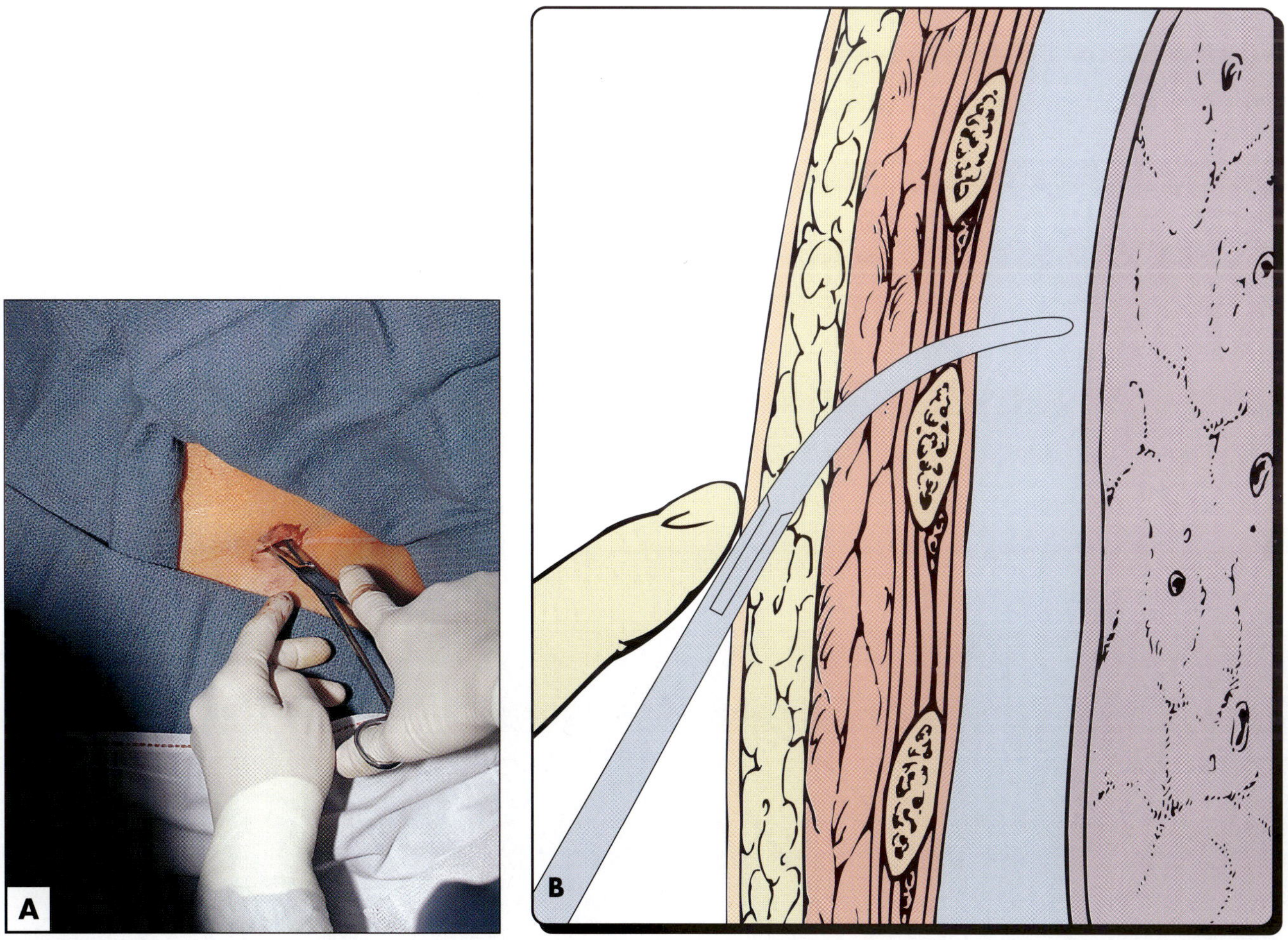

Figure 11-11. Chest tube (thoracostomy tube) insertion. The chest tube is inserted in the fourth or fifth intercostal space at the anterior axillary line: This should be between the pectoralis major and latissimus dorsi muscles. The second intercostal space in the midclavicular line has been used and is efficient for drainage of an apical pneumothorax; however, any dependent fluid will not be well drained and the scar from insertion in this position is unsightly. The skin and subcutaneous tissues are infiltrated with lidocaine and the intercostal muscle and periosteum are also infiltrated. Thoracocentesis can be performed with the infiltrating needle to confirm positioning and the presence of underlying air. **A** and **B**, The chest tube should be inserted in the lower part of the intercostal space, immediately above the rib below, to avoid damage to the neurovascular bundle that runs along the underside of each rib. A skin incision is made parallel to the rib, below the interspace. A Kelly clamp is used to penetrate the intercostal muscle through to the pleural space. The Kelly clamp is then opened and closed to secure a route for chest tube insertion. It is important that the pointed trocar, supplied with some chest tubes, is not used to penetrate the intercostal muscle [5]: Significant force is required and there may be a sudden give with penetration of underlying organs. (*Continued on next page*)

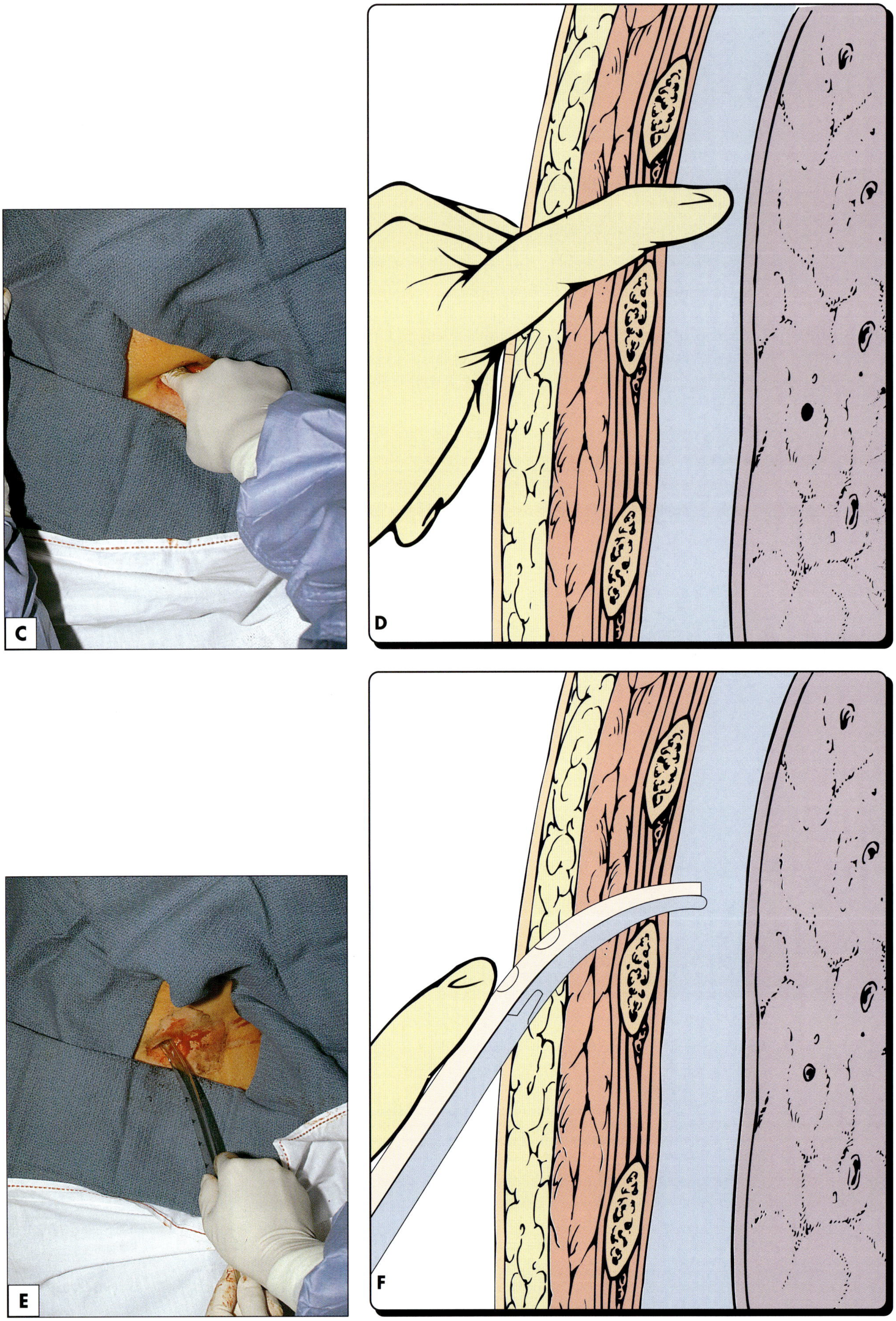

Figure 11-11. (*Continued*) **C** and **D**, A finger is inserted to confirm both the position in the pleural cavity and the absence of adhesions that would cause the lung to stick to the parietal pleura. **E** and **F**, A 24F to 28F chest tube is then gently inserted. The Kelly clamp may be used to assist insertion. The tube should be directed anteriorly and superiorly to evacuate a pneumothorax. The tube is connected to a Heimlich flap valve or a water-sealed drainage system. Suction may be applied to the drainage system to aid re-inflation. There is risk of re-expansion pulmonary edema after rapid re-inflation of a lung that has been collapsed for a prolonged period. (From Civetta and coworkers [6].)

CARDIAC TAMPONADE

CAUSES OF PERICARDIAL EFFUSION
Chest trauma
Cardiac surgery
Central line insertion
Myocardial rupture after myocardial infarction
Dressler's syndrome
Postcardiomyotomy
Postmyocardial infarction
Malignancy
Uremia
Connective tissue disorders
Radiotherapy

Figure 11-12. Rapid accumulation of pericardial fluid causing acute cardiac tamponade during anesthesia is most frequently caused by bleeding into the pericardial space secondary to trauma or after cardiac surgery. In Dressler's syndrome an autoimmune reaction to myocardial damage occurs causing pericarditis and sometimes effusion. Onset is usually weeks after either cardiac surgery or a myocardial infarction. Fluid may accumulate in the pericardial space in chronic conditions such as uremia, malignancy, and connective tissue disorders. This less frequently leads to acute decompensation with tamponade [7] because there is time for stretching of the pericardium to occur. Patients with pericardial effusion may suffer cardiovascular collapse on induction of anesthesia [8]. Radiotherapy may cause fibrosis and constriction of the pericardium, compressing the heart. A reactive effusion may develop after radiotherapy.

DIAGNOSIS OF CARDIAC TAMPONADE
Hypotension
Muffled heart sounds
Elevated central venous pressure
Kussmaul's sign
Oliguria
Pulsus paradoxus
Equalization of pressures
Low-voltage electrocardiographic complexes
Electrical alternans on the electrocardiogram
Enlarged heart shadow on chest radiography
Echocardiography

Figure 11-13. The diagnosis of cardiac tamponade is usually made clinically. Beck's triad of hypotension, muffled heart sounds, and elevated central venous pressure are characteristic signs at presentation, although tension pneumothorax as a cause of elevated central venous pressure and hypotension should be considered and excluded before pericardiocentesis is attempted. Kussmaul's sign may be seen; this is an inspiratory increase in jugular venous pressure. Pulsus paradoxus (*see* Fig. 11-15) and equalization of diastolic pressures across the right heart (*see* Fig. 11-16) are strongly suggestive of cardiac tamponade. The urine output is almost invariably reduced. The heart is insulated by the effusion and electrocardiograph size may be reduced.

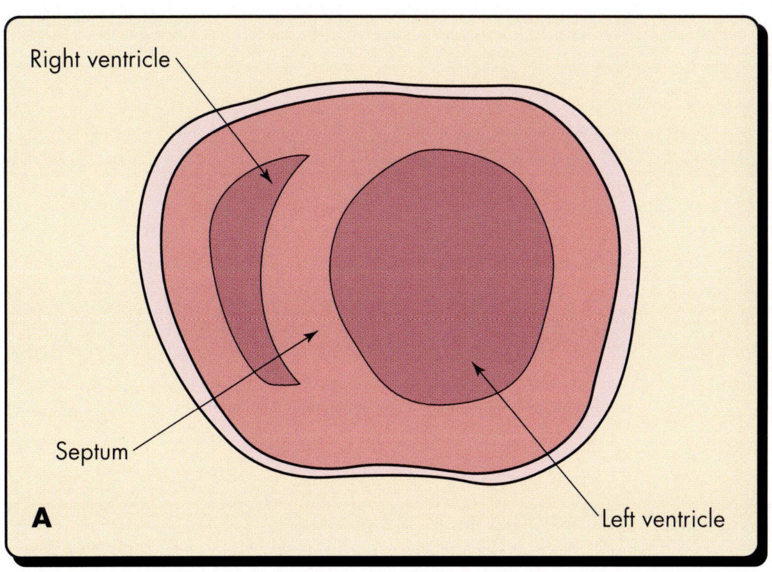

Figure 11-14. Cross section of the heart with the septum bulging from right to left. The pericardium is relatively inelastic, and increasing volume in the pericardial space rapidly results in an increase in pericardial pressure. The increasing pressure is able to compress the heart chambers having the lowest pressure. Right atrial filling is compromised first; then, as pressure further increases, the right ventricle is compressed and diastolic filling is reduced. Although left ventricular function may be preserved, cardiac output decreases because of decreasing preload to the left heart. Increased right ventricular pressure can alter the normal pressure differential between the left and right ventricles during diastole. This results in shift of the interventricular septum to the left. The left ventricular outline, which is normally circular in cross section (**A**), is compressed by the flattened or bulging septum (*Continued on next page*)

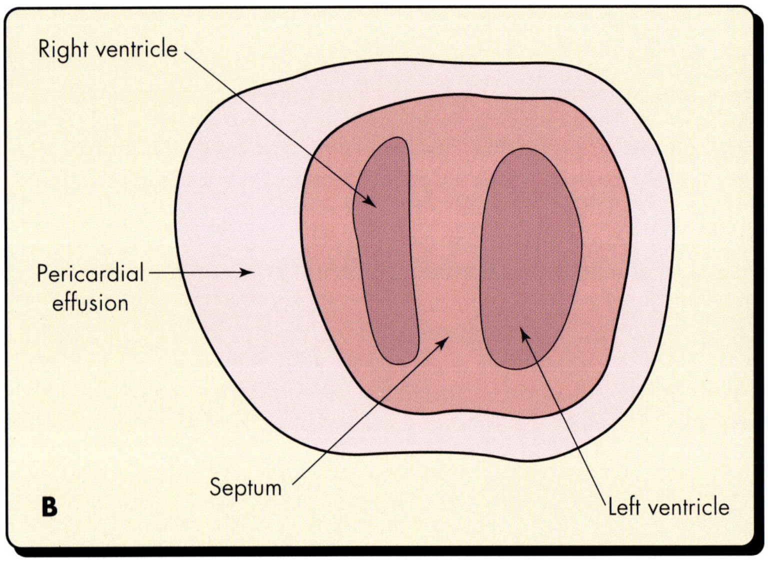

Figure 11-14. (*Continued*) (B), further compromising left ventricular function.

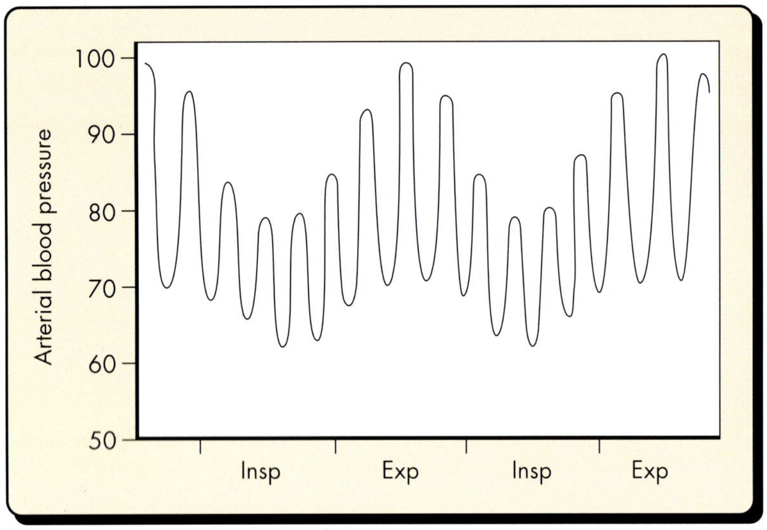

Figure 11-15. Tracing of systemic arterial pressure showing pulsus paradoxus of 20 mm Hg. Pulsus paradoxus is said to occur when there is a decrease in systolic pressure over 10 mm Hg during inspiration. In cardiac tamponade reduction in stroke volume occurs, and pulse pressure is usually less than 40 mm Hg. In spontaneous breathing there is an increase in venous return to the right heart during inspiration because of the decrease in intrathoracic pressure, causing distention of the right ventricle. The right ventricle cannot expand its free wall because of the fixed pericardial volume. Therefore, bulging of the interventricular septum occurs, compromising left ventricular filling (*see* Fig. 11-14). Pulsus paradoxus results because of this further reduction in left ventricular stroke volume during inspiration. The changes seen in pulsus paradoxus are an exaggeration of the normal changes seen during respiration. Pulsus paradoxus is assessed with a blood pressure cuff by inflating above peak systolic pressure and slowly deflating the cuff listening for Korotkoff sounds. When an occasional Korotkoff sound is heard during expiration with long gaps in between (about 100 mm Hg in this example), the pressure is noted. As the cuff is slowly deflated the number of Korotkoff sounds heard during each expiration becomes greater, with smaller gaps in between. When the sounds are heard throughout the respiratory cycle, without gaps, the second systolic pressure is noted (80 mm Hg in this case), and the difference between the two pressures is the amount of paradox (*ie*, 20 mm Hg). Paradox is easily measured directly from a tracing from an intra-arterial blood pressure line.

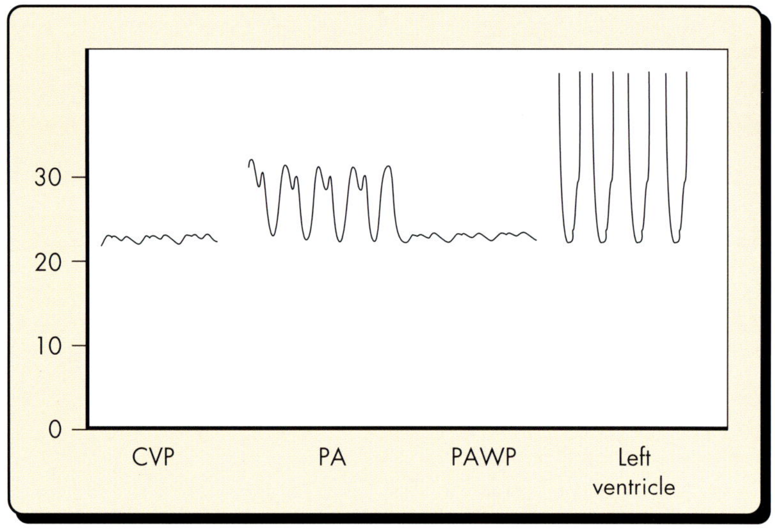

Figure 11-16. Equalization of end-diastolic blood pressures in cardiac tamponade occurs when the central venous pressure (*CVP*), pulmonary artery (PA) diastolic pressure, and pulmonary artery wedge pressure (*PAWP*) are raised and equal. The pressure reached at these sites is indicative of the pressure in the pericardial space, this pressure being transmitted to all chambers of the heart normally at a lower pressure.

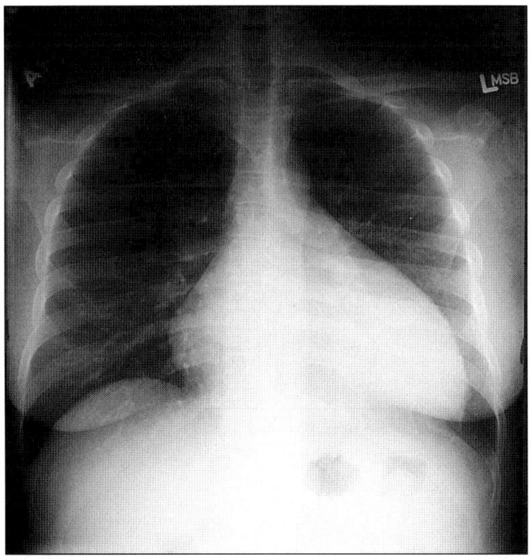

Figure 11-17. Chest radiograph of a large pericardial effusion. The cardiac diameter is markedly enlarged and the cardiac silhouette has a characteristic globular shape. This picture is seen in slowly developing chronic effusions when there is time for the pericardium to stretch. In an acute cardiac tamponade caused by bleeding into the pericardium the chest radiograph may show little or no cardiac enlargement.

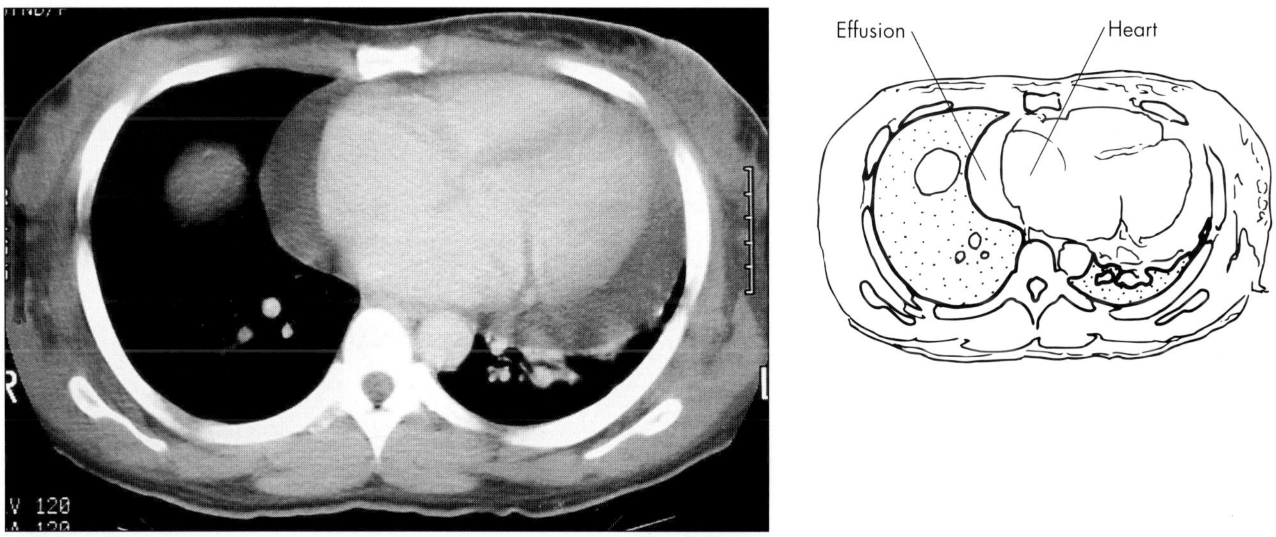

Figure 11-18. Chest computed tomographic scan of the same patient as in Figure 11-16. The enlargement of the cardiac shadow is confirmed as being caused by a pericardial effusion. A homogenous area of fluid density is seen surrounding the myocardium.

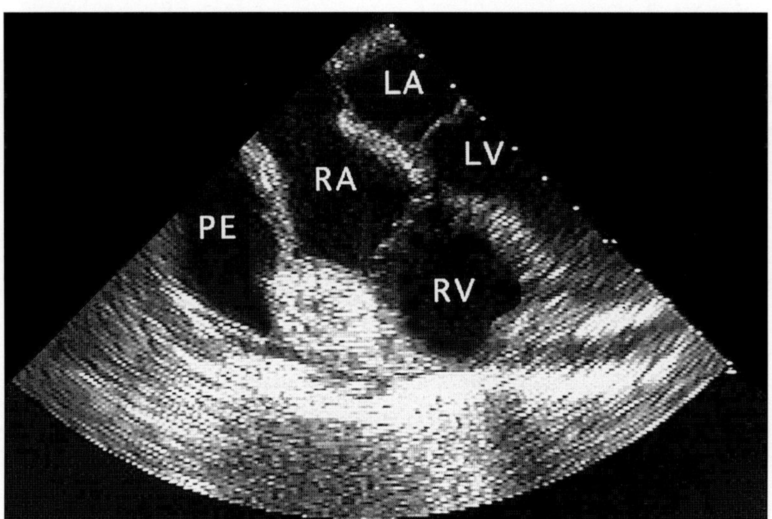

Figure 11-19. Transesophageal echocardiogram of a pericardial effusion in a patient with cardiac tamponade who had bleeding into the pericardium after cardiac surgery. This is a four-chamber view of the heart. A fluid-filled space can be seen adjacent to the right side of the heart. The right atrium (*RA*) is being compressed by the pericardial effusion (*PE*) and the free wall is bulging inward. LA—left atrium; LV—left ventricle; RV—right ventricle.

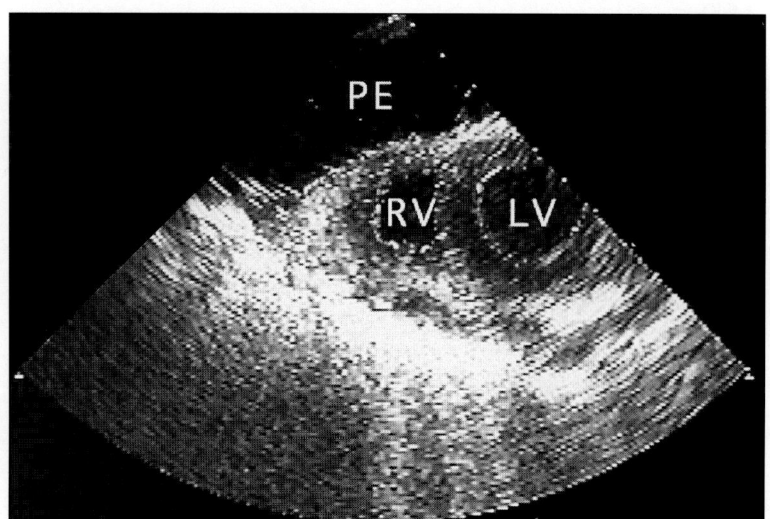

Figure 11-20. A short axis (cross-section) view of the heart in the same patient as in Figure 11-19, demonstrating the pericardial effusion (*PE*) lying posterior and lateral to the right and left ventricles (*RV* and *LV*). The presence of cardiac compromise from tamponade can be confirmed with echocardiography by showing diastolic collapse of the atria and right ventricle.

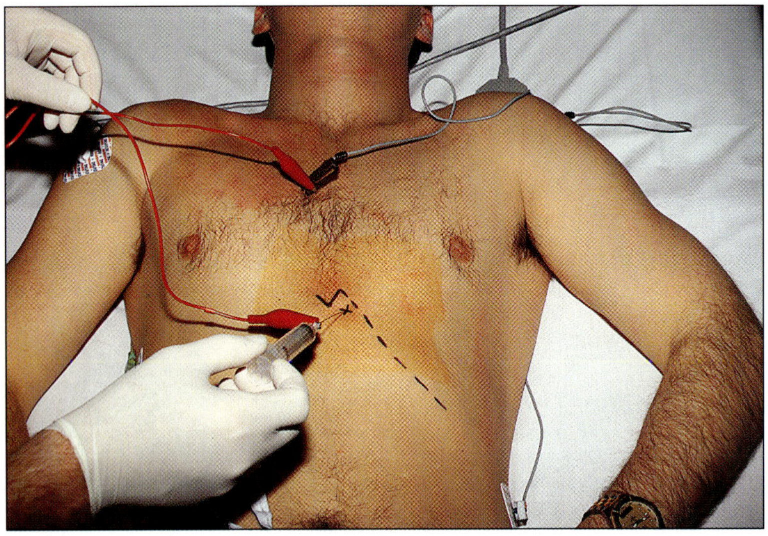

Figure 11-21. Pericardiocentesis is considered when cardiac tamponade is causing life-threatening hemodynamic compromise. The considerable risk of complications should limit its use electively [9]. A parasternal approach can be used; however, it is more likely to cause pneumothorax or coronary artery laceration and is not recommended unless surface echocardiography has demonstrated easier localization of the effusion by this route. The subxiphoid approach may prove more effective in draining the effusion when it is encouraged to pool inferiorly by having the patient in a 45° head-up position [10]. After infiltration with local anesthesia, an 18- to 23-gauge spinal needle is inserted just below and to the left of the xiphoid process. The needle is directed at a 45° angle to the skin and aimed toward the midclavicular point. The needle is advanced until pericardial fluid can be aspirated. If the fluid appears to be blood, then it is examined for clotting: Blood in the pericardium is usually defibrinated and will not clot. The development of clot suggests that blood has been aspirated from the ventricle. The action of a beating heart contracting on the fixed tip of a needle may result in myocardial or coronary artery laceration. The risk of the procedure may be reduced by ultrasound guidance, which may facilitate location of the effusion. Guidance by electrocardiogram (ECG) can also be used to identify cardiac penetration. The V lead of the ECG is connected to the needle with an alligator clip, as shown in this figure. As the needle is advanced through the subcutaneous tissues, a normal QRS complex is seen. S-T segment elevation is seen on penetration of the myocardium; if the ventricle is entered, then the ECG changes with the development of deep Q waves (the normal intraventricular pattern). Ectopic beats may also be seen if the myocardium is contacted. Chronic effusions may recur and require surgical formation of a pericardial window.

PULMONARY EMBOLISM

CAUSES OF PULMONARY EMBOLUS
Thrombus
Air
Fat
Amniotic fluid
Tumors
Kidney
Trophoblast

Figure 11-22. Massive pulmonary embolism causing cardiovascular collapse has a number of etiologies. Thrombus arising from a peripheral deep vein thrombosis may break off and pass to the lungs. Small thrombi may lodge peripherally in the pulmonary vasculature and cause release of mediators that can produce a marked rise in pulmonary vascular resistance. A large thrombus may lodge in the pulmonary artery at its bifurcation point (called a *saddle embolus*) and obstruct outflow from the right ventricle. Air may be entrained into the veins at the operative site or may enter through venous cannulae, particularly if the intravenous infusion has been pressurized. Fat emboli can arise during orthopedic procedures or after fracture of a long bone. Amniotic fluid embolism may occur during delivery. Tumors, including trophoblast, may have intravascular extension that can be dislodged during surgery and cause pulmonary embolism. Renal tumors are capable of extension into the inferior vena cava and may embolize in this manner.

DIAGNOSIS OF PULMONARY EMBOLISM

Pleuritic chest pain
Hemoptysis
Pleural rub
Hypoxia
Tachycardia
Hypotension from reduction in cardiac output
Dyspnea
Decreased end-tidal carbon dioxide
Right ventricular failure
- Pulmonary hypertension
- Raised central venous pressure
- Gallop rhythm

Electrocardiography
- Tachycardia
- S_1, Q_3, T_3
- Right bundle branch block
- Transesophageal echocardiography

Chest radiography
- Pulmonary oligemia
- Atelectatic areas from previous emboli

Pulmonary angiography
Ventilation-perfusion (V/Q) scan

Figure 11-23. In massive pulmonary embolism (PE) causing hemodynamic collapse, the signs of peripheral emboli (dyspnea, pleuritic chest pain, hemoptysis, and pleural rub) may be absent. During anesthesia the first sign may be a dramatic decrease in end-tidal carbon dioxide levels, to less than 15 to 20 mm Hg. This is soon followed by the development of hypoxia shown by pulse oximetry. Hypotension may have developed by the next time the noninvasive blood pressure cycles, and examination of the electrocardiogram (ECG) may show tachycardia or even bradycardia if the embolus is large enough to be seriously life threatening. Signs of right ventricular failure may occur, including marked jugular venous distention. A pulmonary artery catheter may show pulmonary hypertension resulting from obstruction by the embolus and from intense pulmonary vasoconstriction owing to mediator release. The pulmonary artery wedge pressure will be very low, differentiating pulmonary embolism from tension pneumothorax and cardiac tamponade. In chronic pulmonary embolism the ECG may show tachycardia, an S wave in lead 1, a Q wave in lead 3, and a T wave inversion in lead 3 (S_1, Q_3, T_3). Right heart strain may be demonstrated as right bundle branch block or T-wave inversion in the right ventricular leads V_1 to V_3. Transesophageal echocardiography has been used to diagnose PE occurring after induction of anesthesia [11]. A chest radiograph may show little abnormality although pulmonary oligemia can be seen and areas of plate atelectasis may be present from previous emboli. In the less-acute situation the diagnosis can be confirmed by pulmonary angiography or ventilation/perfusion (*V/Q*) lung scan.

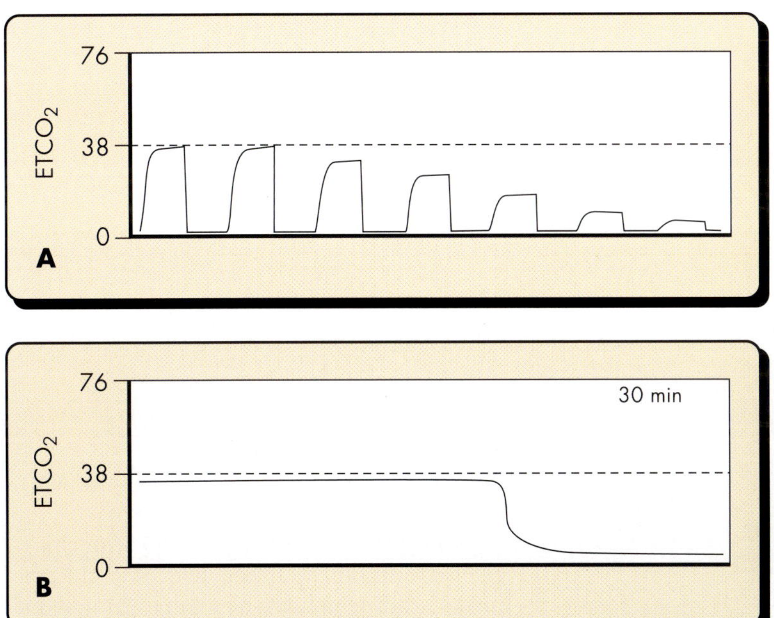

Figure 11-24. A, Rapid decrease in end-tidal carbon dioxide ($ETCO_2$) levels as a result of massive pulmonary embolism. B, Trended display showing an abrupt decline in $ETCO_2$. Capnography may provide early evidence of pulmonary embolism under anesthesia. The $ETCO_2$ decreases to a level that may be so low as to give the impression of a partial disconnection of the sampling tubing. A sudden decrease of this nature should always raise suspicion of massive pulmonary embolus or of a sudden catastrophic decrease in cardiac output. The decrease in $ETCO_2$ is not a reflection of the partial pressure of CO_2 in arterial blood ($PaCO_2$), which may increase if minute ventilation remains unchanged. The $PaCO_2$-$ETCO_2$gradient increases because of the dead-space effect of ventilated but unperfused lung caused by the pulmonary embolism.

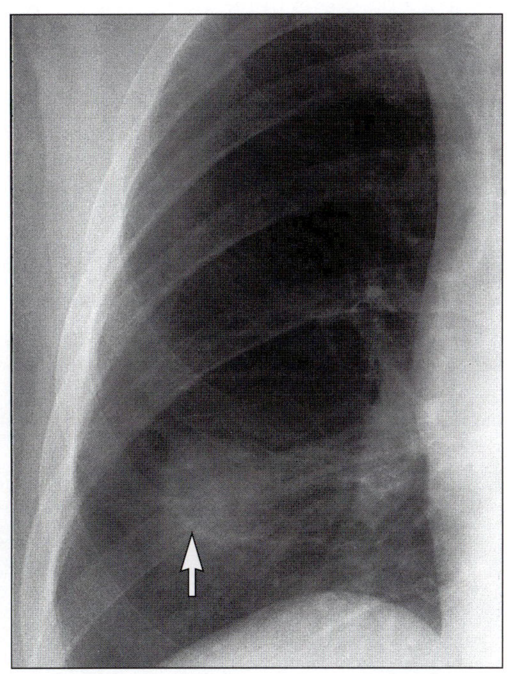

Figure 11-25 Chest radiograph of a patient with pulmonary embolus. There is an area of opacification in the lower right zone of the lung (*arrow*).

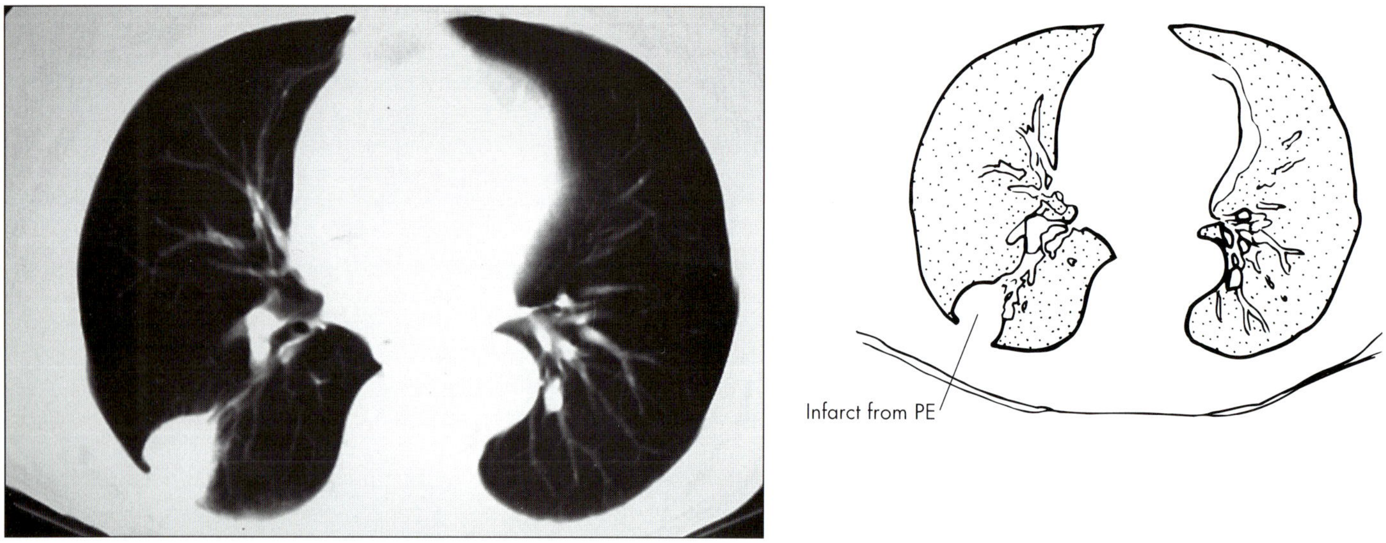

Figure 11-26. Computed tomography scan of the chest of the patient in Figure 11-25 who has a pulmonary embolus (PE). This slice, at lung density, clearly shows the right-sided wedge shaped infarct with a sharp apex pointing toward the hilum.

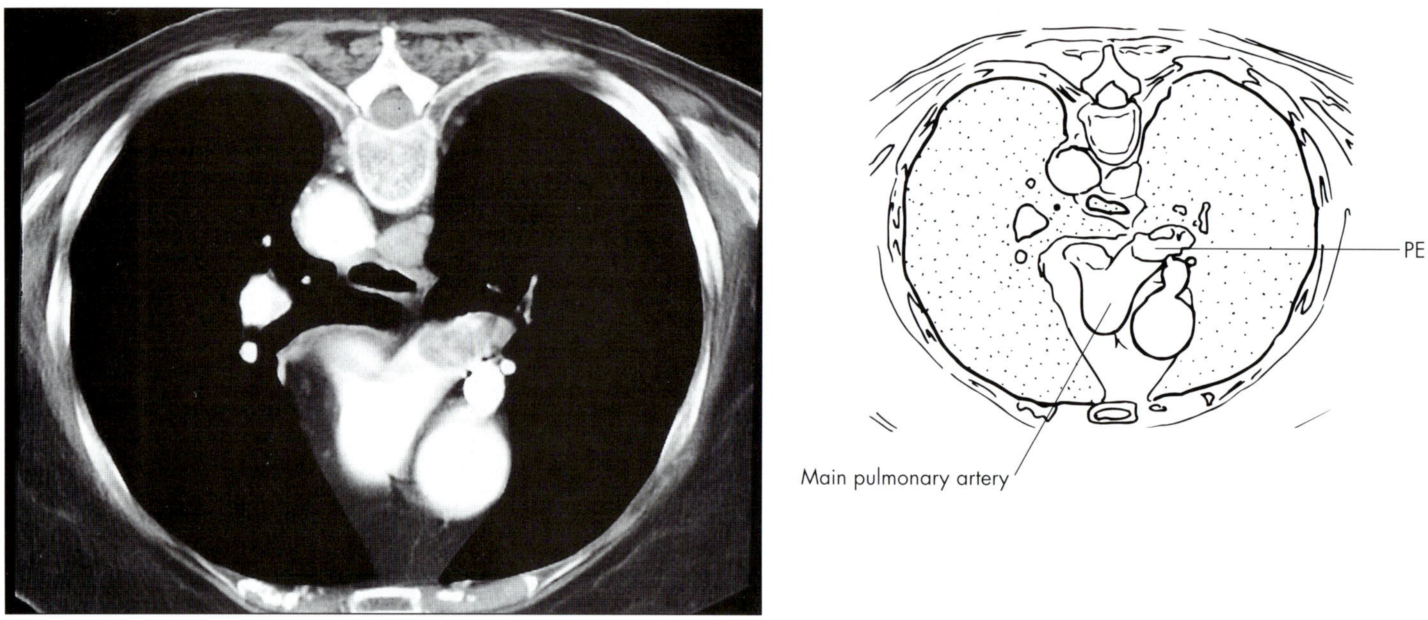

Figure 11-27. Computed tomographic scan of the chest of the patient in Figures 11-25 and 11-26. The pulmonary vessels are white with the darker embolus sitting at the bifurcation of the pulmonary trunk.

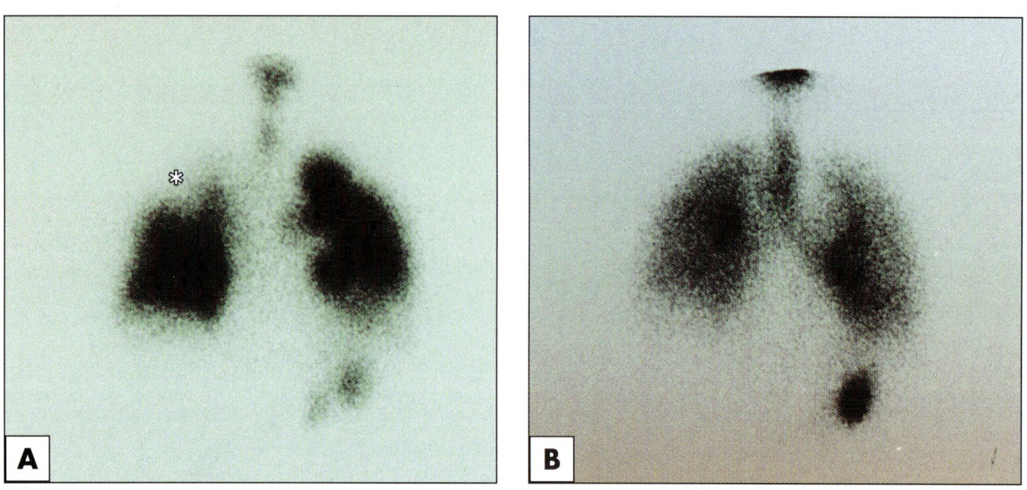

Figure 11-28. Ventilation-perfusion (V/Q) scan of the lungs showing pulmonary embolism (PE). The positive V/Q scan characteristically shows filling defects on the perfusion scan, which are normally ventilated. **A**, Filling defect in the right upper lobe on perfusion. **B**, This area has no filling defect on ventilation. However, there are a large number of false-positive results, and scans with "low" probability for PE still have a 25% to 40% incidence of PE on pulmonary angiography [12].

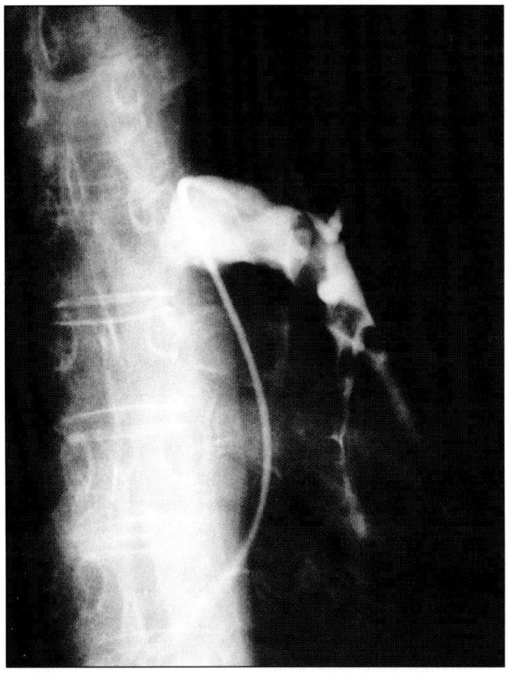

Figure 11-29. Pulmonary angiogram showing thrombus as a dark filling defect in the left pulmonary artery. The pulmonary angiogram is the definitive examination for the diagnosis of pulmonary embolism.

CRITERIA FOR FAT EMBOLISM

Major features
Respiratory difficulty leading to acute respiratory distress syndrome
Cerebral involvement
Disorientation, lethargy, and irritability
Petechial rash
In 50% to 60% of patients
Upper trunk, axillary folds, conjunctivae, and fundi
Minor features
Pyrexia, tachycardia, retinal changes, anemia, and thrombocytopenia
Increased fibrin degradation products, although disseminated intravascular coagulation is rare
Inconsistent lipiduria
Fat globules in sputum
Diffuse alveolar infiltrate on chest radiography
S-T segment changes and right ventricular strain on electrocardiography

Figure 11-30. Fat embolism characteristically occurs about 2 to 3 days after fractures of a long bone. Patients present with pyrexia, tachypnea, and tachycardia. Other signs include mental status changes, such as confusion and lethargy, hypoxia that may progress to acute respiratory distress syndrome (*ARDS*), and a petechial rash seen on the torso and in the axillae. Fat globules can be seen in retinal vessels, in the sputtern, and occasionally in the urine. A diffuse infiltrate may be seen on chest radiography and this may progress to the picture of frank ARDS. If the pulmonary effects are prominent, then right ventricular strain may be seen on the ECG. A mild coagulopathy may develop. During orthopedic surgery, particularly total hip arthroplasty, when then femoral prosthesis is inserted using methyl methacrylate cement, loose particles of cement, clot, air, and bone may be forced into the circulation. This can result in hemodynamic collapse caused by pulmonary embolism and in vasodilatation from the methyl methacrylate monomer.

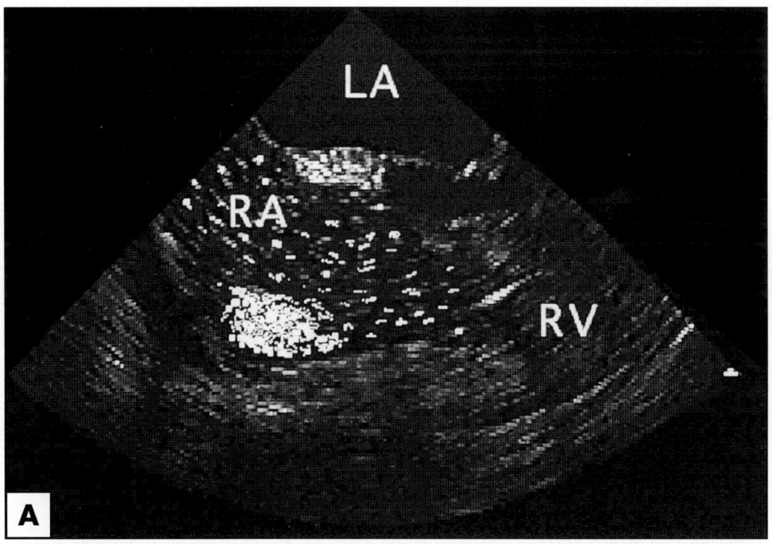

B. CAUSES OF AIR EMBOLUS

Surgery
- Operative site above the heart
  - Craniotomy in the sitting position
  - Spine surgery in the prone position
  - Pelvic surgery in steep Trendelenberg
- Cerebral venous sinuses
- Open heart operations

Intravenous lines
- Central line insertion
- Air in intravenous tubing
- Pressurized intravenous infusions

Figure 11-31. A, Echocardiogram of air in the right heart. The right atrium (*RA*) is filled with numerous air bubbles. Air bubbles in any fluid-filled space appear as very bright points on ultrasonography. The gas–fluid interface is extremely echogenic and often causes artefactual extension of the echo perpendicular to the ultrasound beam. This gives air bubbles their characteristic wings, making them appear like bright fireflies on the two-dimensional echocardiogram. This impression is accentuated by their dancing movement. **B**, Air embolism may occur during anesthesia owing to entry of air at the surgical site or through intravenous (IV) lines. Entrainment of air during surgery is most likely to occur when the surgical site is above the level of the heart, (*eg*, craniotomy in the sitting position, spine surgery in the prone position, or pelvic surgery in a steep Trendelenberg position). Surgical entrainment of air is also prone to occur when veins are held open by surrounding structures and not allowed to collapse, (*eg*, the cerebral venous sinuses or open heart surgery). Air entry through IV cannulae may occur during insertion of central venous lines if the cannula is left in the vein unconnected to a flushed IV line. The risk is reduced by positioning the patient head-down to increase venous pressure. In any IV line, care should be taken to ensure that air is cleared from the tubing and is not allowed to enter the patient. The risk is greatest when the IV bag is pressurized for rapid transfusion. A large amount of air can be forced in rapidly, with potentially fatal consequences. LA—left atrium; RV—right ventricle.

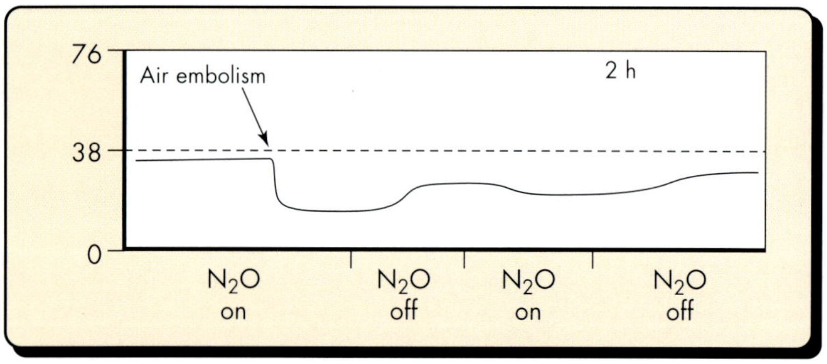

Figure 11-32. Trend display from a capnogram during neurosurgery with the patient in the sitting position. An air embolism caused rapid decline in the end-tidal carbon dioxide ($ETCO_2$). Nitrous oxide (*N_2O*) was being used and was turned off. Over approximately the next 20 minutes, the $ETCO_2$ increased as the air was being absorbed. The N_2O was turned back on, when it was felt that the patient was recovering from the air embolus. Doing so caused a further decline in $ETCO_2$ levels owing to movement of the N_2O into the remaining air bubbles in the pulmonary circulation, increasing their size. Massive air embolism causes foaming of air in the right ventricle and pulmonary artery with cessation of cardiac output. This can be rapidly fatal and should be managed by aspiration of the air through central venous or pulmonary artery catheters. Placing the patient in a left lateral position may aid aspiration by encouraging the air to float upward into the right atrium. It must be remembered that a rapid decrease in $ETCO_2$ will be produced by any catastrophic drop in cardiac output and is therefore not diagnostic of pulmonary embolism.

MANAGEMENT OF PULMONARY THROMBOEMBOLISM
ABCs of resuscitation:
Oxygenation
Cardiac massage
Volume expansion
Inotropic agents
Cardiopulmonary bypass
Anticoagulation
Thrombolytic agents
Pulmonary embolectomy on cardiopulmonary bypass
Greenfield filter in interior vena cava

Figure 11-33. The management of massive pulmonary thromboembolism [12] commences with the initiation of resuscitation. Intubation and ventilation with 100% oxygen are started. If no pulses are felt cardiopulmonary resuscitation is initiated. Fluid loading is recommended, despite the increased central venous pressure, to increase left ventricular preload. Inotropic support may be needed. Pulmonary vasodilators such as isoproterenol or prostaglandin E_1 may be beneficial; however, all vasodilators can also cause systemic effects and worsen hypotension. Inhaled nitric oxide has an extremely short duration of effect, which minimizes systemic vasodilatation; however, its use is not widespread. Thromboembolism causing severe right heart failure may require urgent cardiopulmonary bypass (CPB) surgery as the only method to provide systemic circulation. Pulmonary embolectomy can then be perfomed. The characteristic finding on exposure of the heart is a tense bulging right ventricle and a slack flaccid left ventricle that is not receiving its normal preload from the pulmonary vasculature. Anticoagulation or thrombolytic therapy is used to promote breakdown of the thrombus in the less severe situation. However, recent surgery often precludes the use of thrombolytic therapy. In recurrent thromboembolism, a Greenfield filter may be placed in the interior vena cava. This may help prevent additional emboli from reaching the pulmonary circulation.

ANAPHYLAXIS

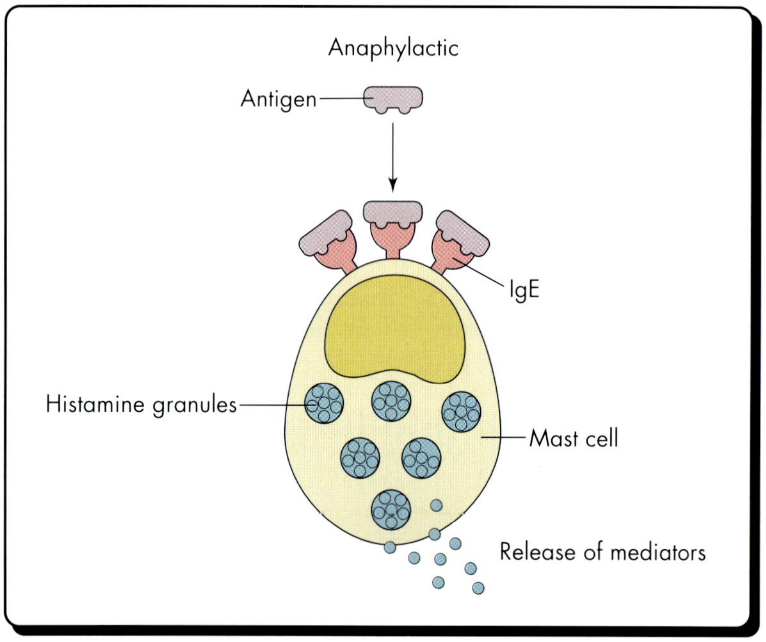

Figure 11-34. Anaphylaxis. In an anaphylactic reaction, antigen binds to immunoglobulin E (*IgE*) on the surface of mast cells, causing degranulation of inflammatory mediators. The terms *anaphylaxis*, *anaphylactic reaction*, *anaphylactoid*, *allergic*, and *hypersensitivity* are often used interchangeably. The terms *anaphylaxis* and *anaphylactic reaction* should be reserved for the situation in which IgE is involved. This reaction requires prior sensitization to the antigen involved or a related antigen.

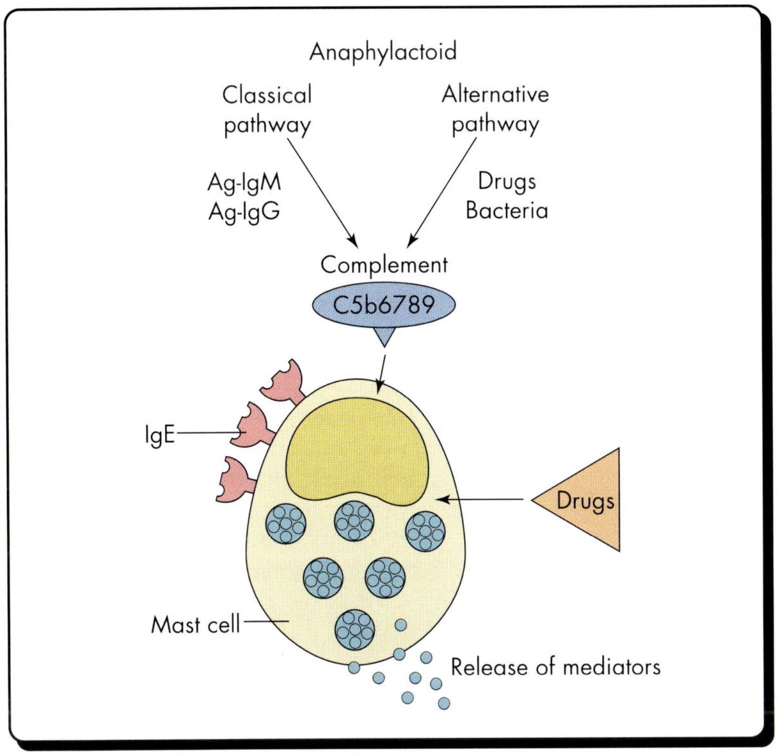

Figure 11-35. Anaphylactoid refers to reactions that involve other mechanisms apart from immunoglobulin E (*IgE*)–antigen binding [13]. Complement may be activated through the classical pathway by antigen–IgG or antigen–IgM (*Ag-IgM* or *Ag-IgG*) complexes, heparin-protamine complexes, or plasmin. The alternate pathway of complement activation may be initiated by polyanionic drugs or certain bacterial elements. Complement activation by either pathway results in the formation of the membrane attack unit C5b6789, which causes release of mediators from the mast cell. Drugs such as thiopental, succinylcholine, tubocurarine, atracurium, and morphine are capable of causing direct release of histamine from mast cells. Propofol, etomidate, the steroid neuromuscular blocking agents, and *cis*-atracurium are thought not to cause histamine release in this manner. Anaphylactic and anaphylactoid reactions produce clinically indistinguishable syndromes. The severity of the reaction is no guide to the mechanism of its initiation. The term *histaminoid reaction* has been used to denote either anaphylactic or anaphylactoid reactions [13].

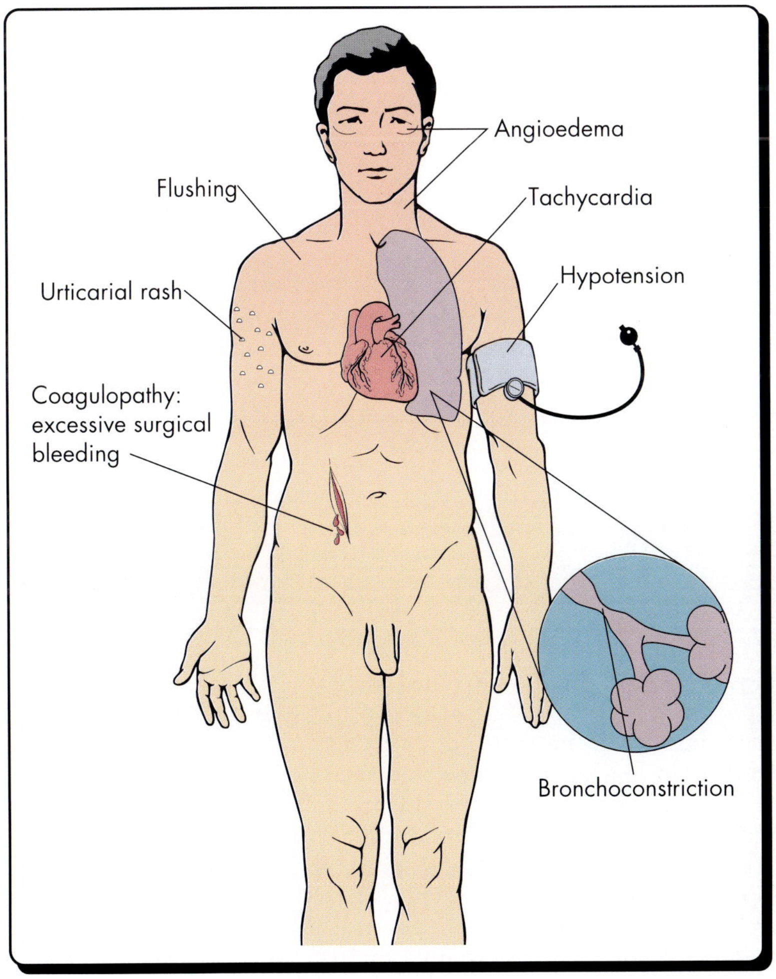

Figure 11-36. During anesthesia, anaphylactic or anaphylactoid reactions may present anywhere on a spectrum from mild evidence of histamine release to life-threatening cardiovascular collapse. Histaminoid reactions may present at any point after induction of anesthesia. A common first sign under anesthesia is an increase in ventilating pressure caused by bronchoconstriction. Severe hypotension may occur because of marked vasodilatation. Skin signs may consist of urticaria and flushing. Angioedema may cause upper airway obstruction and swelling around the eyes. Anesthesia is particularly prone to cause histaminoid reactions because of the rapidity of administration of intravenous (IV) agents. Slow IV anesthetic administration may mean injection over 1 second, and the resulting high plasma levels of drugs are capable of provoking histamine release. This is especially true if precipitate is injected (*eg*, after mixture of thiopental and a nondepolarizing neuromuscular blocker in the IV line). If a severe anaphylactoid reaction occurs after induction, it may be prudent to cancel surgery because coagulopathy or even disseminated intravascular coagulation may occur.

MANAGEMENT OF SEVERE ANAPHYLACTIC OR ANAPHYLACTOID REACTIONS

Stop the triggering agent
ABCs of resuscitation:
- Oxygenation
- Volume expansion

Epinephrine
Other vasoconstrictors, *eg*, norepinephrine
Bronchodilators
- Nebulized albuterol
- Aminophylline

Corticosteroids
Antihistamines
Immunologic follow-up

Figure 11-37. If a severe histaminoid reaction occurs during anesthesia, administration of potentially triggering agents should be stopped immediately. Resuscitation is begun, and cardiopulmonary resuscitation may be required. The patient should be ventilated using 100% oxygen. Cardiovascular collapse is from intravascular volume loss and vasodilatation. Intravenous fluids should be administered. When shock is not corrected by simple fluid administration, epinephrine, 1-mL increments of 1 in 10,000 (0.1 mg), should be administered early and given until hemodynamic stability is restored. Large doses or an epinephrine infusion may be required. Other vasoconstrictors or inotropes may be used; however, epinephrine is the only agent that has been demonstrated to be of benefit in anaphylactoid reactions. Calcium should not be used as a vasopressor because it may increase mediator release from mast cells [13]. Epinephrine may help reduce bronchoconstriction, and other more selective agents may be helpful. Steroids such as hydrocortisone have little effect in the acute reaction; however, they may inhibit the late phase of reactions and immunoglobulin E expression. Antihistamine use is controversial because some effects of histamine are beneficial and blockade may reduce the inotropic effect on the heart. There is concern that histamine blockade reduces the homeostatic negative feedback that further reduces histamine release. Patients should be referred for immunologic follow-up to try to establish the mechanism of the reaction and identify the triggering agent so it can be avoided in the future.

ARRHYTHMIAS

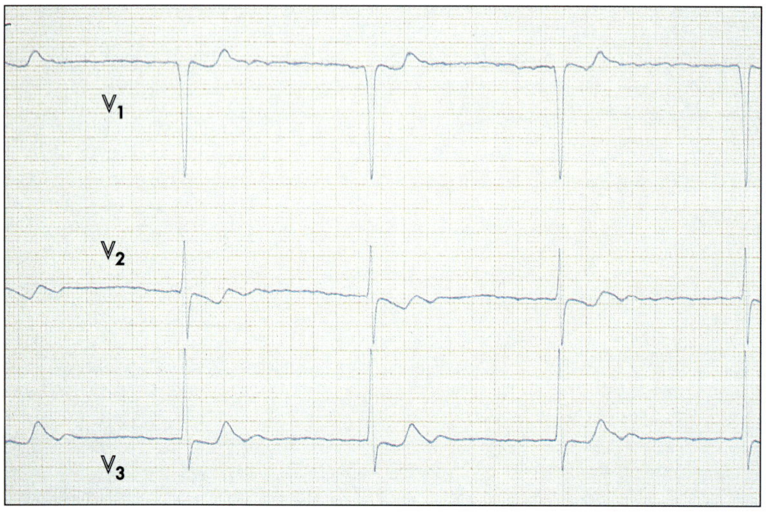

Figure 11-38. Severe bradycardia (heart rate 36 bpm) in a patient with complete heart block caused by digoxin toxicity.

CAUSES OF BRADYCARDIA UNDER ANESTHESIA

Sinus node disease
- Vagal reflex
  - Oculocardiac
  - Carotid sinus stimulation
  - Peritoneal stimulation
  - Cervical dilatation
  - Light anesthesia
  - Increased intracranial pressure
- Sick sinus syndrome
- Drugs

Atrioventricular node disease
- Myocardial infarction
- Drugs
- Rheumatic fever
- Amyloidosis
- Sarcoidosis
- Idiopathic fibrosis

Figure 11-39. Bradyarrhythmia as a cause of cardiovascular collapse during anesthesia is usually easy to recognize. Bradycardia may occur because of sinus node problems or atrioventricular node problems (heart block). Sinus node block may occur because of vagal reflexes, as commonly seen in patients under anesthesia. In sick sinus syndrome, sinus bradycardia and supraventricular tachycardias arising from the sinus nodes may occur. Succinylcholine may cause bradycardia by imitating the action of acetylcholine at the vagal receptors. Drugs such as beta blockers, calcium channel antagonists, and digoxin may cause sinus node or atrioventricular block. Inferior myocardial infarction not infrequently causes complete heart block if the AV node has been involved. The cardiac conduction system can be directly involved in disease processes such as amyloidosis, sarcoidosis, and idiopathic fibrosis.

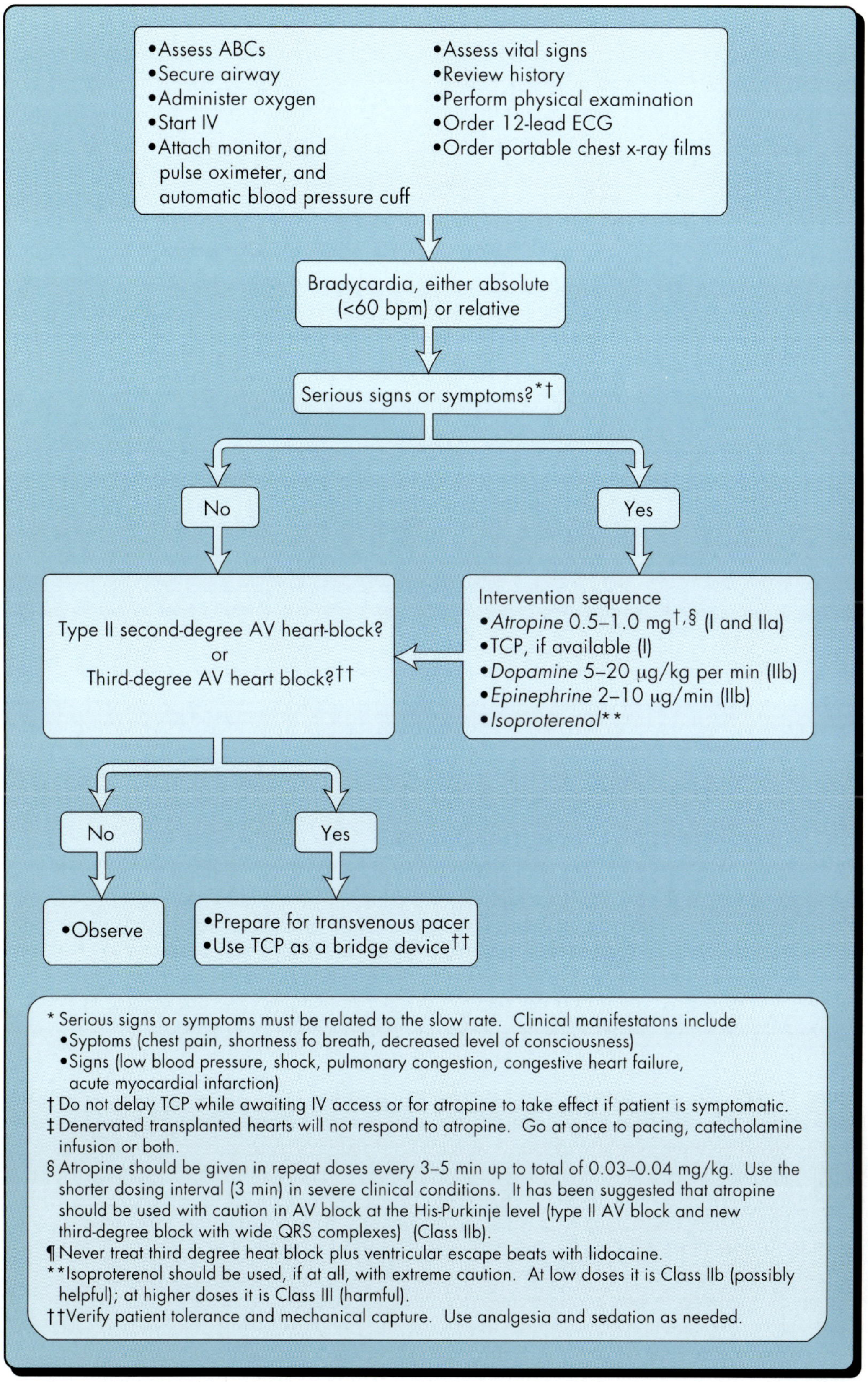

Figure 11-40. The Advanced Cardiac Life Support (ACLS) bradycardia algorithm [14] is followed in any bradycardic situation as long as the patient is not in cardiac arrest. Interventions in ACLS are graded as follows: Class I: definitely helpful; Class IIa: acceptable, probably helpful; Class IIb: acceptable, possibly helpful; and Class III: not indicated, may be harmful. Dopamine and epinephrine can be used after atropine, especially if the patient is also hypotensive and very symptomatic. In the past, isoproterenol was commonly used; however, its use has been downgraded because of its ability to increase myocardial oxygen demand to an extent that may be detrimental to patients with coronary heart disease. Transcutaneous pacing (*TCP*) is recommended while transvenous pacing is being established. AV—atrioventricular; bpm—beats per minute; ECG—electrocardiogram; IV—intravenous. (*From* Essentials of ACLS [14].)

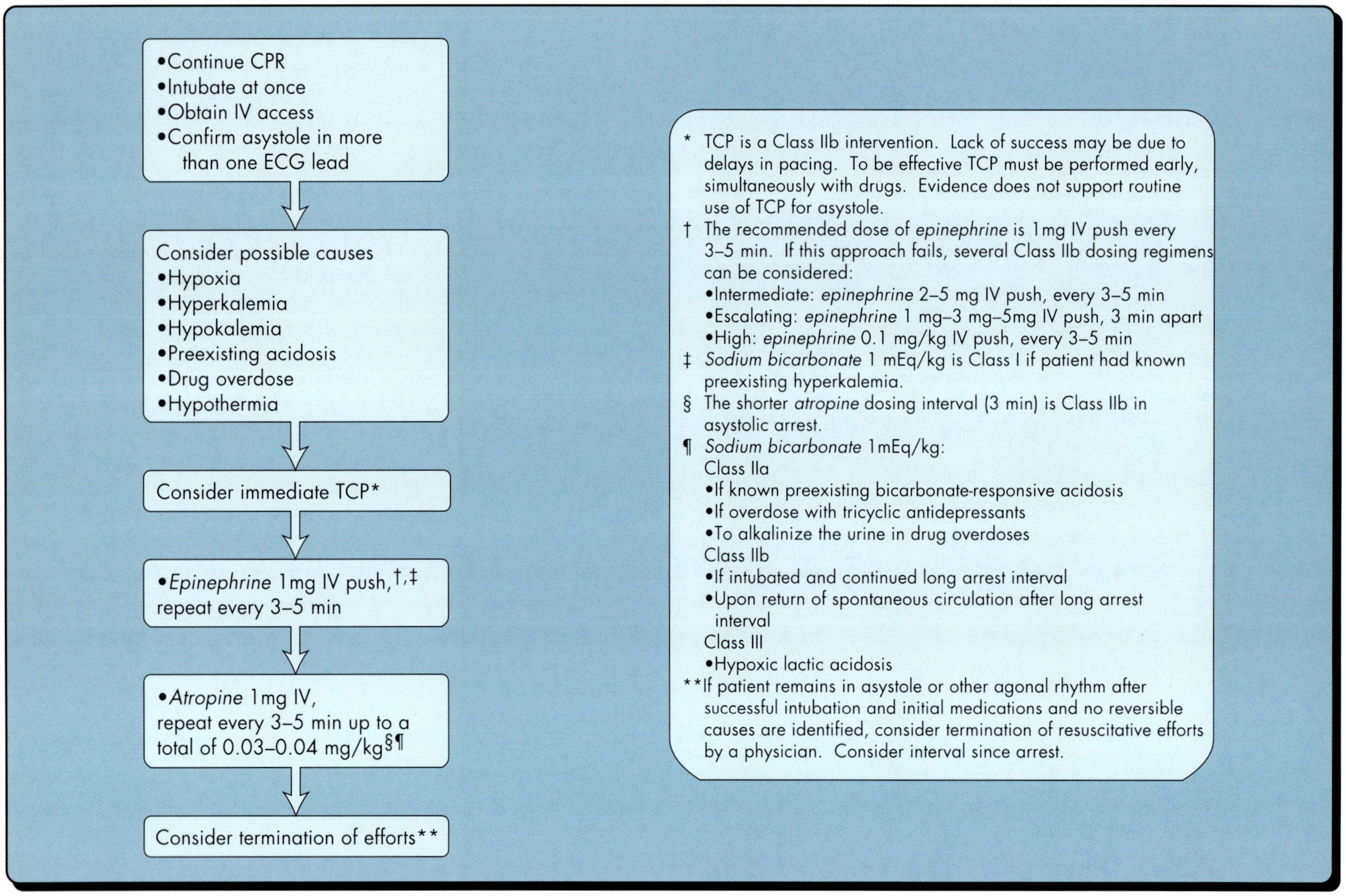

Figure 11-41. Advanced cardiac life support (ACLS) algorithm for treatment of asystole [14]. Obviously, the immediate treatment of asystole is to establish cardiopulmonary resuscitation (CPR). It is important to confirm that asystole is the true rhythm: A detached electrocardiogram (*ECG*) lead may easily mimic asystole. If there is any doubt as to the true rhythm during an arrest, cardioversion should be considered. Unless asystole is from a rapidly correctable underlying cause, the prognosis may be very poor. Pacing is only rarely successful for asystole outside the operating room; however, when rapidly initiated, it may be beneficial in the situations of vagal arrest, Stokes-Adams attacks, bradyasystolic arrest, or after defibrillation of ventricular fibrillation. IV—intravenous; TCP—transcutaneous pacing. (*From* Essentials of ACLS [14].)

METHODS FOR EMERGENCY PACING
Transvenous
Fluoroscopy-directed
Balloon-directed
Pacing pulmonary artery catheter
Epicardial
Transcutaneous
Esophageal

Figure 11-42. When treatment of bradycardia with pharmacologic means such as atropine or beta agonists fails, electrical pacing may be necessary. A variety of transvenous methods of pacing exists. A simple pacing wire can be inserted but requires fluoroscopic control because passage through the tricuspid valve into the right ventricle may be difficult. A special pacing pulmonary artery catheter with an extra lumen opening in the right ventricle may be passed in the usual manner. A fine pacing wire is passed through the lumen and comes into contact with the endocardium of the right ventricle. There can be difficulty in achieving capture with this method because the wire is very flimsy and may not achieve solid contact with the heart. Balloon-directed pacing wire is our preferred method for emergency pacing in the operating room or intensive care unit. Epicardial wires can be inserted directly into the external surface of the myocardium. This is only practicable when the chest is already open, (*eg*, in cardiac surgery). The transcutaneous routes can also be used. Transesophageal atrial pacing has recently been developed [15]. An esophageal stethoscope with electrodes embedded in it is inserted in the normal manner, and if intra-operative bradycardia occurs then the atrium can easily be paced at the desired rate. Obviously, atrial pacing is ineffective for complete heart block of the atrioventricular node.

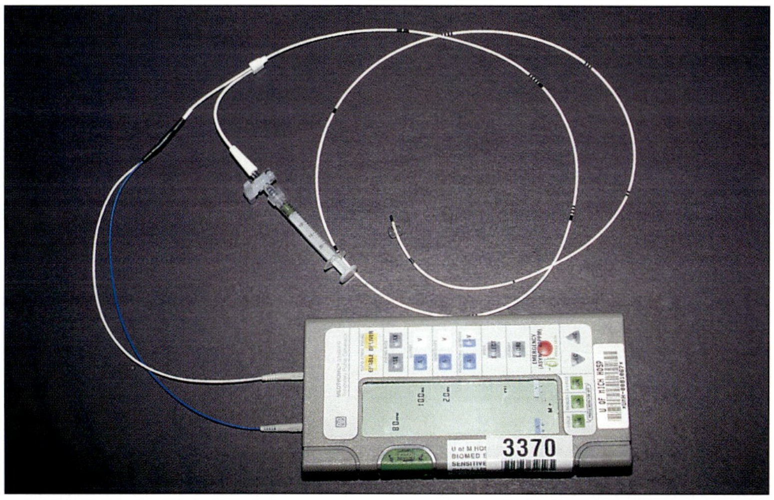

Figure 11-43. A balloon-directed pacing wire and pacemaker (Arrow, Reading, PA). The balloon is inflated and flow-directed through the tricuspid valve in the same manner as is a pulmonary artery catheter. The balloon is then deflated and the wire lodged into the apex of the right ventricle. (Courtesy of Arrow International, Inc, Reading, PA, and Medtronic, Inc, Minneapolis, MN.)

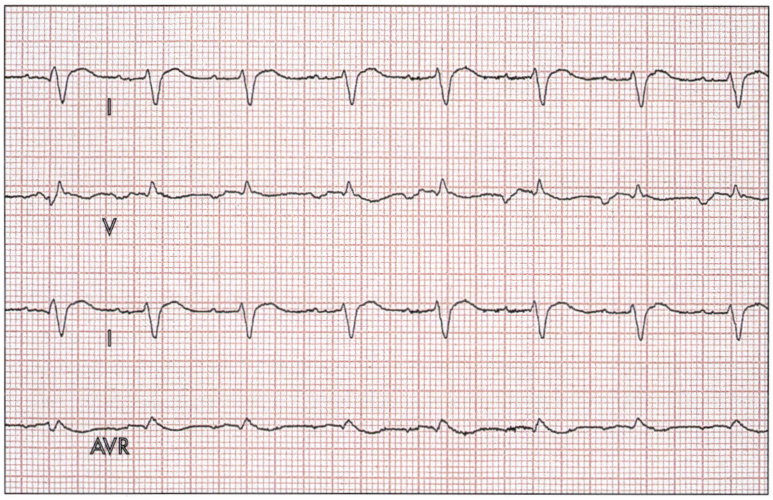

Figure 11-44. Balloon-directed pacing wire insertion under electrocardiogram (ECG) control. The V lead of the ECG is connected to the distal electrode of the pacing wire with an alligator clip. In this figure the second waveform (*V*) is from the pacing wire. The wire is in the superior vena cava and small-sized P and QRS complexes are seen.

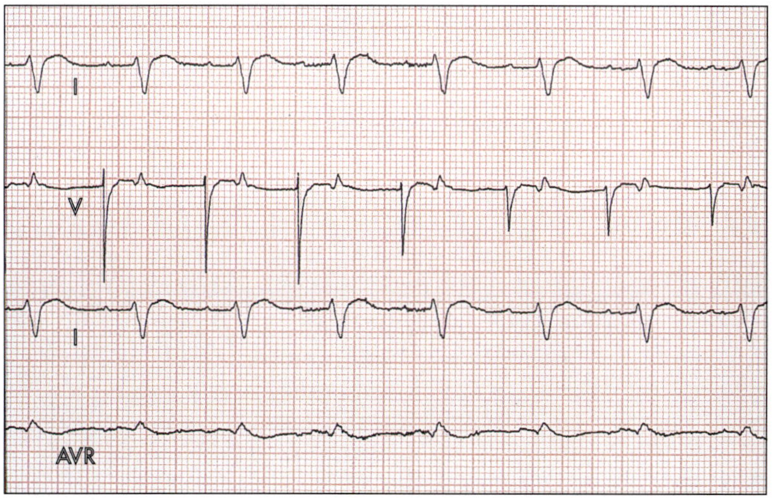

Figure 11-45. The wire has passed into the right atrium. A typical atrial electrocardiogram is seen with very large P waves and small QRS complexes.

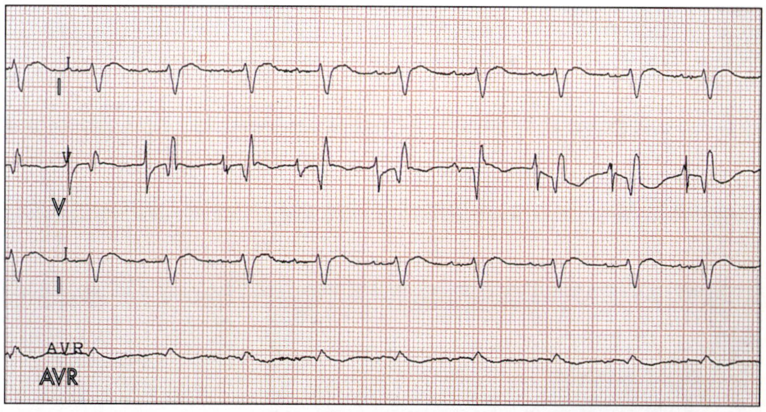

Figure 11-46. The pacing wire passing through the tricuspid valve into the right ventricle. The P waves are still of moderate size; however, the QRS complex has increased in size and has deep Q waves characteristic of an intraventricular cavity electrocardiogram (ECG). At this point the balloon is deflated, the wire advanced a small amount to lodge in the right ventricle, and the ECG disconnected. The pacing box is connected to see if there is capture.

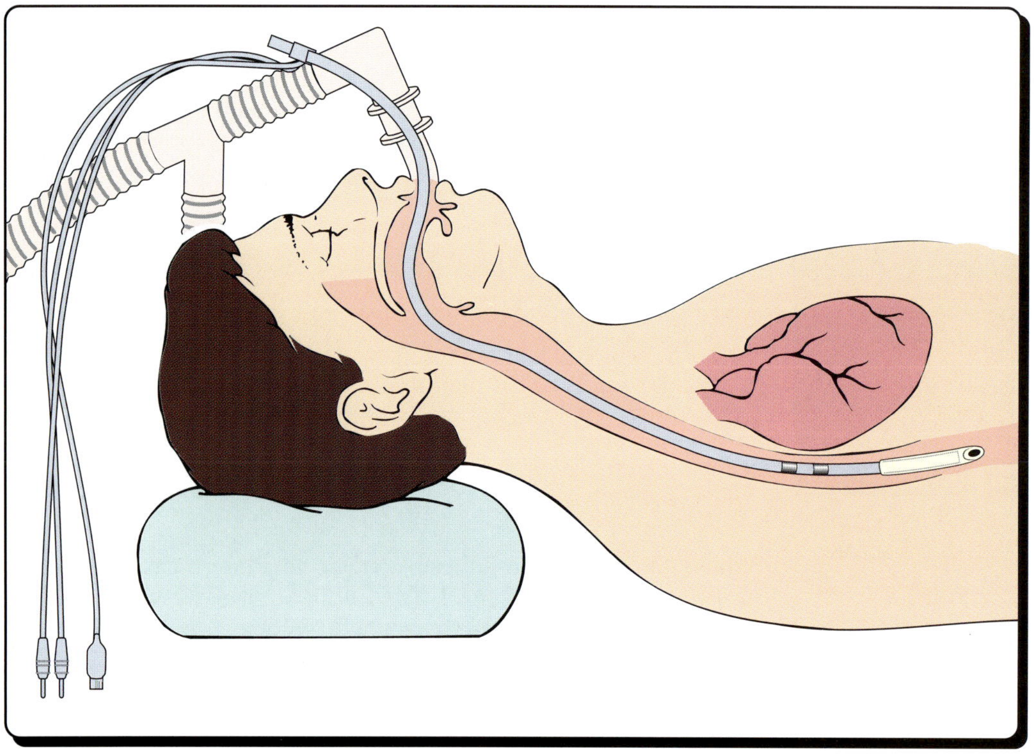

Figure 11-47. Transesophageal atrial pacer [15]. An esophageal stethoscope with embedded electrodes is inserted in the normal manner. If intraoperative bradycardia occurs, then the atrium can easily be paced at the desired rate. Obviously, atrial pacing is ineffective for complete heart block at the atrioventricular node. (Courtesy of Arzco, Tampa, FL.)

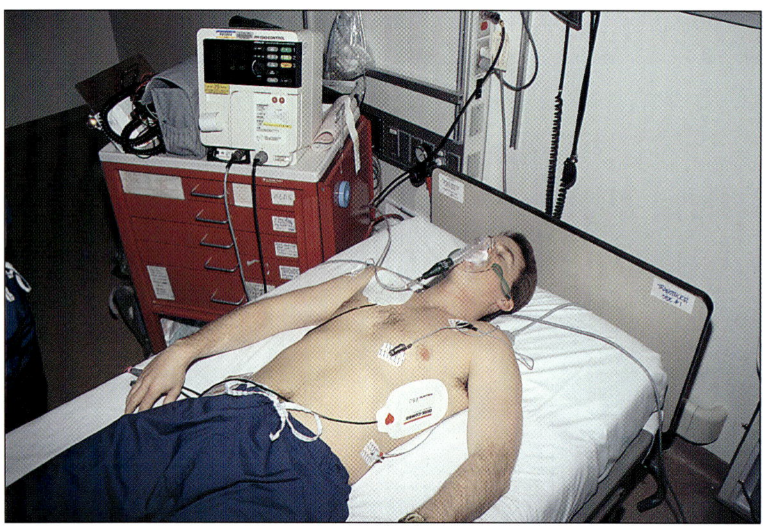

Figure 11-48. Transcutaneous pacing. In emergency situations, without time for placement of a percutaneous intravenous pacing wire, a transcutaneous pacing system can be used. Adhesive patches that can also be used for hands-off DC (Direct Current) cardioversion are attached to the patient's chest. They should be placed well apart, one on the right upper chest and one on the left lateral chest beyond the apex of the heart. Alternatively, one patch can be placed on the back between the scapulae and one on the front of the chest over the sternum.

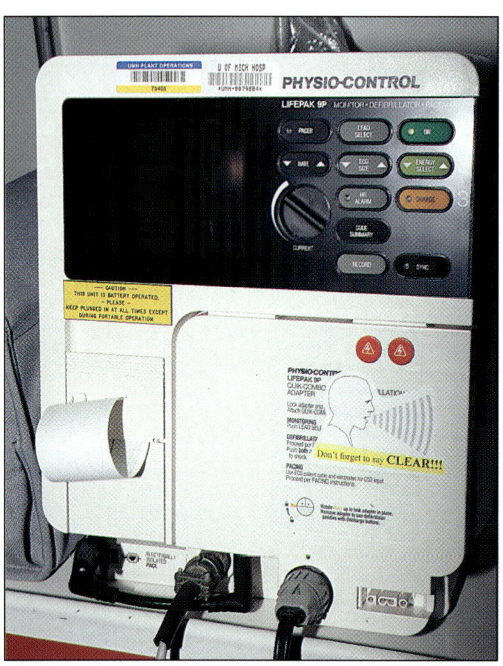

Figure 11-49. The transcutaneous pacer is turned on and the heart rate set by a control on the front of the defibrillator. The current is dialed up until the heart is captured. Determination of capture on the electrocardiogram may be difficult because of muscle artefact. A pulse wave on an arterial line is the best way to assess cardiac contraction at the paced rate. Skin and muscle stimulation can make transcutaneous pacing very uncomfortable or even painful; however, it may be life saving in the emergency situation as a temporary measure while a transvenous wire is being placed. (Courtesy of PhysioControl, Redmond, WA.)

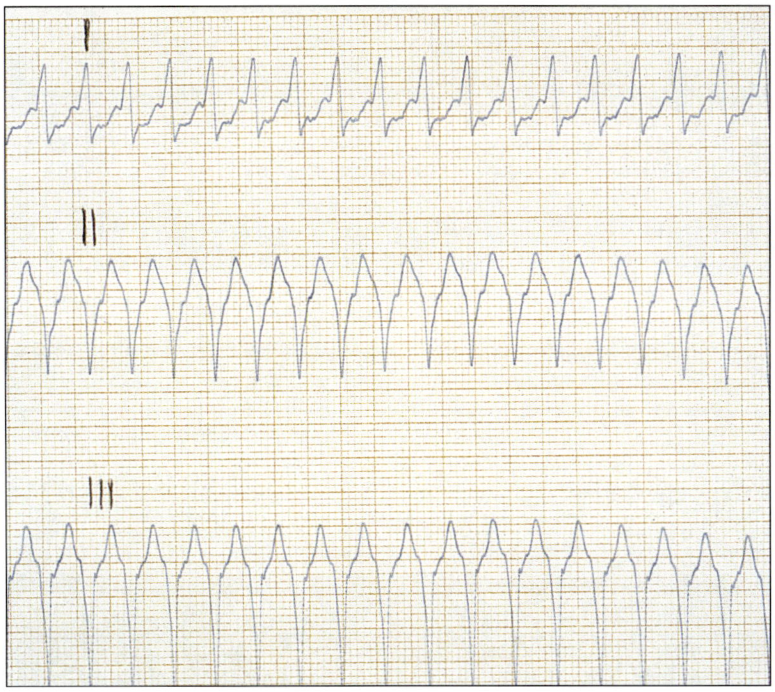

Figure 11-50. Electrocardiogram showing supraventricular tachycardia (SVT), with a rate of 300 bpm. This narrow-complex tachycardia is caused by atrial flutter with one-to-one conduction. The advanced cardiac life support (ACLS) algorithm [14] for tachycardia should be followed to manage narrow- and wide-complex tachyarrhythmias [16]. A key point in this algorithm is that if the patient is unstable and the rate is over 150 bpm, then immediate cardioversion should be considered. A wide-complex tachycardia is most commonly ventricular tachycardia, and lidocaine (1 mL/kg) should be used initially. If there is no response to repeated doses, then a diagnostic trial of adenosine (6 mg; if ineffective, repeat with 12 mg) can be used to establish whether it is SVT with aberrant conduction. Failure of medical treatment may subsequently require cardioversion, even in a relatively stable patient.

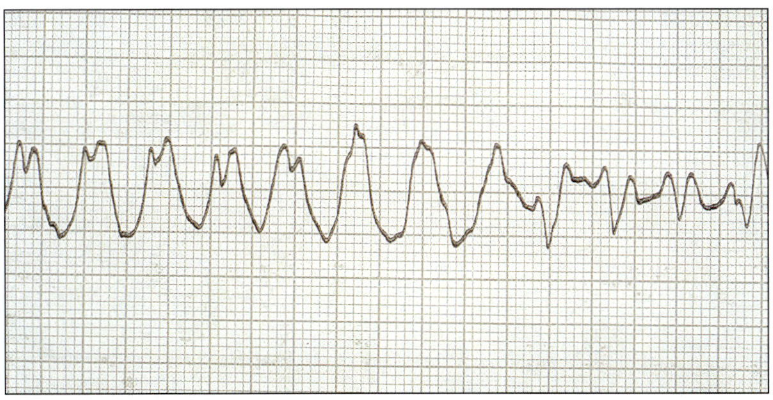

Figure 11-51. Electrocardiogram of torsade de pointes ventricular tachycardia (VT). Lidocaine was ineffective at preventing recurrence of this VT. Correction of the patient's hypokalemia led to cessation of the abnormal rhythm. The advanced cardiac life support (ACLS) algorithm [14] for ventricular fibrillation/pulseless ventricular tachycardia (VF/VT) is followed for cardiac arrest owing to ventricular arrythmias [16]. Early and repeated defibrillation is key in this algorithm. Epinephrine is given early to cause vasoconstriction and improve the efficacy of cardiopulmonary resuscitation. If the recommended drug sequence of lidocaine, bretylium, procainamide is ineffective at stopping the arrhythmia, then it may be followed by intravenous amiodarone, as a fourth-line agent, which has recently been licensed for use in the United States.

PULSELESS ELECTRICAL ACTIVITY

Includes
- Electromechanical dissociation
- Pseudo–electromechanical dissociation
- Idioventricular rhythms
- Ventricular escape rhythms
- Bradyasystolic rhythms
- Postdefibrillation idioventricular rhythms

Possible causes (possible treatment)
- Hypovolemia (volume infusion)
- Hypoxia (ventilation)
- Cardiac tamponade (pericardiocentesis)
- Tension pneumothorax (needle decompression)
- Hypothermia (rewarm)
- Massive pulmonary embolism (surgery, thombolytics)
- Drug overdoses; vasodilators and negative inotropes
- Hyperkalemia
- Acidosis
- Massive acute myocardial infarction

Figure 11-52. The advanced cardiac life support (ACLS) [14] pulseless electrical activity (PEA) algorithm [16] summarized here brings us back to the overall theme of hemodynamic collapse during anesthesia. The ABCs of resuscitation are carried out and supportive measures such as epinephrine or atropine considered while a diligent search for any treatable underlying cause is made. Common scenarios under anesthesia are hypovolemia (*see* Fig. 11-6), tension pneumothorax (*see* Fig. 11-7), cardiac tamponade (*see* Fig. 11-11), and pulmonary embolism (*see* Fig. 11-20).

REFERENCES

1. Guyton AC: Heart Muscle: The Heart as a Pump. In *Human Physiology and Mechanisms of Disease*. Philadelphia: WB Saunders; 1987:80–89.
2. Bartlett RH: Blood Volume and Hemodynamics. In *Critical Care Physiology*. Boston: Little, Brown; 1995:24–47.
3. Cronen MC, Cronen PW, Arino P, Ellis K: Delayed pneumothorax after subclavian vein catheterization and positive pressure ventilation. *Br J Anaesth* 1991, 67:480–482.
4. Engdahl O, Toft T, Boe J: Chest radiograph: a poor method for determining the size of a pneumothorax. *Chest* 1993, 103:26–29.
5. Symbas PN: Chest drainage tubes. *Surg Clin North Am* 1989, 69:41.
6. Yeston NS, Grote RL, Niehopp JM: Important Intensive Care Unit Procedures. In *Critical Care*. Edited by Civetta JM, Taylor RW, Kirby RR. Philadelphia: JB Lippincott; 1992:190–193.
7. White JB, Macklin S, Studley JG, Marshall RD: Cardiac tamponade: a review of diagnosis and anaesthetic and surgical management illustrated by three case reports. *Ann R Coll Surg England* 1988, 70:386–391.
8. Cyna AM, Rodgers RC, McFarlane H: Hypotension due to unexpected cardiac tamponade. *Anaesthesia* 1990, 45:140–142.
9. Warrel RJ, Portal RW: Pericardial Aspiration. In *Procedures in Practice*. Edited by S Lock. London: British Medical Association; 1981:59–61.
10. Palatianos GM, Thurer RJ, Pompeo MD, Kaiser GA: Clinical experience with subxiphoid drainage of pericardial effusions. *Ann Thoracic Surg* 1989, 48:381–385.
11. Marti RA, Ricou F, Tassonyi E: Life-threatening pulmonary embolism at induction of anesthesia: utility of transesophageal echocardiography. *Anesthesiology* 1994, 81:501–503.
12. Dehring DJ Arens JF: Pulmonary thromboembolism: disease recognition and patient management. *Anesthesiology* 1990, 73:146–164.
13. McKinnon RP, Wildsmith JAW: Histaminoid reactions in anaesthesia. *Br J Anaesth* 1995, 74:217–228.
14. Essentials of ACLS. In *Textbook of Advanced Cardiac Life Support*. Edited by RO Cummins. Dallas: American Heart Association; 1994:1-1–1-71.
15. Atlee JL, Pattison CZ, Mathews EL, Hedman AG: Transesophageal atrial pacing for intraoperative sinus bradycardia or AV junctional rhythm: feasibility as prophylaxis in 200 anesthetized adults and hemodynamic effects of treatment. *J Cardiothoracic Vascular Anesthesia* 1993, 7:436–441.
16. Melker RJ, Kirby RR: In-Hospital Caradiopulmonary Resuscitation: Emphasis on ICUs. In Miller RD: *Atlas of Anesthesia*, Vol. 1. Edited by Kirby RR. New York: Churchill Livingstone, 1997; 5.1–5.22.

INDEX